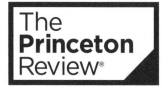

MCAT®

Elite, 2nd Edition

Advanced Strategies to Reach Your Highest Score

The Staff of The Princeton Review

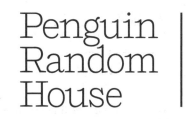

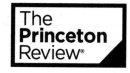

The Princeton Review
555 W. 18th St
New York, NY 10018
E-mail: editorialsupport@review.com

Published in the United States by Penguin Random
House LLC, New York, and in Canada by Random House
of Canada, a division of Penguin Random House Ltd.,
Toronto.

ISBN: 978-1-101-92061-9
ISSN: 2150-878X

Sr. Author: Judene Wright
Editor: Selena Coppock
Production Artist: Craig Patches
Production Editor: Liz Rutzel

10 9 8 7 6 5 4 3 2 1

Editorial
Rob Franek, Senior VP, Publisher
Casey Cornelius, VP Content Development
Mary Beth Garrick, Director of Production
Selena Coppock, Managing Editor
Meave Shelton, Senior Editor
Colleen Day, Editor
Sarah Litt, Editor
Aaron Riccio, Editor
Orion McBean, Editorial Assistant

Penguin Random House Publishing Team
Tom Russell, VP, Publisher
Alison Stoltzfus, Publishing Director
Jake Eldred, Associate Managing Editor
Ellen Reed, Production Manager
Suzanne Lee, Designer

ACKNOWLEDGMENTS

The Princeton Review would like to acknowledge the very significant contributions of the following individuals:

Judene Wright, M.S., M.A.Ed. - Senior Author

Bethany Blackwell, M.S.—General Chemistry
Jon Fowler, M.A.—Physics
Tom Kurtovik, M.A.—Psychology and Sociology
Jason Osman, Ph.D.—Organic Chemistry
Jennifer Wooddell—Critical Analysis and Reasoning Skills

Without their unfailing dedication to this project and endless hours of work, this book, quite literally, would not have been written.

The author would also like to acknowledge the contributions of the members of the MCAT Development teams for not only some of the text of the book, but more importantly, for the writing and editing of the practice sections:

MCAT Biology and Biochemistry:
Chris Fortenbach, Ph.D., Andrew D. Snyder, M.D., Jenkang Tao, B.S., B.A., Kendall Wong, B.A., Sarah Woodruff, M.S., Judene Wright, M.S., M.A.Ed.

MCAT G-Chem:
Bethany Blackwell, M.S., Jonathan Edwards, M.D., Bill Ewing, Ph.D., Chris Fortenbach, Ph.D., Katherine Miller, M.S., Jenkang Tao, B.S., B.A.

MCAT O-Chem:
Bethany Blackwell, M.S., Bill Ewing, Ph.D., Brandon Kelley, Ph.D., Jason Osman Ph.D.

MCAT Physics:
Jon Fowler, M.A., Babak Hassanzadeh, Huan Lee, Chris Pentzell, M.S., Felicia Tam, Ph.D.

MCAT Psychology and Sociology
Sarah A. Kass, Ph.D., Tom Kurtovic, M.A., Christine Lindwall, B.A., M.A., J.D., Jennifer A. McDevitt, Ph.D., Jonathan Nasrallah, B.S., Andrew D. Snyder, M.D.

MCAT CARS:
Jessica Burstrem, M.A., Gina Granter, M.A., Christopher Hinkle, Th.D., Jennifer Wooddell

Special thanks to Adam Robinson, who conceived of and perfected the Joe Bloggs approach to standardized tests, and many of the other successful techniques used by The Princeton Review.

Periodic Table of the Elements

1 H 1.0																	2 He 4.0
3 Li 6.9	4 Be 9.0											5 B 10.8	6 C 12.0	7 N 14.0	8 O 16.0	9 F 19.0	10 Ne 20.2
11 Na 23.0	12 Mg 24.3											13 Al 27.0	14 Si 28.1	15 P 31.0	16 S 32.1	17 Cl 35.5	18 Ar 39.9
19 K 39.1	20 Ca 40.1	21 Sc 45.0	22 Ti 47.9	23 V 50.9	24 Cr 52.0	25 Mn 54.9	26 Fe 55.8	27 Co 58.9	28 Ni 58.7	29 Cu 63.5	30 Zn 65.4	31 Ga 69.7	32 Ge 72.6	33 As 74.9	34 Se 79.0	35 Br 79.9	36 Kr 83.8
37 Rb 85.5	38 Sr 87.6	39 Y 88.9	40 Zr 91.2	41 Nb 92.9	42 Mo 95.9	43 Tc (98)	44 Ru 101.1	45 Rh 102.9	46 Pd 106.4	47 Ag 107.9	48 Cd 112.4	49 In 114.8	50 Sn 118.7	51 Sb 121.8	52 Te 127.6	53 I 126.9	54 Xe 131.3
55 Cs 132.9	56 Ba 137.3	57 *La 138.9	72 Hf 178.5	73 Ta 180.9	74 W 183.9	75 Re 186.2	76 Os 190.2	77 Ir 192.2	78 Pt 195.1	79 Au 197.0	80 Hg 200.6	81 Tl 204.4	82 Pb 207.2	83 Bi 209.0	84 Po (209)	85 At (210)	86 Rn (222)
87 Fr (223)	88 Ra 226.0	89 †Ac 227.0	104 Rf (261)	105 Db (262)	106 Sg (266)	107 Bh (264)	108 Hs (277)	109 Mt (268)	110 Ds (281)	111 Rg (272)	112 Cn (285)	113 Uut (286)	114 Fl (289)	115 Uup (288)	116 Lv (293)	117 Uus (294)	118 Uuo (294)

*Lanthanide Series:

58 Ce 140.1	59 Pr 140.9	60 Nd 144.2	61 Pm (145)	62 Sm 150.4	63 Eu 152.0	64 Gd 157.3	65 Tb 158.9	66 Dy 162.5	67 Ho 164.9	68 Er 167.3	69 Tm 168.9	70 Yb 173.0	71 Lu 175.0
90 Th 232.0	91 Pa (231)	92 U 238.0	93 Np (237)	94 Pu (244)	95 Am (243)	96 Cm (247)	97 Bk (247)	98 Cf (251)	99 Es (252)	100 Fm (257)	101 Md (258)	102 No (259)	103 Lr (260)

†Actinide Series:

CONTENTS

Register Your

1 Go to **PrincetonReview.com/cracking**

2 You'll see a welcome page where you should register your book or boxed set of books using the ISBN. If you have a book, the ISBN can be found above the bar code on the back cover. If you have a boxed set, the ISBN can be found on the back of the box above the bar code. Type in 9781101920619 and create a username and password so that next time you can log into www.PrincetonReview.com easily.

3 After placing this free order, you'll either be asked to log in or to answer a few simple questions in order to set up a new Princeton Review account.

4 Finally, click on the "Student Tools" tab located at the top of the screen. It may take an hour or two for your registration to go through, but after that, you're good to go.

NOTE: If you are experiencing book problems (potential content errors), please contact EditorialSupport@review.com with the full title of the book, its ISBN number, and the page number of the error.

Experiencing technical issues? Please e-mail TPRStudentTech@review.com with the following information:

- your full name
- e-mail address used to register the book
- full book title and ISBN
- your computer OS (Mac or PC) and Internet browser (Firefox, Safari, Chrome, etc.)
- description of technical issue

Book Online!

Once you've registered, you can...

- take 2 full-length practice MCAT exams
- find useful information about taking the MCAT and applying to medical school
- check to see if there have been any updates to this edition

Offline Resources

If you are looking for more review or medical school advice, please feel free to pick up these books in stores right now!

- *Medical School Essays That Made a Difference*
- *The Best 167 Medical Schools*
- *The Princeton Review Complete MCAT*

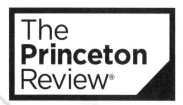

Part I

MCAT Overview

Chapter 1
Welcome to *MCAT Elite*

If you're buying this book, you already have some experience with the MCAT. You've studied using your school science textbooks, perhaps even used test preparation books or took preparation courses, you have a solid grasp of science content, and you've done reasonably well on the practice tests and problems you've been given. But you're not satisfied. You want to do better than "reasonably well." You want to improve and get those last few points. You want to take your MCAT score to the next level.

Succeeding on the MCAT requires a combination of content knowledge, critical reasoning, and reading comprehension skills. Be aware that this book is not intended as content review...we assume you know your science content and CARS strategies. (However, if you need to review any of the science content areas or CARS strategies, consider our books in the *MCAT Review* series.) *MCAT Elite* is designed to help you brush up on your passage reading and analysis skills, and hone your test-taking abilities and learn how to analyze the results of your practice exams to identify your weaknesses so you can improve. By learning how to identify problem areas, you can make your MCAT preparation as efficient and effective as possible. You can bring your score up a few crucial notches and enter the realm of the MCAT Elite.

WHAT IS THE MCAT...REALLY?

Most test takers approach the MCAT as though it were a typical college science test, where they just have to regurgitate facts and knowledge in order to do well. They study for the MCAT the same way they did for their college tests, by memorizing facts and details, formulas and equations. And when they get to the MCAT they are surprised...and disappointed in their scores.

It's a myth that the MCAT is purely a test of knowledge. If medical school admission committees want to see what you know from college, all they have to do is look at your transcripts. What they really want to see, though, is how you *think*. Especially, how you think under pressure. And *that's* what your MCAT score will tell them.

The MCAT is really a test of your ability to apply basic knowledge to different, possibly new, situations. It's a test of your ability to reason out and evaluate arguments. Do you still need to know your science content? Absolutely. But not at the level that most test takers think they need to know it. Furthermore, your science knowledge won't help you on the CARS section. So how do you study for a test like this?

You study for the science sections by reviewing the basics and then applying them to MCAT practice questions. You study for the CARS section by learning how to adapt your existing reading and analytical skills to the nature of the test. And once you've done that, you hone your skills by reviewing your practice tests and analyzing your weaknesses to target your ongoing study to your specific needs.

The book you are holding will teach you how to review and analyze your practice tests. It also includes hundreds of the most difficult MCAT questions designed to make you think about the material in a deeper way, and it includes full explanations to clarify the logical thought processes needed to get to the answer. And, since the MCAT is a computer-based test, this book also comes with online access to two full-length practice exams to further hone your skills. After all, what better way to practice for a computer-based test?

Chapter 2
MCAT Nuts and Bolts

OVERVIEW

The MCAT is a computer-based test (CBT) that is *not* adaptive. Adaptive tests base your next question on whether or not you've answered the current question correctly. The MCAT is *linear*, or *fixed-form*, meaning that the questions are in a predetermined order and do not change based on your answers. However, there are many versions of the test, so that on a given test day, different people will see different versions. The following table highlights the features of the MCAT exam.

Registration	Online via www.aamc.org. Begins as early as six months prior to test date; available up until week of test (subject to seat availability).
Testing Centers	Administered at small, secure, climate-controlled computer testing rooms.
Security	Photo ID with signature, electronic fingerprint, electronic signature verification, assigned seat.
Proctoring	None. Test administrator checks examinee in and assigns seat at computer. All testing instructions are given on the computer.
Frequency of Test	Many times per year distributed over January, April, May, June, July, August, and September.
Format	Exclusively computer-based. NOT an adaptive test.
Length of Test Day	7.5 hours
Breaks	Optional 10-minute breaks between sections, with a 30-minute break for lunch.
Section Names	1. Chemical and Physical Foundations of Biological Systems (Chem/Phys) 2. Critical Analysis and Reasoning Skills (CARS) 3. Biological and Biochemical Foundations of Living Systems (Bio/Biochem) 4. Psychological, Social, and Biological Foundations of Behavior (Psych/Soc)
Number of Questions and Timing	59 Chem/Phys questions, 95 minutes 53 CARS questions, 90 minutes 59 Bio/Biochem questions, 95 minutes 59 Psych/Soc questions, 95 minutes
Scoring	Test is scaled. Several forms per administration.
Allowed/ Not Allowed	No timers/watches. Noise reduction headphones available. Unopened package of foam earplugs is allowed. Scratch paper and pencils given at start of test and taken at end of test. Locker or secure area provided for personal items.
Results: Timing and Delivery	Approximately 30 days. Electronic scores only, available online through AAMC login. Examinees can print official score reports.
Maximum Number of Retakes	As of April 2015, the MCAT can be taken a maximum of three times in one year, four times over two years, and seven times over the lifetime of the examinee. An examinee can be registered for only one date at a time.

Registration

Registration for the exam is completed online at www.aamc.org/students/applying/mcat/reserving. The AAMC opens registration for a given test date at least two months in advance of the date, often earlier. It's a good idea to register well in advance of your desired test date to make sure that you get a seat.

Sections

There are four sections on the MCAT exam: Chemical and Physical Foundations of Biological Systems (Chem/Phys), Critical Analysis and Reasoning Skills (CARS), Biological and Biochemical Foundations of Living Systems (Bio/Biochem), and Psychological, Social, and Biological Foundations of Behavior (Psych/Soc). All sections consist of multiple-choice questions.

Section	Concepts Tested	Number of Questions and Timing
Chemical and Physical Foundations of Biological Systems	Basic concepts in chemistry and physics, including biochemistry; scientific inquiry; reasoning; research and statistics skills.	59 questions in 95 minutes
Critical Analysis and Reasoning Skills	Critical analysis of information drawn from a wide range of social science and humanities disciplines.	53 questions in 90 minutes
Biological and Biochemical Foundations of Living Systems	Basic concepts in biology and biochemistry, scientific inquiry, reasoning, research and statistics skills.	59 questions in 95 minutes
Psychological, Social, and Biological Foundations of Behavior	Basic concepts in psychology, sociology, and biology, research methods and statistics.	59 questions in 95 minutes

Most questions on the MCAT (44 in the science sections, all 53 in the CARS section) are **passage-based**; the science sections have 10 passages each and the CARS section has 9. A passage consists of a few paragraphs of information on which several following questions are based. In the science sections, passages often include equations or reactions, tables, graphs, figures, and experiments to analyze. CARS passages come from literature in the social sciences and humanities, and they do not test content knowledge in any way.

Some questions in the science sections are *freestanding questions* (FSQs). These questions are independent of any passage information and appear in several groups of about four to five questions, interspersed throughout the passages. 15 of the questions in the science sections are freestanding, and the remainder are passage-based.

Each section on the MCAT is separated by either a 10-minute break or a 30-minute lunch break.

Section	Time
Test Center Check-In	Variable, can take up to 40 minutes if center is busy.
Tutorial	10 minutes
Chemical and Physical Foundations of Biological Systems	95 minutes
Break	10 minutes
Critical Analysis and Reasoning Skills	90 minutes
Lunch Break	30 minutes
Biological and Biochemical Foundations of Living Systems	95 minutes
Break	10 minutes
Psychological, Social, and Biological Foundations of Behavior	95 minutes
Void Option	5 minutes
Survey	5 minutes

The survey includes questions about your satisfaction with the overall MCAT experience, including registration, check-in, etc., as well as questions about how you prepared for the test.

Scoring

The MCAT is a scaled exam, meaning that your raw score will be converted into a scaled score that takes into account the difficulty of the questions. There is no guessing penalty. All sections are scored from 118–132, with a total scaled score range of 472–528. Because different versions of the test have varying levels of difficulty, the scale will be different from one exam to the next. Thus, there is no "magic number" of questions to get right in order to get a particular score. Plus, some of the questions on the test are considered "experimental" and do not count toward your score; they are just there to be evaluated for possible future inclusion in a test.

At the end of the test (after you complete the Psychological, Social, and Biological Foundations of Behavior section), you will be asked to choose one of the following two options, "I wish to have my MCAT exam scored" or "I wish to VOID my MCAT exam." You have five minutes to make a decision, and if you do not select one of the options in that time, the test will automatically be scored. If you choose the VOID option, your test will not be scored (you will not now, or ever, get a numerical score for this test), medical schools will not know you took the test, and no refunds will be granted. You cannot "unvoid" your scores at a later time.

So, what's a good score? The AAMC is centering the scale at 500 (i.e., 500 will be the 50th percentile), and recommends that application committees consider applicants near the center of the range. To be on the safe side, aim for a total score of around 510. Remember that if your GPA is on the low side, you'll need higher MCAT scores to compensate, and if you have a strong GPA, you can get away with lower MCAT scores. But the reality is that your chances of acceptance depend on a lot more than just your MCAT scores. It's a combination of your GPA, your MCAT scores, your undergraduate coursework, letters of recommendation, experience related to the medical field (such as volunteer work or research), extracurricular activities, your personal statement, etc. Medical schools are looking for a complete package, not just good scores and a good GPA.

Section Score	Percentile Rank, Chem/Phys*	Percentile Rank, CARS*	Percentile Rank, Bio/Biochem*	Percentile Rank, Psych/Soc*
132	100	100	100	100
131	99	99	99	99
130	98	97	97	97
129	95	93	92	92
128	90	87	87	86
127	83	79	78	78
126	74	68	67	67
125	62	57	56	55
124	49	45	44	44
123	37	33	33	32
122	25	22	22	22
121	14	13	13	13
120	7	7	7	7
119	3	3	3	3
118	1	1	1	1

Total Score	Percentile Rank*	Total Score	Percentile Rank*	Total Score	Percentile Rank*
528	100	506	73	490	20
523–527	> 99	505	70	489	18
521–522	99	504	67	488	16
519–520	98	503	63	487	13
518	97	502	60	486	12
517	96	501	56	485	10
516	95	500	53	484	8
515	94	499	49	483	7
514	92	498	45	482	5
513	90	497	42	481	4
512	88	496	39	480	3
511	86	495	35	478–479	2
510	84	494	32	476–477	1
509	82	493	29	472–475	< 1
508	79	492	26		
507	76	491	23		

*Data from **https://students-residents.aamc.org/advisors/article/percentile-ranks-for-the-mcat-exam/**

PREPARATION

Academic preparation for the MCAT should include one year each of physics, general chemistry, organic chemistry, and biology, and one semester each of biochemistry, psychology, and sociology. Specific topic lists for each subject can be found in their respective chapters in this book; you should peruse these lists and if you find any subject in which your knowledge is deficient, you should review that material. Note, however, that this book does not include content review. We recommend The Princeton Review's *MCAT Review* series for science content review. Since the CARS section is not content-based, there is no specific coursework to take to prepare yourself; however, any course that requires you to read difficult social science or humanities material can help prepare you for the type of reading you will be doing in the CARS section. Again, The Princeton Review's *MCAT CARS Review* provides in-depth coverage of strategies and techniques for this section.

Chapter 3
General MCAT
Strategies

3.1 QUESTION TYPES

In the science sections of the MCAT, the questions fall into one of three main categories.

1) Memory questions: These questions can be answered directly from prior knowledge and represent about 25 percent of the total number of questions.
2) Explicit questions: These questions are those for which the answer is explicitly stated in the passage. To answer them correctly, for example, may just require finding a definition, reading a graph, or making a simple connection. Explicit questions represent about 35 percent of the total number of questions.
3) Implicit questions: These questions require you to apply knowledge to a new situation; the answer is typically implied by the information in the passage. These questions often start "if…then…" (For example, "If we modify the experiment in the passage like this, then what result would we expect?") Implicit style questions make up about 40 percent of the total number of questions.

In the CARS section, the questions fall into four main categories:

1) Specific questions: These either ask you for facts from the passage (Retrieval questions) or require you to deduce what is most likely to be true based on the passage (Inference questions).
2) General questions: These ask you to summarize central themes (Main Idea and Primary Purpose questions) or evaluate an author's opinion (Tone/Attitude questions).
3) Reasoning questions: These ask you to describe the purpose of, or the support provided for, a statement made in the passage (Structure questions) or to judge how well the author supports his or her argument (Evaluate questions).
4) Application questions: These ask you to apply new information from either the question stem itself (New Information questions) or from the answer choices (Strengthen, Weaken, and Analogy questions) to the passage.

More detail on question types and strategies can be found in the specific subject chapters.

3.2 MCAT PASSAGES

Passages in the science sections consist of a few paragraphs of text and often include descriptions of experiments and experimental data. Many of the passages are "blended" topics, meaning that they are not, for example, purely Physics, or not purely General Chemistry; this is especially true of passages in the Chem/Phys section. Often, specific subject concepts are tested within the context of a biological setting: for example, pressure and fluid flow in blood vessels, or acid-base balance within the context of the respiratory system, or torque and other forces around the ankle joint. Biochemistry is often woven into General Chemistry, Organic Chemistry, or Biology passages, and Biology questions show up everywhere: in Chem/Phys, in Bio/Biochem (obviously), and in the Psych/Soc section. A total of four to six questions will be associated with each passage, and there are 10 passages in each science section.

Passages in the CARS section may be on any subject in the humanities and social sciences. Passage topics may include philosophy, ethics, archaeology, economics, history, political science, literature and literary theory, psychology, sociology, anthropology, cultural studies, geography, population health, and art history and theory. This range of topics may seem overwhelming. However, unlike the other sections of the test, CARS passages do not test your outside knowledge of any subject. In fact, using your own factual knowledge or opinions of the subject can lead you to pick incorrect answers; the questions require you to use only the information provided in the passage. Clearly you can't prepare for or approach this section of the test in the same way as the sciences!

3.3 GENERAL LAYOUT AND TEST-TAKING STRATEGIES

Layout of the Test

In each section of the test, the computer screen is divided vertically, with the passage on the left and the range of questions for that passage indicated above it (e.g., "Passage 1 Questions 1–5"). The scroll bar for the passage text appears in the middle of the screen. A single question appears on the right, and you need to click "Next" to move to each subsequent question.

In the science sections, the freestanding questions are found in groups of 4–5, interspersed with the passages. The screen is still divided vertically; on the left is the statement "Questions [X–XX] do not refer to a passage and are independent of each other," and each question appears on the right, as described above.

CBT Tools

There are a number of tools available on the test, including highlighting, strike-outs, the Mark button, the Review button, the Periodic Table button, and of course, scratch paper. The following is a brief description of each tool.

1) **Highlighting:** This is done in the passage text (including table entries and some equations, but excluding figures and molecular structures) and in the question stems by left-clicking and dragging the mouse across the words you wish to highlight; the selected words will then be highlighted in blue. When you release the mouse, a highlighting icon will appear; clicking on the icon will highlight the selected text in yellow. To remove the highlighting, left-click on the highlighted text.

2) **Strike-outs:** Right-clicking on an answer choice causes the entire text of that choice to be crossed out. The strike-out can be removed by right-clicking again. Left-clicking selects an answer choice; note than an answer choice that is selected cannot be struck out. When you strike out a figure or molecular structure, instead of being crossed out, the image turns grey.

3) **Mark button:** This allows you to flag the question for later review. When clicked, the flag on the "Mark" button turns red and says "Marked."

4) **Review button:** Clicking this button brings up a new screen showing all questions and their status (either "completed," "incomplete," or "marked"). You can choose to: "review all," "review incomplete," or "review marked." You can also double-click any question number to quickly return to that specific question. You can only review questions in the section of the MCAT you are currently taking, but the Review button can be clicked at any time during the allotted time for that section; you do NOT have to wait until the end of the section to click it.

5) **Periodic Table button:** Clicking this button will open a periodic table. Note that the periodic table is large; however, it can be resized to see the questions and a portion of the periodic table at the same time.

6) **Scratch paper:** You will be given four pages (8 faces) of scratch paper at the start of the test. You can ask for more at any point during the test, and your first set of paper will be collected before you receive fresh paper. Scratch paper is only useful if it is kept organized; do not give in to the tendency to write on the first available open space! Good organization will be very helpful when/if you wish to review a question. Indicate the passage number and the range of questions for that passage in a box near the top of your scratch work, and indicate the question you are working on in a circle to the left of the notes for that question. Draw a line under your scratch work when you change passages to keep the work separate. Do not erase or scribble over any previous work. If you do not think it is correct, draw one line through the work and start again. You may have already done some useful work without realizing it.

General Strategy for the Science Sections

Passages vs. FSQs in the Science Sections: What to Start With

Since the questions are displayed on separate screens, it is awkward and time consuming to click through all of the questions up front to find the FSQs. Therefore, go through the section on a first pass and decide whether to do the passage now or to save it for later, basing your decision on the passage text and the first question. Tackle the FSQs as you come upon them. More details are below.

Here is an outline of the procedure:

1) For each passage, write a heading on your scratch paper with the passage number, the general topic, and its range of questions (e.g., "Passage 1, thermodynamics, Q 1–5" or "Passage 2, enzymes, Q 6–9"). The passage numbers do not currently appear in the Review screen, thus having the question numbers on your scratch paper will allow you to move through the section more efficiently.

2) Skim the text and rank the passage. If a passage is a "Now," complete it before moving on to the next passage (also see Attacking the Questions below). If it is a "Later" passage, first write "SKIPPED" in block letters under the passage heading on your scratch paper and leave room for your work when you come back to complete that passage. (Note that the specific passages you skip will be unique to you; in the Bio/Biochem section, you might choose to do all Biology passages first, then come back for Biochemistry. Or in Chem/Phys, you might choose to skip the experiment-based or analytical passages. Know ahead of time what type of passage you are going to skip and follow your plan.) More details on mapping the passage will be presented in the individual subject sections.

3) If you have decided to skip the passage, click on the "Review" button at the bottom to get to the review screen. Double-click on the first question of the next passage; you'll be able to identify it because you know the range of questions from the passage you just skipped. This will take you to the next passage, where you will repeat steps 1–3.

4) Once you have completed the "Now" passages, go to the Review screen and double-click the first question for the first passage you skipped. Answer the questions, and continue going back to the Review screen and repeating this procedure for other passages you have skipped.

Attacking the Questions

As you work through the questions, if you encounter a particularly lengthy question, or a question that requires a lot of analysis, you may choose to skip it. This is a wise strategy because it ensures you will tackle all the easier questions first, the ones you are more likely to get right. If you choose to skip the question (or if you attempt it but get stuck), write down the question number on your scratch paper, click the Mark button to flag the question in the Review screen, and move on to the next question. At the end of the passage, click back through the set of questions to complete any that you skipped over the first time through, and make sure that you have filled in an answer for every question.

General Strategy for the CARS Section

Ranking and Ordering the Passages: What to Start With

Ranking and Ordering: There will always be some easy, some medium level, and some very difficult passages in the CARS section. You will maximize your score by doing easier (what we call "Now") passages early on, leaving the medium to hard ones ("Later" and "Killer") until later in the section and making sure that any passages you do not complete are among the hardest (that is, "Killer") ones. As with the science passages, since each question is displayed on a separate screen it is too awkward and time consuming to click through all of the questions before deciding to do a passage now, later, or never. Therefore, rank the passage and decide whether or not to do it on the first pass through the section based only on the passage text, skimming and paraphrasing the first 2–3 sentences.

Here is an outline of the basic "Two Pass" Ranking and Ordering procedure to follow.

1) For each passage, write a heading on your scratch paper with the passage number and its range of questions (e.g., "Passage 1 Q 1–7"). The passage numbers do not currently appear in the Review screen, thus having the question numbers on your scratch paper will allow you to move through the section more efficiently.

2) Skim the first 2–3 sentences and rank the passage. If the passage is a "Now," complete it before moving on to the next. If it is a "Later" or "Killer," first write either "Later" or "Killer" and "SKIPPED" in block letters under the passage heading on your scratch paper and leave room for your work if you decide to come back and complete that passage. Then click through each question, marking each one and filling in random guesses, until you get to the next passage. If you aren't sure at this stage whether it is a Later or a Killer passage, leave that decision until later, once you have done your easier first pass passages and are coming back through for your second pass.

3) Once you have completed the "Now" passages, come back for your second pass and complete the "Later" passages, leaving your random guesses in place for any "Killer" passages that you choose not to complete. Go to the Review screen and use your scratch paper notes on the question numbers; double-click on the number of the first question for that passage to go back to that question and proceed from there. Alternatively, if you have consistently marked all the questions for passages you skipped in your first pass, you can use "Review Marked" from the Review screen to find and complete your "Later" passages.

4) Regardless of how you choose to find your second pass passages, unmark each question after you complete it, so that you can continue to rely on the Review screen (and the "Review Marked" function) to identify questions that you have not yet attempted.

Previewing the Questions

The formatting and functioning of the tools facilitates effective previewing. Having each question on a separate screen will encourage you to really focus on that question. Even more importantly, you can highlight in the question stem (but not in the answer choices).

Here is the basic procedure for previewing the questions:

Start with the first question, and if it has lead words referencing passage content, highlight those words. You may also choose to jot them down on your scratch paper. Once you reach and preview the last question for the set on that passage, THEN stay on that screen and work the passage (your highlighting appears and stays on every passage screen, and it persists through the whole 90 minutes).

Attacking the Questions

Once you have worked the passage and defined the Bottom Line, work **backward** from the last question to the first. The question types and the detailed procedure for attacking each type will be discussed later. However, it is important **not** to attempt the hardest questions first (potentially getting stuck, wasting time, and discouraging yourself).

So, as you work the questions from last to first (see Previewing the Questions above), if you encounter a particularly difficult and/or lengthy question (or if you attempt a question but get stuck) write down the question number on your scratch paper (you may also choose to mark it) and move on backward through the rest of the questions. Then click **forward** through the questions and complete any that you skipped over the first time through the set, unmarking any questions that you marked that first time through and making sure that you have filled in an answer for every question.

Once you reach and complete the last question for that passage, clicking "Next" will send you to the first question of the next passage. Working the questions from last to first the first time through the set will eliminate the need to click back through multiple screens to get to the first question immediately after previewing, and will also make it easier and more efficient to do the hardest questions last.

Pacing Strategy for the MCAT

Since the MCAT is a timed test, you must keep an eye on the timer and adjust your pacing as necessary. It would be terrible to run out of time at the end only to discover that the last few questions could have been easily answered in just a few seconds each.

In the science sections you will have about one minute and thirty-five seconds (1:35) per question, and in the CARS section you will have about one minute and forty seconds (1:40) per question (not taking into account time reading the passage before answering the questions).

Section	# of Questions in Passage	Approximate Time (including reading the passage)
Chem/Phys, Bio/Biochem, and Psych/Soc	4	6.5 minutes
	5	8 minutes
	6	9.5 minutes
CARS	5	8.5 minutes
	6	10 minutes
	7	11.5 minutes

When starting a passage in the science sections, make note of how much time you will allot for it and the starting time on the timer. Jot down on your scratch paper what the timer should say at the end of the passage. Then just keep an eye on it as you work through the questions. If you are near the end of the time for that passage, guess on any remaining questions, make some notes on your scratch paper, Mark the questions, and move on. Come back to those questions if you have time.

For the CARS section, keep in mind that many people will maximize their score by *not* trying to complete every question or every passage in the section. A good strategy for test takers who cannot achieve a high level of accuracy on all nine passages is to randomly guess on at least one passage in the section, and spend your time getting a high percentage of the other questions right. To complete all nine CARS passages, you have about ten minutes per passage. To complete eight of the nine, you have about 11 minutes per passage. Do keep rough track of the time as you go. However, don't give yourself a strict time limit for each passage or question. Some passages and questions deserve more time than others. Even more importantly, if you are thinking too much at each moment about how much time you are spending, you will be overly distracted. Not only will you miss questions you could/should get right, but you will work through the section less efficiently (that is, more slowly) overall.

To help maximize your number of correct answer choices in any section, do the questions and passages within that section in the order *you* want to do them in. See General Strategy.

Process of Elimination

Process of Elimination (POE) is probably the most useful technique you have to tackle MCAT questions. Since there is no guessing penalty, POE allows you to increase your probability of choosing the correct answer by eliminating those you are sure are wrong.

1) Strike out any choices that you are sure are incorrect or that do not address the issue raised in the question.
2) Jot down some notes to help clarify your thoughts if you return to the question.
3) Use the "Mark" button to flag the question for review. (Note, however, that in the CARS section, you generally should not be returning to rethink questions once you have moved on to a new passage.)

4) Do not leave it blank! For the sciences, if you are not sure and you have already spent more than 60 seconds on that question, just pick one of the remaining choices. If you have time to review it at the end, you can always debate the remaining choices based on your previous notes. For CARS, if you have been through the choices two or three times, have re-read the question stem and gone back to the passage and you are still stuck, move on. Do the remaining questions for that passage, take one more look at the question you were stuck on, then pick an answer and move on for good.

5) Special Note: If three of the four answer choices have been eliminated, the remaining choice must be the correct answer. Don't waste time pondering *why* it is correct, just click it and move on. The MCAT doesn't care if you truly understand why it's the right answer, only that you have the right answer selected.

6) More subject-specific information on techniques will be presented in the next chapter.

Guessing

Remember, there is NO guessing penalty on the MCAT. NEVER leave a question blank!

3.4   TESTING TIPS

Before Test Day

- Take a trip to the test center at least a day or two before your actual test date so that you can easily find the building and room on test day. This will also allow you to gauge traffic and see if you need money for parking or anything like that. Knowing this type of information ahead of time will greatly reduce your stress on the day of your test.
- During the week before the test, adjust your sleeping schedule so that you are going to bed and getting up in the morning at the same times as on the day before and morning of the MCAT. Prioritize getting a reasonable amount of sleep during the last few nights before the test.
- Don't do any heavy studying the day before the test. This is not a test you can cram for! Your goal at this point is to rest and relax so that you can go into test day in a good physical and mental condition.
- Eat well. Try to avoid excessive caffeine and sugar. Ideally, in the weeks leading up to the actual test you should experiment a little bit with foods and practice tests to see which foods give you the most endurance. Aim for steady blood sugar levels during the test: sports drinks, peanut-butter crackers, trail mix, etc. make good snacks for your breaks and lunch.

General Test Day Info and Tips

- On the day of the test, arrive at the test center at least a half hour prior to the start time of your test.
- Examinees will be checked in to the center in the order in which they arrive.
- You will be assigned a locker or secure area in which to put your personal items. Textbooks and study notes are not allowed, so there is no need to bring them with you to the test center.
- Your ID will be checked, a digital image of your fingerprint will be taken, and you will be asked to sign in.
- You will be given scratch paper and a couple of pencils, and the test center administrator will take you to the computer on which you will complete the test. You may not choose a computer; you must use the computer assigned to you.
- Nothing, not even your watch, is allowed at the computer station except your photo ID, your locker key (if provided), and a factory sealed packet of ear plugs.
- If you choose to leave the testing room at the breaks, you will have your fingerprint checked again, and you will have to sign in and out.
- You are allowed to access the items in your locker, except for notes and cell phones. (Check your test center's policy on cell phones ahead of time; some centers do not even allow them to be kept in your locker.)
- Don't forget to bring the snack foods and lunch you experimented with during your practice tests.
- At the end of the test, the test administrator will collect your scratch paper and shred it.
- Definitely take the breaks! Get up and walk around. It's a good way to clear your head between sections and get the blood (and oxygen!) flowing to your brain.
- Ask for new scratch paper at the breaks if you use it all up.

A Note About Flashcards

For most of the exams you've taken previously, flashcards were likely very helpful. This was because those exams mostly required you to regurgitate information, and flashcards are pretty good at helping you memorize facts. However, the most challenging aspect of the MCAT is not that it requires you to memorize the fine details of content knowledge, but that it requires you to apply your basic scientific knowledge to unfamiliar situations: Flashcards alone may not help you there.

Flashcards can be beneficial if your basic content knowledge is deficient in some area. For example, if you don't know the hormones and their effects in the body, flashcards can certainly help you memorize these facts. Or, maybe you don't know the amino acids and their 1- and 3-letter abbreviations; flashcards can help you memorize these. But unless you are trying to memorize basic facts in your personal weak areas, you are better off doing and analyzing practice passages than carrying around a stack of flashcards.

Chapter 4
Journal Article Analysis

4.1   JOURNAL ARTICLE ANALYSIS

MCAT passages often include descriptions of experiments and experimental data to analyze. This can be a daunting part of understanding the passage. You can develop your ability to analyze experiments and data quickly by practicing reading and analyzing the source of this information: journal articles.

The goal in reading journal articles is not to learn content. It's to get comfortable skimming and extracting information from them. Plan to read at least one or two articles a week, rotating through the different MCAT subjects. Start by making a list of topics that interest you, sorted by subject. For example, in Biology you might be interested in multiple sclerosis, or high fat/low carb diets, or epilepsy. For Physics, you might be interested in medical imaging technology like MRI or PET scans. For Organic Chemistry you might be interested in synthesizing aromatic compounds for artificial flavors. Or whatever! Then do an online search for journal articles using those topics as keywords. Finding articles about topics in which you already have an interest will make them easier to read. Keep the following in mind while reading the articles.

1. You should know:

- what distinguishes a control group from an experimental group,
- how to determine whether results are statistically significant,
- how to increase the power of the study (generally by increasing the number of participants), and
- how to read a graph and a data table.

More information on controls, statistical significance, and reading graphs and tables can be found in the subject-specific sections of this book.

2. Try to summarize the purpose and the methods of the study in four or five sentences. Consider:

- How is the study designed? (I.e., is the experimenter conducting research on humans or on animals or on bacteria in a petri dish, or something else? Are there multiple experimental groups or just one? Is there a control group? Is the control group given some sort of placebo or nothing at all? Etc.)
- Was this study conducted over a long period of time, collecting data at multiple points in time?
- Did this study have a large N or a small N?
- Was this a blinded study? If so, was it double blind or single blind?
- How do the experimental groups differ from the control? If there are multiple experimental groups, how do they differ from each other?
- Is this study attempting to determine cause-and-effect or is this a correlational study?

3. Consider the data:

- How are the data presented? Are you given tables, figures, images, or none of the above? What are the independent variables? What is the dependent variable?
- What types of statistical analyses were used? Is anything considered statistically significant or statistically insignificant? Why?
- Try interpreting the data on your own before reading the results section.

4. Consider the discussion:

- Are the conclusions of the authors supported by the data? What potential weaknesses or flaws do you see in the study's design? Are these addressed in the discussion section?
- How might this study be biased?
- Do you agree with the conclusions drawn by the investigators?
- How might this study be improved? What would be the next most logical study?

Let's analyze a Biology journal article on proton pump inhibitors:

Eosinophilic esophagitis (EoE) is an increasingly recognized disorder. Diagnosis of EoE is based on histologic demonstration of eosinophilic inflammation, with ≥15 eosinophils per high power field (hpf) being the cutoff most commonly used, in the absence of pathologic reflux as evidenced by a normal pH monitoring study or persistent inflammation on high-dose proton pump inhibitor (PPI) treatment [1]. Symptoms include feeding issues, vomiting, chest or abdominal pain, dysphagia and food impaction [2].

Eosinophils contain multiple toxic granules, whose content include basic proteins, cytokines, chemokines, lipid mediators, and oxygen radicals. Free-lying granules serve as a surrogate marker for released eosinophil products that promote tissue damage, inflammation, remodeling, and fibrosis [3]. Eotaxin-3 is a chemokine stimulated by T-helper cytokines to recruit and activate eosinophils. PPI's have been shown to block eotaxin-3 release, suggesting a role independent of acid production [4]. We previously reported improvement of symptoms in children with EoE on long-term PPI monotherapy despite persistent eosinophilic inflammation [5]. We hypothesized that symptomatic improvement in our patients was due to a PPI effect in eotaxin 3- induced degranulation. Therefore, we sought to determine whether the improvement with PPI monotherapy was associated with decreased eosinophil degranulation.

We reviewed the records and biopsies from ten patients previously described [5] with EoE who improved clinically on PPI monotherapy. All patients were between 1 month and 18 years old, were on an unrestricted diet, were diagnosed with EoE based on standard criteria [1] with persistence of eosinophils on follow-up biopsies 3 months after diagnosis while on PPI, and had undergone follow-up endoscopy at least one year after diagnosis.

Hematoxylin and eosin-stained sections were reproduced from formalin fixed paraffin-embedded, endoscopically-obtained esophageal biopsies and evaluated to quantify eosinophils and assess degranulation. Immunohistochemical staining with tryptase for mast cells, and S100 for Langerhans cells using standard methodology was performed to evaluate their presence and possible role in eosinophil recruitment.

Using 400X magnification, all intraepithelial eosinophils were counted in three separate fields that had the highest density of eosinophils in each slide. The average number of eosinophils for these three fields was reported. The same method was used to quantify mast cells (tryptase) and Langerhans cells (S-100).

Using 600X magnification, areas with the highest concentration of scattered eosinophil granules were photographed using a Nikon Digital Sight DS-Fi1 microscope camera. Each image was printed on standard short bond paper (21.5 cm x 28 cm, representing a microscopic field of 7752 μm^2). A 5.3 cm x 6.8 cm rectangular frame (corresponding to a microscopic area of 1938 μm^2) was used to designate the areas with the highest density of free-lying eosinophil granules. All free-lying granules within this framed area in three separate fields were counted, and the mean was reported.

Comparison of results between presentation and most recent endoscopy was performed using paired t-test. Results are expressed as mean ± SD.

This study was reviewed and approved by the Institutional Review Board of the North Shore - LIJ Health System.

The mean age of the patients was 6.6 ± 4.8 years with 7 males. Presenting complaints were dysphagia (4), failure to thrive (3), abdominal pain (1) and vomiting (2). The patients had a second follow-up biopsy 17.1±8.5 months following initiation of PPI. The mean PPI dose was 1.5 ± 0.6 mg/kg. Nine patients were treated with lansoprazole and one child with esomeprazole. All patients were either asymptomatic (n=9) or significantly improved (n=1) on PPI monotherapy.

There was no significant difference in eosinophil count between initial and follow-up endoscopies. Compared to the initial endoscopy, the granule count decreased by the 3-month follow-up endoscopy and significantly decreased by the 1-year follow-up (Table 1).

	Mean ± SD	p value*
Eosinophils/hpf		
Initial endoscopy	106.2 ± 38.6	
3-month endoscopy	76.7 ± 60.1	NS
One-year endoscopy	67.6 ± 75.6	NS
Granule count		
Initial endoscopy	105.5 ± 58.1	
3-month endoscopy	72.0 ± 28.2	NS
One-year endoscopy	48.7 ± 43.3	p<0.05
Mast cells/hpf		
Initial endoscopy	6.4 ± 12.9	
3-month endoscopy	3.4 ± 2.7	NS
One-year endoscopy	4.7 ± 5.7	NS
Langerhans cells/hpf		
Initial endoscopy	3.7 ± 2.5	
3-month endoscopy	6.8 ± 3.5	p<0.01
One-year endoscopy	5.5 ± 2.1	NS

*p values are comparing 3-month and 1-year endoscopy to initial endoscopy.

Table 1 Comparison of histological markers in Eosinophilic Esophagitis.

Compared to initial endoscopy, the mast cell number was not different at the 3-month or 1-year follow-up endoscopy. The Langerhans cell number was increased at the 3-month follow-up endoscopy, but was not significantly different from the initial endoscopy at the 1-year follow-up (Table 1).

There was no statistically significant difference in eosinophil number between proximal and distal biopsies for all endoscopies. There was no difference in granule number between proximal and distal biopsies on the initial and 3-month follow-up endoscopies. However, at the 1-year follow-up endoscopy, the granule number in the proximal biopsy (50.8±41.8) was significantly increased compared with the distal biopsy (25.1±28.7, p<0.05, Table 2).

	Proximal esophagus (mean ± SD)	Distal esophagus (mean ± SD)	p value
Initial endoscopy	139.2±84.2	151.0 ± 10.5	p=NS
3-month endoscopy	61.4 ± 30.2	46.0 ± 41.7	p=NS
One year endoscopy	50.8 ± 41.8	25.1 ± 28.7	p<0.05

Table 2 Granule counts in proximal and distal esophagus.

Our case series suggests that children diagnosed with EoE treated with PPI monotherapy for at least one year have decreased eosinophil degranulation despite persistent eosinophilic inflammation. The persistence of eosinophils in these patients is not surprising since the criteria used for diagnosing EoE is lack of histologic response to PPI therapy. However, the finding of decreased degranulation despite the persistence of eosinophilic inflammation with only PPI therapy has not been previously described.

The decline in granules and improvement in symptoms may be due to an effect of PPI on eosinophil function. Zhang et al. [4] demonstrated that omeprazole significantly inhibited IL-4 stimulated eotaxin-3 protein secretion and m-RNA expression in EoE esophageal cells. Eotaxin-3 is known to be a potent eosinophil chemoattractant, but it also plays a role in activation and degranulation of eosinophils [4]. Although the studies suggest that PPI has an in-vitro effect [4] as well as a clinical benefit [5] in EoE, our current study is the first to associate the clinical improvement with the decrease in eosinophil degranulation. Reduced eosinophil degranulation after PPI is a morphologic finding that correlates with reduced eotaxin secretion. One of the novelties of the current paper lies in the fact that it provides a morphologic correlate of the biochemical findings, and allows a visual window into the mechanism involved. It is likely that eosinophil degranulation contributes to clinical symptoms, perhaps by inducing inflammation and fibrosis [3]. Although our patients who were clinically well still had some degree of free-lying esophageal granules, the significant decrease in granule number suggests that the lesser degree of degranulation is the factor leading to the clinical improvement. The lack of effect of PPI therapy on eosinophil number in our study may reflect the fact that eotaxin-3 may have a quicker or earlier effect on eosinophil degranulation than recruitment, and that longer PPI treatment may eventually lead to decreased tissue eosinophilia.

We noted that the granule number in distal biopsies at 1-year follow-up was significantly more decreased than the granule count in proximal biopsies. It is known that patients with EoE have dysmotility [2] which may predispose them to reflux-induced disease. One may postulate that the acid-suppressive effect of PPI contributes to improvement in eosinophil degranulation noted in the distal biopsies.

The inflammatory cascade may play a role in EoE [2]. In this study, we found that the mast cell number did not differ between initial and follow-up endoscopies in the EoE group. Langerhans cells were increased at the 3-month biopsy compared with the initial biopsies; however, the numbers were not different between initial and 1-year biopsies.

Eosinophils contain many different toxic granules and it is unclear which specific granule is responsible for the inflammation, remodeling and fibrosis seen in EoE. Free-lying granules serve as a surrogate marker for all released eosinophil products. Therefore, in this study we did not attempt to identify the specific protein seen within the released granules.

This paper examines the extracellular localization of the eosinophil granules in the epithelium, not the protein content of the granules. The tinctural properties of these granules are stable after fixation. Although formalin fixation may theoretically have an effect on eosinophil degranulation at the moment the tissue is placed into formalin, all tissues were treated the same way. Once embedded in paraffin the tissues are stable in a state of "suspended animation" reflecting their morphology at the time of fixation. Degranulation cannot occur once the tissue is embedded in paraffin.

The patients studied were all maintained on a regular unrestricted diet, and therefore, any differences could not be due to changes in dietary exposure. The patients in our EoE group are distinct from those patients who are thought to have a newly described entity called PPI-responsive esophageal eosinophilia. In that group, patients have increased esophageal eosinophilia but respond histologically to PPI monotherapy [1].

Prospective studies are needed to confirm our findings, to evaluate the precise mechanism in which PPIs decrease eosinophilic degranulation, and the role granules play to explain symptomatic improvement.

Adapted from Levine J, Lu Y, Carreon CK, Edelman M, *Proton-Pump Inhibitor Treatment in Eosinophilic Esophagitis is Associated with Decreased Eosinophil Degranulation*, Journal of Gastrointest Digestive Systems 5: 259, 2015.

Let's try to answer the questions posed at the beginning of this chapter.

Try to summarize the purpose of the experiment and the methods in 4–5 sentences. Consider:

- *How is the study designed? Is the experimenter conducting research on humans or on animals or on bacteria in a petri dish, or something else? Are there multiple experimental groups or just one? Is there a control group? Is the control group given some sort of placebo or nothing at all?*
- *Was this study conducted over a long period of time, collecting data at multiple points in time?*
- *Did this study have a large N or a small N?*
- *Was this a blinded study? If so, was it double blind or single blind?*
- *How do the experimental groups differ from the control? If there are multiple experimental groups, how do they differ from each other?*
- *Is this study attempting to determine cause-and-effect or is this a correlational study?*

This is a correlational study on humans with an age range of 1 month to 18 years of age designed to determine if proton-pump inhibitor therapy is related to a decrease in eosinophil degranulation in the esophagus. The researchers had previously determined that patients on proton-pump therapy showed an improvement in the symptoms of esophageal inflammation, despite continued presence of large numbers of eosinophils. They hypothesized that this may be due to less degranulation (release of granules that promote tissue damage and inflammation). This is a small study that looks at data from only 10 individuals over a 12 month period; observations were made at 3 months and at 12 months. There is no control group. All patients except one were treated with the same proton pump inhibitor.

Consider the data:

- *How are the data presented? Are you given tables, figures, images, or none of the above? What are the independent variables? What is the dependent variable?*
- *What types of statistical analyses were used? Is anything considered statistically significant or statistically insignificant? Why?*
- *Try interpreting the data on your own before reading the results section.*

The data are presented in two tables, one comparing the changes in the numbers of inflammatory mediators (eosinophil, mast cell, Langerhans cell counts, and granule counts) in esophageal biopsies at 3 months and 12 months after the start of proton pump inhibitor therapy, and one showing the differences in granule counts between proximal and distal biopsies, also at 3 months and 12 months after the start of therapy. The independent variable (if anything) is time and the dependent variables are the cell counts and granule counts. The results were analyzed by determining means and standard deviations, and a p-test was used to determine statistical significance.

From the data, it appears that cell counts do not change significantly, but granule counts overall decrease significantly by 12 months, and granule counts in the distal esophagus decrease more than in the proximal esophagus. The data seem to be showing correlation between proton pump inhibitor therapy and a reduction in eosinophilic degranulation.

Consider the discussion:

- *Are the conclusions of the authors supported by the data? What potential weaknesses or flaws do you see in the study's design? Are these addressed in the discussion section?*
- *How might this study be biased?*
- *Do you agree with the conclusions drawn by the investigators?*
- *How might this study be improved? What would be the next most logical study?*

The authors concluded that proton pump inhibitor therapy decreased eosinophilic degranulation over time and that this improved symptoms. They postulated that this was due to the inhibition by PPIs of eotaxin secretion, and eotaxin is associated with degranulation. Thus, if the release of eotaxin is inhibited, degranulation is reduced. However, this was only a correlational study, meaning that they did not show specifically that PPIs inhibited eotaxin release, or that the reduced eotaxin release specifically prevented degranulation; correlation does not imply causation. They addressed this in the discussion section by saying things like "It is likely that…" or "the…decrease in granule number suggests that…" Also, this study included only a very small number of participants; with larger numbers there may be less of a correlation (or more). The researchers imply the next most logical study: They suggest that longer PPI treatment may ultimately lead to reduced cell counts (in addition to reduced degranulation), thus the logical follow up would be to look at the same data but perhaps after 2 or 3 years of proton pump inhibitor therapy.

Let's analyze another article. This one is on racial diversity in practicing physicians.

The geographic distribution of the physician workforce in the United States has important implications for patients and their ability to access care. Many federal incentive programs have been established to mitigate the effect of regional shortages and to improve the recruitment and retention of health care providers in underserved areas. Additionally, many training models and recruitment strategies intended to improve geographic distribution of the physician workforce have been studied. However, few studies focus on the role of racial and ethnic composition of the physician workforce in establishing a more equitable distribution of physicians. For example, prior research indicates that physicians underrepresented in medicine are important for the delivery of primary care, the provision of care to underserved populations, and to improve access to health care services in medically underserved areas. Although the nation is experiencing a significant demographic shift towards more racial and ethnic diversity, the physician workforce has not kept pace.

This *Analysis in Brief (AIB)*, the second in a two-part series exploring racial and ethnic diversity in the physician workforce, examines geographic distribution to determine whether a more racially and ethnically diverse physician workforce could positively contribute to a more equitable distribution of the U.S. physician workforce. Medical schools can use this information to inform their efforts to foster a geographically well-distributed physician workforce that is responsive to the nation's evolving health care needs.

The 2012 American Medical Association (AMA) Physician Masterfile was used to study the characteristics and distribution of direct patient care physicians who graduated from medical school between 1980 and 2010. The sample was limited to these physicians because racial and ethnic data for medical school graduates was not systematically or reliably collected prior to 1980. Physician race and ethnicity information was obtained from the AAMC Student Records System and the AAMC Minority Physicians Database. The variation in physician practice locations by physician race and ethnicity was analyzed. Specifically, physician practice locations that were identified as rural (2003 Urban Rural Continuum Codes), areas with 20 percent or more of the population living in poverty (2011 American Community Survey Five-year Estimate), federally designated 2012 Primary Care Health Professional Shortage Areas (HPSAs), and Medically Underserved Areas/Populations (MUA/P) were studied. Bivariate measures of association were performed to study the relationship between physician race/ethnicity and their practice location.

The sample was comprised of 507,622 direct patient care physicians, reflecting 73 percent of the total direct patient care physicians in the nation as of 2012. Less than one percent of these physicians identified as American Indian, Alaskan Native, or Hawaiian/Pacific Islander; roughly five percent of these physicians identified as black or African American; five percent identified as Hispanic/Latino; 11 percent identified as Asian; 17 percent identified as "other" or were listed as unknown race/ethnicity, and 62 percent identified as white. Together, the groups underrepresented in medicine (URM) comprise roughly ten percent of the physicians, which is substantially lower than their percentage in the overall U.S. population (30 percent). It is worth noting that although the Asian group appears to be overrepresented in the physician pool, many studies have pointed out that combining Asian subgroups can mask subtle differences within certain groups.

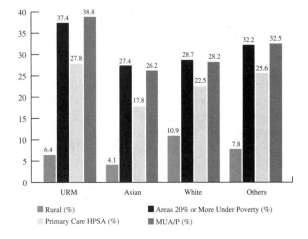

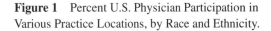

Figure 1 Percent U.S. Physician Participation in Various Practice Locations, by Race and Ethnicity.

In terms of practice in rural areas, results show significant differences among racial and ethnic groups (see Figure 1). Nine percent of physicians in the study sample practiced in rural areas, but significant differences exist between racial and ethnic groups (p < .001): four percent of Asian physicians, six percent of URM physicians, and 11 percent of white physicians were practicing in rural areas. Results also show significant differences (p < .001) between physicians based on race and ethnicity practicing in areas high in poverty. Compared to the 27 percent of Asian physicians and 29 percent of white physicians practicing in these areas, results show that 37 percent of URM physicians practice in these locations.

Similarly, significant associations exist between physician race, ethnicity and practice locations in primary care HPSAs and MUA/Ps (p < 0.001). Twenty-eight percent of URM physicians were practicing in a HPSA, compared to 18 percent of Asian physicians and 23 percent of white physicians. Similar patterns were found for practice locations in MUA/Ps, with URM physicians being more likely to practice in a MUA/P than Asian and white physicians. Results show that while 33 percent of Asian physicians and 38 percent of white physicians practice in either a HPSA or MUA/P, nearly half of URM physicians practice in these areas.

These results show that there are significant associations between physician practice location and their racial and ethnic composition. Physicians identifying as American Indian, Alaska Native, or Hawaiian/Pacific Islander; black or African American; and/or Hispanic/Latino were more likely to practice in impoverished areas, and areas federally designated as medically underserved or experiencing health professional shortages. American Indian, Alaska Native, or Hawaiian/Pacific Islander physicians as a group are significantly more likely to practice in rural areas when compared to the overall physician pool. These finding suggest that increasing the racial and ethnic diversity of the physician workforce—in particular, increasing representation from American Indian, Alaska Native, or Hawaiian/Pacific Islander; black or African American; and Hispanic/ Latino groups—may help improve the distribution of the physician workforce, and could have a profound impact on improving access to physicians in underserved areas. Furthermore, diversifying the physician workforce also may be key in addressing health disparities among racial and ethnic minority groups.

In light of the nation's evolving racial and ethnic landscape, physician workforce diversity is becoming an increasingly urgent matter. As part I of this AIB series discussed, eliminating disparities in K-12 education, enhancing pipeline programs and college-level interventions, and transforming medical school admissions are some ways to increase physician racial and ethnic diversity and ultimately promote excellence in health care. Future workforce interventions should consider the role of racial and ethnic diversity in the physician workforce, and the positive impact of this diversity on the geographic distribution of the physician workforce.

Adapted from Xierali, I., Castillo-Page, L., Conrad, S., Nivet, M., *Analyzing Physician Workforce Racial and Ethnic Composition Associations: Geographic Distribution (Part II),* Association of American Medical Colleges, 14:9, 2014.

Try to summarize the purpose of the experiment and the methods in 4–5 sentences. Consider:

- *How is the study designed? Is the experimenter conducting research on humans or on animals or on bacteria in a petri dish, or something else? Are there multiple experimental groups or just one? Is there a control group? Is the control group given some sort of placebo or nothing at all?*
- *Was this study conducted over a long period of time, collecting data at multiple points in time?*
- *Did this study have a large N or a small N?*
- *Was this a blinded study? If so, was it double blind or single blind?*
- *How do the experimental groups differ from the control? If multiple experimental groups, how do they differ from each other?*
- *Is this study attempting to determine cause-and-effect or is this a correlational study?*

This is a correlational study on practicing physicians to see if their race and ethnicity was correlated to the location of practice. There is no control group and no real experiment, this is just data analysis and postulation. It has a large N; a dataset including over half a million physicians was analyzed, representing approximately 75% of the total direct patient care physicians in the United States. Of this group, over 60% identified as white, while a little less than 40% identified as non-white (black, Latino, Asian, American Indian, etc.).

Consider the data:

- *How are the data presented? Are you given tables, figures, images, or none of the above? What are the independent variables? What is the dependent variable?*
- *What types of statistical analyses were used? Is anything considered statistically significant or statistically insignificant? Why?*
- *Try interpreting the data on your own before reading the results section.*

The data are presented as a bar graph showing each of four different physician population: underrepresented in medicine minority groups, Asian, white, and other (those who did not identify as a listed ethnicity). Each population was then categorized according to the percentage of physicians practicing in four areas: rural areas, health professional shortage areas, areas of high poverty, and medically underserved areas/populations. A p-test was used to determine statistical significance, and in all cases, differences among percentages of populations serving in these areas were statistically significant.

Consider the discussion:

- *Are the conclusions of the authors supported by the data? What potential weaknesses or flaws do you see in the study's design? Are these addressed in the discussion section?*
- *How might this study be biased?*
- *Do you agree with the conclusions drawn by the investigators?*
- *How might this study be improved? What would be the next most logical study?*

The authors concluded that there is a significant association with a physician's race and ethnicity and the location in which they practice. A much higher percentage of non-white physicians practice in rural, underserved, and impoverished areas than white physicians. They postulate that increasing diversity may "help improve the distribution of the physician workforce"; however, they do not clarify specifically what that means. One might infer that a greater diversity of physicians might increase numbers in these typically underserved areas (i.e., if we have more black, Latino, American Indian etc. doctors overall, there will be more doctors in underserved areas), but this assumes that the current percentage trends would continue if there were more URM physicians.

The study might be improved by clarifying the data; the four categories clearly overlap (as indicated by the total percent of URMs serving in the different areas—adding up the numbers shows them at a little over 110%!), yet this is not addressed, and that makes the data harder to interpret. It would be useful if the degree of overlap were addressed, for example, by stating what percentage of rural communities were also counted as HPSAs.

The next most logical study would be to see if medical schools have increased their diversity since 2012 (when this study was done), if that diversity actually translated to a more diverse physician population, and if that improved access to health care in rural and impoverished areas.

Chapter 5
Test Analysis Overview

Every time you take an exam, you should be sure to review your results thoroughly. Most people know to review the questions they got wrong in order to learn why their answer choice was incorrect and why the correct answer was a better choice. However, it is also important to review the questions you got right to reinforce proper thought processes. This is especially important for questions you happen to have gotten right but were unsure about or guessed on. Going back will help you solidify knowledge you may be weak in. After you complete a practice passage or take a Princeton Review practice exam, you can perform a detailed review of your results using a couple of different tools. If the practice passage or test happened to be an online test, you will have additional tools built into the online environment to help you analyze your results.

5.1 ONLINE SCORE REPORT

Generally, tests taken online come with an online score report. This is true of both Princeton Review tests as well as other products (for example, the AAMC Practice tests).

Princeton Review score reports will come with a total score, as well as a breakdown of the individual section scores. You can review each section separately to get information about the questions within that section of the test, as well as the breakdown of topics and subtopics. When viewing the section as a whole, you can see quickly which questions you got right or wrong (or left blank), and you can look at each individual question to see it in context with its passage and its explanation. Remember to register your book (at PrincetonReview.com/cracking) to access all of your online Student Tools, including the aforementioned score report.

In the next chapter we'll walk through an example of a score report—your actual report may look slightly different visually, but your process of reviewing your report should be similar to the one we'll go through.

The category view for each section sorts the questions into their main subjects (or question types for CARS) as well as providing the topics and subtopics for each primary subject. This provides you with very granular information about the concepts each question is testing.

Even if the online exam you took was not a Princeton Review test, it should come with similar analysis tools. For example, the AAMC provides online practice exams for purchase and has score reports with comparable types of section breakdown and examination.

5.2 WORKSHEET SELF-ANALYSIS

While the online tools are useful for identifying content deficiencies in the sciences, often what holds students back from getting higher scores in these sections is not a lack of content knowledge, but instead a difficulty in dealing with certain question types. Therefore, it is important to review your test not only for content errors and weaknesses, but also to see how the questions you missed fall into the categories described below. You also need to think about what led you to the wrong answer choice. For CARS, an online report will likely give you a breakdown based on question type. However, that breakdown is not enough; you need to figure out **why** you are having trouble with certain question types as well as to identify other reasons, aside from the question type, why you might be missing questions. The Question Review Worksheet on pages 35 and 36 will help you diagnose reasons for your mistakes in all four sections by asking you to first categorize the question and then to decide why you got it right or wrong. Let's look in more detail at this worksheet.

5.3 OVERVIEW OF THE QUESTION REVIEW WORKSHEET

Question Type

As stated previously, in the science sections of the MCAT, the questions fall into one of three main categories:

1. **Memory questions** are answered directly from prior knowledge without any use of the passage.
2. In **Explicit questions**, the correct answer is explicitly stated in the passage or requires making a simple connection between passage information and prior knowledge. To answer them correctly, for example, may just require finding a definition, or reading a graph, and connecting that to what you already know.
3. **Implicit questions** require you to apply your existing knowledge to a new situation, or require more complex connections between passage information and prior understanding. The correct answer is typically implied by the information in the passage; you need to think logically and carefully to arrive at it.

There are four main CARS categories:

1. **Specific questions** ask you for specific information from the passage, such as a fact, an inference, or a definition.
2. **General questions** ask you to summarize the main theme or purpose of the passage, or to evaluate the author's overall attitude.
3. **Reasoning questions** ask you to either describe how parts of the author's argument relate to each other or evaluate how well the author constructs or supports his or her argument.
4. **Application questions** ask you to apply new information from the question stem or from the answer choices to the passage. These questions may ask you how the author would react to some fact or event, what would weaken or strengthen the author's claims, or what new situation or relationship is most logically similar to something described in the passage.

Result Code

This code helps you identify why you got a question right or wrong.

1. **Correct, easy:** You understood this. It was very clear, you have no concerns or worries, and you were absolutely sure the answer was right when you chose it.
2. **Correct, the hard way:** You read every single word of every single answer choice, pondered, debated, calculated, and struggled, but got the right answer.
3. **Correct, got it down to two:** You eliminated two answer choices as wrong, guessed between the remaining two, and got lucky.
4. **Wrong, got it down to two:** You eliminated two answer choices as wrong, guessed between the remaining two, and didn't get lucky.
5. **Wrong, eliminated the right answer:** Oops. (Kudos for trying to use POE, though!)
6. **Guessed randomly (right or wrong):** You had no clue and guessed. Randomly. Picked the "letter of the day."

Most codes have an action associated with them; note below that the ONLY code with no action is the one for correct/easy. Again, in order to maximize your MCAT score, you must review not only the incorrect answers, but the correct ones as well in order to recognize and reinforce the correct thought processes.

1. Action for Code 2: Review for shortcuts, POE strategies, deductions, etc. You got this question right, and that's great, but there may be an easier way to do it. Did you miss something in the passage? Forget to use proportionality? Miss a connection?
2. Action for Codes 3 and 4: Read the question solution and think about what led you to your answer choice. Try to follow the logic of the explanation and apply that to future similar questions.
3. Action for Code 5: Review for comprehension. In other words, did you fully understand the question before you tried to answer it? If it was a CARS question, did you ID it properly? Would it be better if you slowed down a bit and read the question/answer choices more carefully?
4. Action for Code 6: Make sure that any questions you guessed on were the super-tough ones you really had no clue on.

Notes/Subtopic

Here you can list the specific reason you got the question wrong, strategies you may want to employ next time, the subtopic of science questions, etc.

Key:

- **Test or Book/pg #**: This is the diagnostic exam you are reviewing or the passage you have completed.
- **Section**: Either CP (chem/phys), CARS (critical analysis), BB (bio/biochem), or PS (psych/soc)
- **P# and Q #**: Passage number and Question number
- **Q type**: Question type; for the science sections this is either M (memory), E (explicit), or I (implicit). For CARS this is either R, (retrieval), I (inference), MI/PP (main idea/primary purpose), T (tone or attitude), S (structure), E (evaluate), ST (strengthen), WK (weaken), NI (new information), or A (analogy). For CARS, also enter codes for two question formats: ELN(Except/Least/Not) and RN (Roman numeral).

Result Code:

Code	Question Result	Action
1	correct, easy	none
2	correct, the hard way	review for shortcuts—POE strategies, deductions, etc.
3	correct, got it down to two	review, look for WHY you picked the correct answer, compare remaining, decide why the correct answer was better, consider what you will do next time
4	wrong, got it down to two	review, look for WHY you picked the incorrect answer, compare remaining, decide why the correct answer was better, consider what you will do next time
5	wrong, eliminated the right answer	review for comprehension—did you ID the question correctly? Did you RTFQ (read the full question)? Misapply POE strategies?
6	guessed randomly (letter of the day)	review for difficulty—did you attempt the easiest questions and passages?

Test or Book/pg #	Content Section	P#	Q#	Q type	Result Code	Notes

Test or Book/pg #	Content Section	P#	Q#	Q type	Result Code	Notes

What's the Point?

Filling out the Question Review Worksheet allows you to see patterns, the types of questions you usually get right, the types of questions you usually get wrong, and why. It helps you target your future study and practice according to your specific areas of weakness. Feel free to copy the worksheet as many times as you need to review your practice passages and tests.

5.4   ANALYZING THE SCIENCE SECTIONS

If you find you are missing a lot of science Memory questions, it might indicate a content area weakness, and you should review material in that subtopic. However, MCAT students typically have more trouble with the second two science categories, Explicit and Implicit questions, because they expect that they should be able to answer the questions based purely off information they already know. This is not the case, since the MCAT is not a test of your science recall. One of the most important things to remember when taking the MCAT is that if you are unsure of how to approach a question, look to the passage for help; it is likely that you are dealing with a question that requires information from the passage in order to be answered correctly.

If you are consistently missing Explicit questions, it might be because you are relying too heavily on memory and not enough on passage retrieval. Make sure you have an effective passage map (passage mapping will be discussed in more detail in the subject sections) to help clarify where information is located in the passage. As you are doing practice problems, force yourself to actively refer to the passage more frequently for relevant information, even on questions where you think you can use memory alone. On some problems, although you may have inherent knowledge of the topic being tested, it's possible that the passage mentions a more specific or anomalous example related to the topic. Therefore, what you know may not apply, and you must retrieve the new information from the passage in order to answer the question correctly.

Implicit questions also involve a fair amount of passage retrieval; they are often based on analogous examples to those given in the passage. Of all of the question types, Implicit questions rely most heavily on critical reasoning skills. If you consistently miss Implicit questions, you should carefully consider what the question is asking, go back to the passage for relevant information, combine that with your knowledge of the topic, and formulate a possible answer in your head before reading through the answer choices. Often the process of formulating the answer in your head first helps the correct answer choice stand out when you see it. You will also have to spend time carefully reviewing the explanations for Implicit questions to make sure you understand the logic required to get to the correct answer. If you can determine where your logic failed, you won't make the same mistake in the future.

5.5 ANALYZING THE CARS SECTION

We will discuss CARS in more detail with particular CARS question types later in the book. For now, let's go over some more general patterns to look for when analyzing a full practice test section.

Pacing

The two obvious pacing issues are: Were you going too fast? Or were you going too slowly? MCAT students who are already scoring at or above average often finish every question on the test. And if you are already doing well, it can be difficult to accept the idea of slowing down and randomly guessing on a certain number of questions. However, if you are writing a lot of comments in your Worksheet along the lines of, "I didn't read it carefully enough," "I didn't go back to the passage when I should have," or "I misunderstood what the question was asking," you may improve your score even more by:

- slowing down where you need to on harder questions,
- reading more carefully,
- using the passage text more actively, and
- randomly guessing on a full passage (or at least on a couple of questions in the last passage you get to).

If you are missing one or two questions on every passage because of careless errors, or if you often crash and burn on one passage and get most of those questions wrong, you should definitely slow down and work harder to be more accurate on the problems you attempt.

On the other hand, if you are completing seven or eight of the nine passages in the section and getting almost every question right, you can improve significantly only by picking up the pace. If you find yourself using Code 2 ("Correct the Hard Way") on a lot of the questions on the Worksheet, you may be overthinking the answers or not using POE enough. Go back and review those questions and ask yourself, "Where did I do more work than necessary to get this question right?" and "How could I have worked the passage and answered this question more efficiently?" For your Code 3 or 4 questions ("Correct, Got it Down to Two," "Incorrect, Got it Down to Two") ask yourself, "What difference between these two answers could I have identified in order to more quickly get it down to the correct choice?"

Question Type Categories

Look for patterns in categories of question types that you tend to miss. If you are missing a high percentage of General questions, did you have a good idea of the main idea or bottom line of the passage? If not, it means that you need to work the passage more effectively. Or, are you consistently picking answers that are too narrow? If so, you need to keep the scope of the whole question more clearly in mind. Are you missing lots of Specific questions? If so, you most likely need to read more carefully and go back to the passage more consistently. Finally, if you are missing a lot of Reasoning or Application questions (which tend to require a bit more work), you need to translate the question more carefully to get a better understanding of what it is really asking you about the passage, use the passage information more actively in conjunction with the question task, and have a reasonably good idea of what you are looking for before you start evaluating the answer choices.

5.6 A FEW THINGS TO REMEMBER ABOUT USING THE QUESTION REVIEW WORKSHEET

- Fill it out soon after taking your practice test or drill, so that you remember your reasoning for choosing your answers. The longer you wait, the more likely you are to forget why you chose a particular answer over another.
- For full-length tests, fill out a separate Question Review Worksheet for each section, and tackle each section one at a time.
- After filling out the worksheet, go back and circle the questions you got wrong in red. Also, for the science sections, use colored pencils to color in the different subjects. For example, in the Chem/Phys section, color general chemistry in green, organic chemistry in orange, physics in purple, and biology/biochemistry in blue. This will help you see patterns in your answer choices.
- Expect to spend a few hours per section reviewing with the Question Review Worksheet. It takes time to look at each question and think about your reasoning for the answer. Consider it time well spent, though, since you will gain valuable insight into not only your thought processes, but your areas of weaknesses and strengths. This information will help you tailor your study sessions so that you can boost your total MCAT score to the range you want.

In the next chapter, we'll take a look at how Joe Bloggs used the Online Score Report to help analyze the results of his practice exam. This is based off the MCAT Demo Exam in your *MCAT Elite* Online Companion.[1]

---

[1] We recommend that you take your first practice test (found online and named "MCAT Demo Test" (if you haven't already) before reading through the Test Analysis section. That exam is found online in your Student Tools. This section goes through some of the questions in detail; you don't want to see the analysis of these questions before you take the actual test. And remember, that you have an another practice test on which to hone your test-taking ability.

Chapter 6
Sample MCAT
Practice Test Analysis

6.1   OVERALL ANALYSIS OF THE MCAT DEMO TEST

Here's an example of a score report—your actual report may look slightly different visually, but your process of reviewing your report should be similar to the one described below.

After completing the MCAT Demo Test, Joe logged onto princetonreview.com and viewed his Score Report. He was reasonably happy with his scores: Chem/Phys 127, CARS 127, Bio/Biochem 128, and Psych/Soc 128.

MCAT Demo Test
This test taken: August 23, 2016

Score Summary
Your Total MCAT Score is **510***

	518 ▼
510	
472	528

Chemical and Physical Foundations of Biological Systems	118	127	130	132
Critical Analysis and Reasoning Skills	118	127	129	132
Biological and Biochemical Foundations of Living Systems	118	128	130	132
Psychological, Social, and Biological Foundations of Behavior	118	128	129	132

Next, Joe looked at the "Section" view of the Chem/Phys section. This view showed all of the questions in the section, clearly indicating which were correct and which were wrong. He noted that from this view, he could click on each individual question to see it in context with its passage and its explanation.

Chemical and Physical Foundations of Biological Systems	Critical Analysis and Reasoning Skills	Biological and Biochemical Foundations of Living Systems	Psychological, Social, and Biological Foundations of Behavior

You Scored: **127**

View by   SECTION   CATEGORY

Your Responses   ☑ ✓ 47 CORRECT   ☑ ✗ 12 INCORRECT   ☑ ○ 0 BLANK   ☑ ▮ 0 MARKED

1 P:1	2 P:1	3 P:1	4 P:1	5 P:1	6 P:2	7 P:2	8 P:2	9 P:2	10	11	12	13	14 P:3	15 P:3	16 P:3	17 P:3	18 P:4	19 P:4
✓	✗	✓	✓	✓	✓	✓	✓	✗	✓	✓	✓	✓	✓	✓	✓	✓	✗	✓

20 P:4	21 P:4	22 P:5	23 P:5	24 P:5	25 P:5	26	27	28	29	30 P:6	31 P:6	32 P:6	33 P:6	34 P:6	35 P:7	36 P:7	37 P:7	38 P:7
✓	✓	✓	✗	✗	✓	✓	✓	✓	✓	✗	✓	✓	✓	✓	✓	✓	✓	✓

39 P:7	40 P:8	41 P:8	42 P:8	43 P:8	44 P:8	45	46	47	48	49 P:9	50 P:9	51 P:9	52 P:9	53 P:10	54 P:10	55 P:10	56 P:10	57
✗	✓	✗	✓	✓	✓	✓	✓	✓	✓	✗	✓	✓	✗	✓	✓	✗	✓	✓

58	59
✓	✓

Joe then switched to the "Category" view, which grouped the questions by subject:

Chemical and Physical Foundations of Biological Systems	Critical Analysis and Reasoning Skills	Biological and Biochemical Foundations of Living Systems	Psychological, Social, and Biological Foundations of Behavior

You Scored: 127

View by SECTION **CATEGORY**

Note that in the category view, you will see questions appear in multiple places. This is because some questions test more than one concept. An understanding of each of these is necessary to answer these questions correctly.

> General Chemistry	✔ 13 Correct	✖ 5 Incorrect	○ 0 Blank	◨ 0 Marked
> Physics	✔ 13 Correct	✖ 2 Incorrect	○ 0 Blank	◨ 0 Marked
> Organic Chemistry	✔ 14 Correct	✖ 2 Incorrect	○ 0 Blank	◨ 0 Marked
> Biology	✔ 13 Correct	✖ 4 Incorrect	○ 0 Blank	◨ 0 Marked

A quick glance showed Joe that for him, the two weaker subjects were General Chemistry (5 wrong out of 18) and Biology (4 wrong out of 17). Physics and Organic Chemistry seemed alright (2 wrong out of 15 for Physics and 2 wrong out of 16 for Organic Chemistry). He noticed also that he could get more information for each of the subjects by expanding the subject and looking at the subtopics:

> Organic Chemistry	✔ 14 Correct	✖ 2 Incorrect	○ 0 Blank	◨ 0 Marked
⌄ Biology	✔ 13 Correct	✖ 4 Incorrect	○ 0 Blank	◨ 0 Marked
> Biochemistry	✔ 9 Correct	✖ 0 Incorrect	○ 0 Blank	◨ 0 Marked
⌄ Lab Techniques	✔ 1 Correct	✖ 1 Incorrect	○ 0 Blank	◨ 0 Marked

Gel Electrophoresis 1/1	PCR 0/1
✔ 13	✖ 55 P:10

> Digestive System	✔ 2 Correct	✖ 0 Incorrect	○ 0 Blank	◨ 0 Marked
> Reading Comprehension	✔ 5 Correct	✖ 3 Incorrect	○ 0 Blank	◨ 0 Marked
> Experiment Analysis	✔ 2 Correct	✖ 2 Incorrect	○ 0 Blank	◨ 0 Marked

Joe noticed that he missed almost half the Reading Comprehension questions in Biology. He decided to spend more time with the Chem/Phys Category view after filling out the Question Review Worksheet, but before that, he looked at the Section and Category views of the other sections on the test. All of the Section views were similar; a listing of each question and which ones he got right or wrong. The Category views, however, gave him a little more high level information.

For CARS, the questions were grouped into question types, allowing Joe to see that he was weakest in Application questions (4 wrong out of 12) and Specific question (6 wrong out of 25), and stronger in General questions (only 1 wrong out of 5) and Reasoning questions (all 11 correct!).

Chemical and Physical Foundations of Biological Systems	Critical Analysis and Reasoning Skills	Biological and Biochemical Foundations of Living Systems	Psychological, Social, and Biological Foundations of Behavior

You Scored: 127

View by **SECTION** **CATEGORY**

Note that in the category view, you will see questions appear in multiple places. This is because some questions test more than one concept. An understanding of each of these is necessary to answer these questions correctly.

⌄ CARS	✓ 42 Correct	✗ 11 Incorrect	◯ 0 Blank	▐ 0 Marked
› General	✓ 4 Correct	✗ 1 Incorrect	◯ 0 Blank	▐ 0 Marked
› Reasoning	✓ 11 Correct	✗ 0 Incorrect	◯ 0 Blank	▐ 0 Marked
› Application	✓ 8 Correct	✗ 4 Incorrect	◯ 0 Blank	▐ 0 Marked
› Specific	✓ 19 Correct	✗ 6 Incorrect	◯ 0 Blank	▐ 0 Marked
› Format	✓ 42 Correct	✗ 11 Incorrect	◯ 0 Blank	▐ 0 Marked

Joe looked at the "Format" category a little more closely, since it appeared that all questions were assigned a format of some sort:

⌄ CARS	✓ 42 Correct	✗ 11 Incorrect	◯ 0 Blank	▐ 0 Marked
› General	✓ 4 Correct	✗ 1 Incorrect	◯ 0 Blank	▐ 0 Marked
⌄ Format	✓ 42 Correct	✗ 11 Incorrect	◯ 0 Blank	▐ 0 Marked

Except/Least/Not: Choice Unlike the Others 5/6	Roman Numeral: Correct Item/Combination 1/3	Standard 36/44

Except/Least/Not: Choice Unlike the Others 5/6
✓ 15 P.3 ✓ 28 P.5 ✓ 31 P.5
✓ 43 P.7 ✓ 44 P.8 ✗ 33 P.6

Roman Numeral: Correct Item/Combination 1/3
✓ 13 P.3 ✗ 6 P.1 ✗ 49 P.9

Standard 36/44
✓ 1 P.1 ✓ 2 P.1 ✓ 4 P.1 ✓ 7 P.1 ✓ 8 P.2 ✓ 9 P.2 ✓ 10 P.2 ✓ 12 P.2 ✓ 14 P.2 ✓ 16 P.2
✓ 17 P.3 ✓ 19 P.3 ✓ 20 P.4 ✓ 21 P.4 ✓ 22 P.4 ✓ 25 P.4 ✓ 27 P.5 ✓ 29 P.5 ✓ 30 P.5 ✓ 32 P.6
✓ 34 P.6 ✓ 35 P.6 ✓ 36 P.6 ✓ 37 P.7 ✓ 38 P.7 ✓ 39 P.7 ✓ 40 P.7 ✓ 41 P.7 ✓ 42 P.7 ✓ 45 P.8
✓ 46 P.8 ✓ 48 P.8 ✓ 50 P.9 ✓ 51 P.9 ✓ 52 P.9 ✓ 53 P.9 ✗ 3 P.1 ✗ 5 P.1 ✗ 11 P.2 ✗ 18 P.3
✗ 23 P.4 ✗ 24 P.4 ✗ 26 P.4 ✗ 47 P.8

› Reasoning	✓ 11 Correct	✗ 0 Incorrect	◯ 0 Blank	▐ 0 Marked
› Application	✓ 8 Correct	✗ 4 Incorrect	◯ 0 Blank	▐ 0 Marked
› Specific	✓ 19 Correct	✗ 6 Incorrect	◯ 0 Blank	▐ 0 Marked

He could see that he struggled a little bit with Roman numeral type questions (2 wrong out of 3) but that the other format types seemed to be OK.

In the Bio/Biochem section, Joe was glad to see that the got all of the General Chemistry and Organic Chemistry questions right.

Chemical and Physical Foundations of Biological Systems	Critical Analysis and Reasoning Skills	Biological and Biochemical Foundations of Living Systems	Psychological, Social, and Biological Foundations of Behavior

You Scored: 128

View by SECTION CATEGORY

⚑ Note that in the category view, you will see questions appear in multiple places. This is because some questions test more than one concept. An understanding of each of these is necessary to answer these questions correctly.

> Biology	✔ 42 Correct	✖ 11 Incorrect	○ 0 Blank	⚑ 0 Marked
> General Chemistry	✔ 3 Correct	✖ 0 Incorrect	○ 0 Blank	⚑ 0 Marked
> Organic Chemistry	✔ 3 Correct	✖ 0 Incorrect	○ 0 Blank	⚑ 0 Marked

He expanded the Biology category to see more detail on the Biology topics.

Chemical and Physical Foundations of Biological Systems	Critical Analysis and Reasoning Skills	Biological and Biochemical Foundations of Living Systems	Psychological, Social, and Biological Foundations of Behavior

You Scored: 128

View by SECTION CATEGORY

⚑ Note that in the category view, you will see questions appear in multiple places. This is because some questions test more than one concept. An understanding of each of these is necessary to answer these questions correctly.

∨ Biology	✔ 42 Correct	✖ 11 Incorrect	○ 0 Blank	⚑ 0 Marked
> Respiratory System	✔ 2 Correct	✖ 1 Incorrect	○ 0 Blank	⚑ 0 Marked
> Nervous System	✔ 3 Correct	✖ 2 Incorrect	○ 0 Blank	⚑ 0 Marked
> Immunology	✔ 1 Correct	✖ 3 Incorrect	○ 0 Blank	⚑ 0 Marked
> Biochemistry	✔ 11 Correct	✖ 3 Incorrect	○ 0 Blank	⚑ 0 Marked
> Molecular Biology	✔ 3 Correct	✖ 0 Incorrect	○ 0 Blank	⚑ 0 Marked
> Microbiology	✔ 1 Correct	✖ 0 Incorrect	○ 0 Blank	⚑ 0 Marked
> Cardiovascular System	✔ 2 Correct	✖ 0 Incorrect	○ 0 Blank	⚑ 0 Marked
> Digestive System	✔ 1 Correct	✖ 0 Incorrect	○ 0 Blank	⚑ 0 Marked
> Cell Biology	✔ 1 Correct	✖ 0 Incorrect	○ 0 Blank	⚑ 0 Marked
> Lab Techniques	✔ 2 Correct	✖ 0 Incorrect	○ 0 Blank	⚑ 0 Marked
> Genetics	✔ 1 Correct	✖ 0 Incorrect	○ 0 Blank	⚑ 0 Marked

> Development	✓ 1 Correct	✗ 0 Incorrect	○ 0 Blank	▌0 Marked
> Renal System	✓ 2 Correct	✗ 0 Incorrect	○ 0 Blank	▌0 Marked
> Endocrine System	✓ 4 Correct	✗ 0 Incorrect	○ 0 Blank	▌0 Marked
> Evolution/Speciation	✓ 1 Correct	✗ 0 Incorrect	○ 0 Blank	▌0 Marked
> Reproductive Systems	✓ 1 Correct	✗ 0 Incorrect	○ 0 Blank	▌0 Marked
> Muscular System	✓ 1 Correct	✗ 0 Incorrect	○ 0 Blank	▌0 Marked
> Experiment Analysis	✓ 9 Correct	✗ 1 Incorrect	○ 0 Blank	▌0 Marked
> Reading Comprehension	✓ 18 Correct	✗ 7 Incorrect	○ 0 Blank	▌0 Marked
> General Chemistry	✓ 3 Correct	✗ 0 Incorrect	○ 0 Blank	▌0 Marked
> Organic Chemistry	✓ 3 Correct	✗ 0 Incorrect	○ 0 Blank	▌0 Marked

The first thing Joe noticed is that the topic list for Biology was very broad, with only a few questions in each topic. He only missed questions in Respiratory System, Nervous System, Immunology, and Biochemistry, and of those, it seemed like Immunology was the weakest (3 wrong out of 4 total). The other three topics were about the same (approximately 30% of the questions wrong). He noted that he could get more information about the subtopics within those categories (for example, the Respiratory System questions covered the Conduction Zone, the Respiratory Zone, Ventilation, and pH Regulation):

Note that in the category view, you will see questions appear in multiple places. This is because some questions test more than one concept. An understanding of each of these is necessary to answer these questions correctly.

∨ Biology	✓ 42 Correct	✗ 11 Incorrect	○ 0 Blank	▌0 Marked
∨ Respiratory System	✓ 2 Correct	✗ 1 Incorrect	○ 0 Blank	▌0 Marked

Conduction and Respiratory Zones 1/2	Ventilation and pH Regulation 1/1
✓ 1 P:1 ✗ 3 P:1	✓ 4 P:1

> Nervous System	✓ 3 Correct	✗ 2 Incorrect	○ 0 Blank	▌0 Marked
> Immunology	✓ 1 Correct	✗ 3 Incorrect	○ 0 Blank	▌0 Marked
> Biochemistry	✓ 11 Correct	✗ 3 Incorrect	○ 0 Blank	▌0 Marked
> Molecular Biology	✓ 3 Correct	✗ 0 Incorrect	○ 0 Blank	▌0 Marked
> Microbiology	✓ 1 Correct	✗ 0 Incorrect	○ 0 Blank	▌0 Marked
> Cardiovascular System	✓ 2 Correct	✗ 0 Incorrect	○ 0 Blank	▌0 Marked
> Reading Comprehension	✓ 18 Correct	✗ 7 Incorrect	○ 0 Blank	▌0 Marked

Joe decided to look at his other weak biology subtopics more closely later, but noticed that he missed a fair amount of questions (about a third) tagged as "Reading Comprehension" questions. This was similar to what he saw in the Chem/Phys section, and told Joe that he might not be pulling information out of passages as well as he could be. He made a note of this and decided to wait until after he filled out the Question Review Worksheet to think about it further.

The last section Joe reviewed was the Psych/Soc section:

He quickly realized that Sociology was his weakness here; he missed 5 out of 16 Sociology questions. A look at the subtopics for Sociology showed that his errors were concentrated in Groups (2 wrong out of 5) and Socialization (3 wrong out of 5):

Joe took a quick look at the Psychology topics, but there was no concentrated area of weakness in Psychology. He was happy to note that Psychology, Statistical Methods, and Research Design all seemed fairly strong:

Finally, Joe started his detailed analysis of the individual sections using the Question Review Worksheet. He began with the Chem/Phys "Section" view on the Score Report, looking at each question individually, and filling out the Question Review Worksheet as he went. The rest of this chapter will discuss these sections and the Question Review Worksheet in more detail.

6.2 PRACTICE TEST ANALYSIS—CHEMICAL AND PHYSICAL FOUNDATIONS OF BIOLOGICAL SYSTEMS

After completing the MCAT Demo Test, Joe reviewed each question in the Chem/Phys section. As he reviewed the questions, he filled out his Question Review Worksheet. He noted the subtopic of each question, and tried to recall as best as he could why he chose the answer he did, jotting these thoughts down in the notes column of the worksheet. Then he got out a box of colored pencils. He colored general chemistry in green, organic chemistry in orange, physics in purple, and biology or biochemistry in blue. He also circled all of his wrong answers in red; this helped him look for patterns, to see if his incorrect answers were associated with specific topics or subtopics, or with specific question types. Lastly, he scanned the QRW to see where his red circles aligned with the different subject colors.

Note: As you read through Joe's analysis of his questions, you should have the MCAT Demo Test open for viewing.

Joe noted that he had a fairly even distribution of wrong answers in all of the subtopics. He got four general chemistry questions wrong, four biology/biochemistry questions wrong, and two questions wrong in both physics and organic chemistry. He also noticed that of the twelve questions he got wrong, seven of them were Implicit questions, four of them were Explicit questions, and only one was a Memory question. Since he got almost all the Memory questions right, his first thought was that his content knowledge must be pretty strong, but he decided to make a final decision on that after reviewing each individual question.

Joe also noticed, when reviewing his notes, that he could have used the passage information more effectively in several cases, even on questions he got right. For Questions 6, 9, 23, 30, 35, 41, and 50 he missed critical information in the passage that either would have made answering the question easier, or would have led him to the correct answer instead of the wrong one. He made a mental note that for future tests he would slow down just a little bit when reading the passage, and he should not be afraid to go back to the passage to find information about a question or answer choice.

Lastly, Joe noted that in a few questions, he did not use techniques to his advantage. In Question 15, he could have used the I-II-III technique more effectively to eliminate answers quickly. In Questions 42 and 52, two of the answer choices were true, but there cannot be two correct answers for a question, so they could have been eliminated faster. And in Question 28, he could have saved time by substituting in answer choices rather than trying to figure out the answer algebraically. He decided to keep these (and other techniques) in the front of his mind going forward.

After this general evaluation of his notes and results, Joe looked more closely at the specific subjects. He started with General Chemistry and Biochemistry, since he missed four questions in each of those, then finished up with Physics and Organic Chemistry.

He did not spend a lot of time thinking about any question he coded as a "1," presuming that he knew this material well enough.

Chem/Phys Section Question Review Worksheet

Let's review the abbreviations and types of information you'll see on the worksheet.

- **Test or Book/pg #**: This is the diagnostic exam you are reviewing or the passage you have completed.
- **Section**: Either CP (chem/phys), CARS (critical analysis), BB (bio/biochem) or PS (psych/soc)
- **P # and Q #**: Passage number and question number
- **Q type**: Question type; for the science sections this is either M (memory), E (explicit), or I (implicit). For CARS, this is either R, (retrieval), I (inference), MI/PP (main idea/primary purpose), T (tone or attitude), S (structure), E (evaluate), ST (strengthen), WK (weaken), NI (new information), or A (analogy).

Result Code:

Code	Question Result	Action
1	correct, easy	none
2	correct, the hard way	review for shortcuts—POE strategies, deductions, etc.
3	correct, got it down to two	review, look for WHY you picked the correct answer, compare remaining, decide why the correct answer was better, consider what you will do next time
4	wrong, got it down to two	review, look for WHY you picked the incorrect answer, compare remaining, decide why the correct answer was better, consider what you will do next time
5	wrong, eliminated the right answer	review for comprehension—did you ID the question correctly? Did you RTFQ (read the full question)? Misapply POE strategies?
6	guessed randomly (letter of the day)	review for difficulty—did you attempt the easiest questions and passages?

SAMPLE MCAT PRACTICE TEST ANALYSIS

Since we are unable to depict the color highlighting in this book, a circled number or letter = red = wrong, a boxed text = green = General Chemistry, an oval around text = orange = Organic Chemistry, and grey highlighting = blue highlighting = Biology/Biochemistry. No shading, circling, ovals, or boxes = Physics. The full color version of this worksheet can be seen in your online companion.

Test or Book/pg #	Content Section	P #	Q #	Q type	Result Code	Notes
MCAT Demo Test	CP	1	1	I	1	G-chem
MCAT Demo Test	CP	1	2	(E)	(4)	G-chem - forgot about supercritical fluids, didn't understand this odd graph
MCAT Demo Test	CP	1	3	E	3	G-chem - 2x2, knew mass was constant, easy to elim. C&D; should have relied on P vs. T direct relationship to eliminate B (lucky guess)
MCAT Demo Test	CP	1	4	E	1	G-chem
MCAT Demo Test	CP	2	5	I	1	Physics
MCAT Demo Test	CP	2	6	E	2	Physics - Passage talked about bell versus diaphragm frequency detection
MCAT Demo Test	CP	2	7	M	1	Physics
MCAT Demo Test	CP	2	8	I	1	Physics
MCAT Demo Test	CP	2	9	(I)	(4)	Physics - overthought reasoning, too much reliance on outside knowledge instead of passage wording
MCAT Demo Test	CP	2	10	M	1	Physics
MCAT Demo Test	CP	FSQ	11	M	1	O-chem
MCAT Demo Test	CP	FSQ	12	E	1	Biochem
MCAT Demo Test	CP	FSQ	13	I	1	Biochem
MCAT Demo Test	CP	FSQ	14	E	1	O-chem
MCAT Demo Test	CP	3	15	I	2	G-chem - for RN Q, did not use I-II-III technique well, should have started with II or III to eliminate half the answers
MCAT Demo Test	CP	3	16	M	1	O-chem
MCAT Demo Test	CP	3	17	I	2	O-chem
MCAT Demo Test	CP	4	18	(I)	(5)	G-chem - didn't understand ratio of ring open/closed was relevant, misread graph as titration curve
MCAT Demo Test	CP	4	19	I	1	G-chem
MCAT Demo Test	CP	4	20	E	1	O-chem
MCAT Demo Test	CP	4	21	M	1	G-chem
MCAT Demo Test	CP	5	22	E	1	O-chem

Test or Book/pg #	Content Section	P #	Q #	Q type	Result Code	Notes
MCAT Demo Test	CP	5	23	(I)	(5)	*O-chem - elim. A based on knowledge, failed to relate the passage details "like an imine" and "resists hydrolysis" to the choices to find the least electrophilic hydrazone*
MCAT Demo Test	CP	5	24	(E)	(4)	*O-chem - correctly elim. A and C; wrong POE of OTHER two choices, misunderstood how pH affects reaction*
MCAT Demo Test	CP	5	25	E	1	*O-chem*
MCAT Demo Test	CP	FSQ	26	M	1	*Biochem*
MCAT Demo Test	CP	FSQ	27	M	2	*G-chem - Faraday's law calculation took a long time, approximate more*
MCAT Demo Test	CP	FSQ	28	M	2	*Physics - spent too much time deriving algebraic solution, could have subbed in numbers or used arrows*
MCAT Demo Test	CP	FSQ	29	M	1	*O-chem*
MCAT Demo Test	CP	6	30	(E)	(4)	*Biochem - assumed this was in blood, missed line in passage about it being in hepatocytes*
MCAT Demo Test	CP	6	31	E	1	*Biochem*
MCAT Demo Test	CP	6	32	I	2	*Biology - thought too much about this one*
MCAT Demo Test	CP	6	33	I	1	*Biochem*
MCAT Demo Test	CP	6	34	M	1	*Biology*
MCAT Demo Test	CP	7	35	I	3	*Physics - answer basically in paragraph 2, took too much time trying to reason through B*
MCAT Demo Test	CP	7	36	I	1	*Physics*
MCAT Demo Test	CP	7	37	M	1	*Physics*
MCAT Demo Test	CP	7	38	M	1	*Physics*
MCAT Demo Test	CP	7	39	(M)	(5)	*Physics - forgot the difference between velocity and speed*
MCAT Demo Test	CP	8	40	E	1	*G-chem*
MCAT Demo Test	CP	8	41	I	5	*Biochem - Incorrectly assumed that vegetarians would have less muscle mass than meat eaters, also missed the line in the passage about the synthesis being non-enzymatic*
MCAT Demo Test	CP	8	42	I	2	*Biochem - missed the "trick" of noting that there can't be two "right" answers*
MCAT Demo Test	CP	8	43	M	1	*O-chem*
MCAT Demo Test	CP	8	44	E	1	*Biochem*
MCAT Demo Test	CP	FSQ	45	M	1	*G-chem*

Test or Book/pg #	Content Section	P #	Q #	Q type	Result Code	Notes
MCAT Demo Test	CP	FSQ	46	M	1	*Physics*
MCAT Demo Test	CP	FSQ	47	M	1	*G-chem*
MCAT Demo Test	CP	FSQ	48	M	2	*Physics - spent too much time on all the math instead of just using intuitive proportions*
MCAT Demo Test	CP	9	49	M	1	*Biochem*
MCAT Demo Test	CP	9	50	E	5	*G-chem - RNQ: wanted I and III only, not a choice; missed passage text that $\downarrow pH$ alters equil. (NH_3 changes pH); $[O_2] \rightarrow$ Le Chat. Prin. doesn't change K, just shifts equilibrium*
MCAT Demo Test	CP	9	51	E	1	*G-chem*
MCAT Demo Test	CP	10	52	I	6	*G-chem - missed how to use K values, missed "trick" of noting two identical answers, confused by enzyme/rate connection trap*
MCAT Demo Test	CP	10	53	E	1	*Biochem*
MCAT Demo Test	CP	10	54	M	1	*Biochem*
MCAT Demo Test	CP	10	55	I	5	*Biochem - didn't understand experiments, relied on outside knowledge (belief that all protein synthesis is regulated at the transcriptional level)*
MCAT Demo Test	CP	10	56	I	5	*Biochem - assumed that direct interaction with ATGL meant that it stimulated ATGL. Misunderstood the significance of correlating with insulin levels*
MCAT Demo Test	CP	FSQ	57	M	3	*O-chem - took too long relating pKa table to answer choices, could elim. A and B, ended up guessing correctly in a hurry*
MCAT Demo Test	CP	FSQ	58	M	3	*Physics - guessed right, had trouble using Kirchhoff's rules to figure out what happened to the current through R2.*
MCAT Demo Test	CP	FSQ	59	M	1	*Biochem*

Individual G-Chem Question Analysis

After reviewing the test for the big picture changes he might make, Joe jumped right into his G-Chem review.

- Question 2: Reading the labels in Figure 1 allowed Joe to eliminate A and B quickly—points to the left of the dome were liquid, while points to the right were vapor, respectively. He then assumed that both liquid and vapor were present at the point in question since it was directly above the dome. Upon review of the solution, however, Joe realized that he should be sure to read the text before and after figures before interpreting or analyzing a graph. He missed the passage text that explained that points *below* the curve represented liquid and gas in equilibrium, and that the dome itself translated to one of the lines in a standard P vs. T phase diagram, at the end of which was the critical point. That meant any points *above* the dome maximum represented a supercritical fluid, neither a liquid nor a gas.

- Question 3: While Joe answered this one correctly, he knew it was a lucky guess. While taking the test he realized this was a 2x2 style question, so he quickly eliminated both choices that referenced mass since that property shouldn't change with temperature or volume. However, because he was struggling to make complete sense of the unfamiliar diagram, he quickly picked choice A and moved on. Upon reflection, he saw that a higher temperature should translate to a higher pressure for any gas, and even saw that the passage text hinted that the ideal gas law might be a useful reference to help him deduce this relationship. Joe realized he should have marked this question to review it if he had time at the end of the test, and he made note to use the Mark button more freely in the future.

✳ Do passages in the order that makes the most sense to you.

Joe realized he struggled with this passage because it began by referencing phase diagrams, but then showed a graph of T vs. V, which was different than the P vs. T or even the T vs. heat diagrams that were more familiar to him. Since this passage was the first one he attempted on the entire practice test, it started him on shaky ground; he was therefore a little flustered while answering the first few questions. Joe realized in hindsight that a better strategy for him would have been to skip to passage 2 and begin with something that seemed more straightforward to build some confidence. Joe also made a note to not only start with a more familiar topic, but also to slow down a bit when answering questions that made him apply his understanding in a new context, and scan the passage a bit more closely for useful information. Both Questions 2 and 3 were explicit questions, and Joe had failed to use the passage information to his advantage.

- Question 15: Joe realized he could have saved some time on this question by looking at his answer choice options first. He noted that two choices had Roman numeral II in them, and two had Roman numeral III. Addressing one of those items first would have allowed him to eliminate 50% of his choices rather than spending a long time thinking about the more challenging item of Roman numeral I, only to be able to eliminate one choice upon finding it true.

✳ Strive to use POE strategically!

- Question 18: Joe was surprised by this incorrect answer as he reviewed the test. He was looking for the pK_a of Mito-pH, which he knew was represented by the pH at the half-equivalence point of a titration. Joe therefore jumped to use the last figure in the passage, which had the classical shape of a titration curve and pH labeled on one of the axes. However, upon further review he realized that pH should have been on the vertical axis, not the horizontal one, and that he had picked a good trap answer (choice B) and quickly moved on. Joe now saw that the text right above the figures indicated that the curve showed the normalized ratio of ring forms, so the 50/50 ratio of rings he wanted was at 0.5 on the vertical axis of the graph. For a second time, Joe realized that he needed to rely on his memory less and use the text around figures more while trying to interpret experimental data.

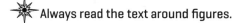 Always read the text around figures.

- Questions 27: As Joe reviewed his scratch paper along with the solutions to the test, he realized he spent a long time working through this calculation when he could have approximated his math a lot more. Using an estimated 7 hours of time made no noticeable difference in the answer he found. Since the answer choices given were very different from each other, he realized this level of rounding was a safe strategy he wasn't using as effectively as he could be.

- Question 50: Joe knew quickly that Roman numeral I should be included since equilibrium constants are temperature dependent. However, after highlighting what he thought important text about positive cooperativity in the passage, he missed the reference to the importance of pH on O_2 binding in hemoglobin and the subsequent connection in the question to NH_3 having a pH-raising effect. Joe also made an incorrect association that the $[O_2]$ would change the K value of the binding rather than just shift an equilibrium that had already been established. When the answer choice he wanted wasn't there (I and III only), he picked choice D and moved on. Joe realized he might need to do a little review on equilibrium and Le Châtelier's Principle.

- Question 52: Joe really struggled to eliminate any answer choices for specific, good reasons for this question as he was unable to parse the difference between them. Joe realized that this question was testing the concepts of thermodynamics and kinetics at the time, but because of the biochemical molecules being used as the context of the question, it just felt more challenging. He decided to try to save himself some time for other questions, and he almost blindly guessed. Unfortunately, he fell into a trap answer that sounded correct (enzymes are associated with stabilizing transition states in molecules, leading to faster reaction rates) but didn't really address the question. Joe was confused by the phrase "overall reaction" in choice A; if he had realized that both choices A and D effectively said the product is more stable, he would have realized both were wrong. As he reviewed this question, Joe found he didn't need to apply the concept of negative cooperativity described in the passage, but he did need to use the K values given in the table and recognize that they were for the reverse process as that described in the question stem. Once he was able to use the passage information appropriately, it made sense that a small K meant an endergonic process.

When you know you're in over your head, just guess and move on. Don't get bogged down.

Summary of Joe's G-Chem Analysis

Joe began to suspect that he has a tendency to rely too heavily on memory, and that he needs to refer to the passage more when he's unsure how to answer a question (Q2, Q18, Q50). Joe also realized that two of the four G-Chem questions he missed were due to his inability to correctly interpret a graph, and that his mistakes were mostly due to overlooking important text associated with the figures before he tried to extract information from them (Q2, Q18). Joe also noted that the passage that heavily tested equilibrium concepts was particularly challenging for him. He thought he might have a content deficiency there, so he planned to brush up on this topic. Joe also decided to practice more calculation problems to become more comfortable with estimating efficiently (Q27).

Individual Biochemistry and Biology Question Analysis

- Question 30: Joe realized that this was a 2x2 question, and that he could eliminate two choices at the same time. He read in the passage that chronic alcohol consumption can lead to GSH depletion, so he knew he could eliminate choices B and D quickly. However, he failed to notice the line in the passage discussing acetaminophen oxidation and how it occurs in hepatocytes, and so he incorrectly assumed these metabolites would be in the bloodstream. Joe saw that his attempt to go quickly backfired on him, and he realized he should slow down just a bit to get more information from the passage.

- Joe answered Question 32 correctly, but he spent a lot of time thinking about it. He was able to eliminate choices B and C fairly quickly, since he knew first that a fair amount of the drug is absorbed, and that most drug breakdown occurred after absorption into the bloodstream. But he struggled with choice A since he knew it to be a true statement; the oral and rectal mucosa are too thick to permit much absorption, and the drug is not absorbed there. After some time he concluded that choice A, while true, did not address the fact that the drug was being absorbed when administered orally or rectally but the plasma concentrations did not rise as high as with IV administration, and he selected choice D. He decided in the future to remember that just because an answer choice is a true statement doesn't make it the correct answer choice.

- Joe got Question 41 wrong by making an incorrect assumption. He assumed that vegetarians, because they consume no meat, would have less muscle mass (and thus produce less creatinine) than meat eaters. However, the amount of meat consumed does not correlate with muscle mass; there are certainly a number of non-meat protein sources, and muscle mass correlates more with body-building exercise than with diet. A meat-eating couch potato may have less muscle mass than a vegetarian exerciser. Also, he realized that he missed the point in the passage about creatinine being formed non-enzymatically, reinforcing the idea that he needs to slow down a bit and pull more info from the passage instead of relying on outside knowledge or assumptions.

Use the information in the passage to help you answer questions!

- Question 43: although Joe got this question right, he realized too late, after spending too much time thinking about it, that he could have answered it quickly using technique. He was able to eliminate choice C quickly, since the product of a dysfunctional enzyme would not be expected to increase. However, both choices A and D were plausible and likely; if the enzyme is dysfunctional, then substrate levels should rise while product level decrease. Finally he realized that neither option was more likely than the other, and since there cannot be two correct answers, both must be eliminated. He then spent too much time trying to justify the remaining answer instead of just selecting it as the only remaining option and moving on. He vowed in future practice tests to remember that two correct answers, if they are equally likely, should be eliminated.

- Joe struggled with Questions 55 and 56, both from a passage he did not understand well. Partly, he did not fully understand the experiments they were running, and he realized he would have to brush up on lab techniques to be able to interpret data like that. Because he did not fully understand the experiments and implications in the results, he relied too heavily on outside knowledge to answer the questions. Joe picked choice C because he believed that all protein synthesis is regulated at the transcriptional level, and while there is a significant amount of transcriptional regulation, there is some regulation at the translational level as well. If he had understood the lab techniques and the experimental data better, he may not have made this error.

- For Question 56, Joe read in the passage that G0S2 interacts directly with ATGL, and he assumed then that G0S2 must stimulate ATGL. He missed the part in the passage about how G0S2 expression correlates with insulin levels; since insulin is released when glucose levels are high (and lipolysis would be inhibited), G0S2 must inhibit ATGL. This was the third biochemistry question Joe got wrong by not reading or by misreading information in the passage. This clearly indicated to him that he needed to slow down and read a little more carefully.

Summary of Joe's Biochemistry and Biology Analysis

In looking over his Question Review Worksheet, Joe realized that he answered all of the freestanding Biology and Biochemistry questions correctly, and also answered all of the Memory questions correctly. He felt reasonably good about his content knowledge (with the exception of perhaps lab techniques), but figured that he would get a better sense of his content area strengths and weaknesses when analyzing the Bio/Biochem section. He did realize, however, that his passage reading skills need a little improvement, since he missed three questions (Q30, Q41, and Q56) by not seeing the relevant information in the passage.

Individual Physics Question Analysis

- Question 6: Joe got this question right, but upon review he realized that he spent too much time thinking it through. He worried about whether artery vibration would be quieter or louder than breathing abnormalities, and he persuaded himself it would be quieter. He knew that frequency and energy go hand-in-hand for light (in the photon model), so he thought that might be true for sound as well. That could argue for choice A, but it's not true: the energy of sound waves depends upon amplitude of the pressure wave, not frequency. More important, choices C and D directly address the text of the first and third passage paragraphs. Essentially, Joe failed to realize that this was an Explicit question and not an Implicit one, so instead of just using the text of the passage to pick the correct choice, he tried to apply outside knowledge and logic and wasted time.

- Joe missed Question 9 because he didn't use POE as thoroughly as he should have. He knew that this was an Implicit Conceptual question—where some answer choices could be eliminated as nonphysical using outside knowledge and others could be eliminated according to the passage—and he used this to eliminate two choices. Joe eliminated choice B because the wires in a stethoscope would be insulated like any wires people regularly handle. He eliminated choice D because he knew that different kinds of waves couldn't interfere with each other, and he'd never heard of electric standing waves (these do exist but are not something Joe needs to worry about for the MCAT!). Joe wasn't sure about choice A, but he knew that human hearing is more sensitive to higher frequencies up to a few thousand Hz. This persuaded him to select choice C, even though the passage didn't address whether electronic amplification increased with frequency. This was his main mistake: Upon rereading the passage, Joe realized that it directly supports choice A in paragraph 2, but it doesn't support choice C. In a case like this, where outside knowledge doesn't completely support a single choice, one should rely more on what the passage does and doesn't say.

- Question 28 was a Memory question, and Joe got it right, but he spent too much time manipulating the lens and magnification equations to solve for m in terms of o and f, then confirming that as object distance decreased, magnification would decrease (eliminating choices A and B). He also solved the lens equation for i in terms of o and f, but then struggled to determine how i would change as o decreased (since o is in both the numerator and denominator). Ultimately, Joe went back to the original equations and reasoned from the lens equation that if $o < f$, then $1/i = 1/f - 1/o < 0$, so i is negative. Moreover, as o decreases, that whole difference on the right side gets increasingly negative (because $1/o$ gets larger), so i decreases in magnitude (gets closer to zero). This means the image is getting closer to the mirror, eliminating choices A and C. Joe had already eliminated choice B, but he also knew from the magnification equation that images closer to the mirror are smaller, so he selected choice D. The lesson for Joe is that he shouldn't spend time getting a complete algebraic solution matching the terms in the answer choices just because he can, as it is often easier to examine the equations in their original form and to use proportions or arrows to follow the trends for how a change in one variable affects another.

- Question 35: Joe got this Implicit Conceptual question right, but again he tried to rely too heavily on outside knowledge when the passage strongly implies the correct answer. He reasoned that torque in the ankle would be greater when the moment arm was greater, since the weight of the dancer (the force down) is the same in either case. This led him to conclude that choice A was better than choice B, because a flat foot extends further beyond the ankle than does a pointed one. However, his reasoning didn't exactly fit the wording of choice A, which makes specific reference to area rather than length. Paragraph 2 does make specific reference to shifting center of mass to maintain balance, however, and choice C fits the idea that keeping the center of mass over the contact area would be easier for a larger area. Joe opted for choice C but he should have eliminated choices A and B faster: If the passage provides a strong reason to pay attention to one group of answers but not another, the best strategy is to eliminate the answers that focus on terms or concepts that aren't mentioned in the passage (or, as is the case here, are mentioned in different contexts than the particular focus of the question, since torque is mentioned in the context of *développé*).

Information in the passage is there to help... don't be afraid to use it!

- Joe was angry to discover he had missed Question 39, a memory question, because of a "dumb mistake," but it's the kind of error one can easily make when a question demands reasoning about more than one physical principle at a time, as a Roman numeral question certainly will. He knew that centripetal forces always point toward the center of the circular motion, which makes Item I false and Item II true (and thus eliminates choices A and D). However, he was fooled into thinking Item III was true (and thus choice C correct) by the mention of "constant speed" in the question stem and the fact that "tangential velocity" is indeed how one finds the instantaneous velocity of a mass in uniform circular motion. The difference between constant speed and constant velocity is important, since speed is a scalar whereas velocity is a vector, and that makes III false. Joe knew this, but he forgot to apply it to this case because item III sounded correct upon first reading. The lesson is that terminology matters and Joe realized that he needs to read more carefully in cases where the question otherwise shouldn't take very long (since this question doesn't rely at all on the information in the passage).

- Question 48: Joe got this memory question right but he did it the long way, recalling all of the possibly pertinent equations (flow rate, Bernoulli's Law, the Big Five kinematics equations for free fall). He started plugging the given values into the equations, and solved for the areas of the pipes using $A = \pi r^2$. Luckily he realized pretty quickly that the Bernoulli equation wasn't going to do him any good because the question asks about the volume of fluid per time, which is flow rate, and the pressure difference wouldn't answer that directly. Still, he wasted time trying to determine the time it took the fluid to reach the ground given the height and then to use that number to find the flow speed. Eventually, after fumbling with these equations, he realized that since everything about the two flows was the same EXCEPT for the distance that water traveled before hitting the ground, the one that went four times further must be coming out four times faster. All the other numerical values were irrelevant because they were identical in the two cases: This was a proportionality problem. $f = Av = V/t$, so t is inversely proportional to v. The lesson is to be suspicious of a question with a lot of numerical information and to look for the hidden proportions for the efficient solution.

- Question 58: Joe also got this Memory question right but felt like he guessed once he got it down to two choices. He knew right away that adding a resistor in parallel always reduces the equivalent resistance of a circuit, so the current coming out of the battery (which is the same as I_1) must increase, eliminating choices C and D. After that, he wasn't sure how to figure out the current I_2. He eventually decided that, since the current would be split up between R_2 and R_3, even though there was more of it, the amount through R_2 would decrease. This reasoning (drawing on Kirchhoff's current rule) does yield the correct answer, but it's not useful if the problem is quantitative or algebraic, so Joe decided to review Kirchhoff's Voltage Rule. Because the battery (which hasn't changed), R_1, and R_2 form a complete loop, the sum of the voltage changes through them must be zero. Thus, since $I_1 R_1$ increases, $I_2 R_2$ decreases, meaning I_2 decreases.

Summary of Joe's Physics Analysis

In the Physics portion of the Chem/Phys section, Joe noticed that he missed only one Memory question (Q39), though he had a bit of trouble with three others (Q28, Q48, and Q58). On the one he missed, he had forgotten to apply a simple definition; on the others, he generally struggled a bit with the math, not taking the simplest possible route to the solution. He decided to review proportions and fractions a little, just to get back in the habit; otherwise he felt confident in his content knowledge. He was more concerned about the fact that he missed one question (Q9) and struggled on two others (Q6 and Q35) because he had not used POE correctly for conceptual questions, and had failed to distinguish between Implicit and Explicit question types in his approach. Joe recognized that all of his studying had prepared him to rely on his outside content knowledge too much, and that he needed to respond more quickly to clues in passages and question stems indicating 1) where a question was asking him to direct his attention, and 2) whether a given choice should be eliminated. Since this issue wasn't specific to physics (he had similar passage-reading issues with biochemistry and general chemistry), Joe decided to review his entire Practice Test Analysis to see whether the patterns recurred and to design a study strategy based on that. He also made a note to review the appropriate sections of Chapter 3 of this text before taking his next practice test.

Individual Organic Chemistry Question Analysis

Joe decided to leave his O-Chem review for last because there were only twelve O-Chem questions in the entire Chem/Phys section. Six of the twelve questions Joe coded as "1" so he did not review them further. Joe coded only one question as "2," getting it right, but the "hard way." He decided to start by reviewing this question, which he noticed was an Implicit question.

- Question 17: Joe was able to locate the correct answer choice by POE but only after exhaustively attempting to deduce taurine's correct structure. His uncertainty in structure drawing left him unclear on why the right answer was right, which led him to doubt his choice, prompting him to return to this question unnecessarily for a second pass. Joe was sure he knew the molecular structure for cysteine, but he struggled to picture taurine next to it; however, more confidently applying POE would have expedited his solution. Upon review, Joe realized that he could deduce the structure of taurine from the larger taurocholic acid structure given in the passage if he looked more closely at its sulfur atom.

There's no need to deliberate over why the right choice is right, when all other the choices are wrong.

Joe then turned his attention to a question where he applied good strategy. He was able to narrow down his answer choices to two options in order to correctly choose the right answer. Joe noticed this question was an FSQ.

- Question 57: While Joe correctly answered this question, he did so in a hurry without feeling certain he was choosing the right answer. Upon review, Joe realized that analyzing the table of pK_a values provided *before* confronting the answer choices was a bad idea because the answer choices didn't always relate back to the table. Joe resolved to avoid pre-analyzing tables or other visual aids too much in the future. On approach, Joe was able to eliminate choices B and D because of his familiarity with pH effects on amino acid side chains and the concept of electrophoretic mobility of amino acids. However, Joe struggled with choice C because he failed to understand why lysine and tyrosine side chains had similar pK_a values when one is a basic side chain and the other is a polar side chain. This confusion led Joe to doubt his knowledge and slowed down his progress. Joe realized he fell into a trap of relying on the table which was unnecessary for the solution.

Joe then examined the question where he got it down to two choices but chose the wrong answer.

- Question 24: Consulting the reaction in Figure 1 allowed Joe to quickly eliminate choices A and C because these two choices are competitive reagents. Joe then knew that pH was a factor so he began to think about conditions that would favor reactions and knew that protonations around carbonyls or leaving groups generally made reactions more favorable. Unfortunately, Joe's assumption led him to jump to a conclusion based on an incomplete assessment of the reaction. Upon review of the solution, Joe realized that he didn't pay close enough attention to is the type of reaction shown in Figure 1. Joe could see how classifying the reaction would have given him room to consider the other pH answer instead.

  Classifying reaction types on the MCAT is a way to remind yourself about details that are easily overlooked!

  Joe decided it would be prudent to be more thorough when reading into reactions because he felt like a detail like this could be easily missed again. Joe decided to review the details of substitution reactions and glance through other O-Chem reactions to apply this thinking so he's ready the next time.

This is the question Joe struggled to answer, which he remembers even after the test for the trouble it caused. Joe coded this question with a "5," which indicates he eliminated the correct answer. This often occurs when moving too quickly or misunderstanding what the question is asking.

- Question 23: Joe had a lot of difficulty understanding this question and how to solve it based on the information given in the passage. He was confused by the answer choices, which looked nothing like the structures anywhere in the passage, moreover, the unfamiliar "hydrazone" term that the passage repeated several times was a curveball. Joe had a lot of practice identifying resonance structures and was able to eliminate choice A immediately. Joe thought he was making a smart move eliminating choice C next,

  Familiar terms are often important clues in a passage!

  but he didn't slow down to think through his understanding in the context of a new type of functional group. Joe missed the detail that a hydrazone "resembles an imine" yet it resists hydrolysis. This information is important because it means the resonance structure that Joe eliminated is in fact the one he needs to choose. Joe made a note to slow down and look for clues that relate unfamiliar language to terms he's more familiar with, and to fully read through the question before he jumps on a choice that looks right to him.

Summary of Organic Chemistry Analysis

Joe missed only two of the twelve O-Chem questions in the Chem/Phys section. Joe felt confident with his understanding of the content because his two mistakes were restricted to a single challenging passage (Q23 and Q24). He was glad to see that he got all of the Memory questions correct, which let him know he was on the right track with his O-Chem knowledge going into the MCAT. Joe noticed one thing in common with the questions he coded to numbers above "1," which is that he struggled more when he needed to relate information given by a question or passage to his knowledge. Joe decided (again, still!) that he needs to slow down and pay closer attention to details instead of falling back on brute knowledge (such as in Q23). Joe resolved to be more careful during the highlighting and mapping periods of his passage review. Joe also noticed that two of the questions (Q24 and Q57) revolved around the topic of pH. He decided to review how pH affects amino acids, and to look closer at the role pH changes may play in organic chemistry reactions.

Remember to...

- fill out the Question Review Worksheet soon after taking your practice test or drill
- fill out a separate Question Review Worksheet for each section, and tackle each section one at a time
- circle the questions you got wrong in red; for the science sections, use colored pencils to shade in the different subjects and make them stand out.
- spend whatever time you need (usually about 2–3 hours per section) reviewing your test

6.3 PRACTICE TEST ANALYSIS—CARS

As with the Chem/Phys section, Joe reviewed each question in the CARS section. As he reviewed the questions, he filled out his Question Review Worksheet, highlighting appropriately. Joe did spend some time thinking about how he got many of the questions coded "1" correct (so that he could identify where and how he successfully implemented his strategy), but he spent most of his time reviewing the questions he struggled with and/or missed. (Note: As you read through Joe's analysis of his questions, you should have the MCAT Demo Test open for viewing.)

CARS Question Review Worksheet

- **Test or Book/pg #**: This is the diagnostic exam you are reviewing or the passage you have completed.
- **Section**: Either CP (chem/phys), CARS (critical analysis), BB (bio/biochem) or PS (psych/soc)
- **P # and Q #**: Passage number and question number
- **Q type**: Question type; for the science sections this is either M (memory), E (explicit), or I (implicit). For the CARS section, this is R (Retrieval), I (Inference), MI/PP (Main Idea/Primary Purpose), T (Tone or Attitude), S (Structure), E (Evaluate), ST (Strengthen), WK (Weaken), NI (New Information), A (Analogy), and when appropriate also ELN (Except/Least/Not) or RN (Roman numeral)

Result Code:

Code	Question Result	Action
1	correct, easy	none
2	correct, the hard way	review for shortcuts—POE strategies, deductions, etc.
3	correct, got it down to two	review, look for WHY you picked the correct answer, compare remaining, decide why the correct answer was better, consider what you will do next time
4	wrong, got it down to two	review, look for WHY you picked the incorrect answer, compare remaining, decide why the correct answer was better, consider what you will do next time
5	wrong, eliminated the right answer	review for comprehension—did you ID the question correctly? Did you RTFQ (read the full question)? Misapply POE strategies?
6	guessed randomly (letter of the day)	review for difficulty—did you attempt the easiest questions and passages?

SAMPLE MCAT PRACTICE TEST ANALYSIS

Since we are unable to depict the color highlighting in this book, a circled number or letter = red = wrong, grey shading = blue coloring = Biochemistry. An oval around the text = green = General or Organic Chemistry. No shading or ovals = Biology. The full color version of this worksheet can be seen in your Online Companion.

Test or Book/pg #	Section	P #	Q #	Q type	Result Code	Notes
MCAT Demo Test	CARS	1	1	MM/PP	1	*Avoided "too narrow" traps by using Bottom Line*
MCAT Demo Test	CARS	1	2	S	1	*Used tone and main points to eliminate wrong answers without going back to passage*
MCAT Demo Test	CARS	1	3	(A)	(5)	*Missed "current" in Q stem & picked B that nicely matched old attitude*
MCAT Demo Test	CARS	1	4	S	1	*Used main point of paragraph to ID correct answer*
MCAT Demo Test	CARS	1	5	(NI)	(5)	*Misread "inconsistent" as "consistent" in question, which led to C*
MCAT Demo Test	CARS	1	6	(R/RN)	(5)	*Picked D (I, II, and III): Remembered II from passage, but didn't check to see that it's specific to novice writers, not all writers*
MCAT Demo Test	CARS	1	7	ST	1	*Went back to passage before POE and identified claim to strengthen—made the question easy (also saw that other answers contradicted passage)*
MCAT Demo Test	CARS	2	8	MI/PP	1	*Used Bottom Line*
MCAT Demo Test	CARS	2	9	S	1	*Went back to passage efficiently to look for evidence*
MCAT Demo Test	CARS	2	10	I	1	*Knew where it was based on Q preview—found it easily in the passage*
MCAT Demo Test	CARS	2	11	(WK)	(4)	*Got stuck between two answers that both appeared inconsistent with passage – picked wrong one*
MCAT Demo Test	CARS	2	12	NI	2	*Got thrown off by length of the question—didn't identify the theme of new info at first*
MCAT Demo Test	CARS	2	13	I/RN	1	*Spent a little bit of time eliminating II, but not too bad*
MCAT Demo Test	CARS	2	14	I	1	*Found it quickly in the passage based on preview of Qs*
MCAT Demo Test	CARS	3	15	I/ELN	3	*Guessed between A and C*
MCAT Demo Test	CARS	3	16	I	2	*Debated too long between A and B*

Test or Book/pg #	Section	P #	Q #	Q type	Result Code	Notes
MCAT Demo Test	CARS	3	17	ST	1	*Down to two, then did good second cut*
MCAT Demo Test	CARS	3	18	Ⓘ	④	*Guessed between A and B*
MCAT Demo Test	CARS	3	19	I	1	*Eliminated A (scope), B (tone), and D (scope) in first cut*
MCAT Demo Test	CARS	4	20	S	1	*Down to A and C—then saw that A = purpose of reference*
MCAT Demo Test	CARS	4	21	I	1	*Back to passage, found info*
MCAT Demo Test	CARS	4	22	A	2	*Hard Q, took too long, but got it finally*
MCAT Demo Test	CARS	4	23	Ⓦⓚ	④	*Lost track of exact issue of question/ passage*
MCAT Demo Test	CARS	4	24	Ⓘ	④	*Didn't use passage enough*
MCAT Demo Test	CARS	4	25	S	3	*A and C: Unsure of direct/indirect*
MCAT Demo Test	CARS	4	26	Ⓐ	④	*Totally lost!*
MCAT Demo Test	CARS	5	27	S (General)	1	*Broke down choices piece by piece*
MCAT Demo Test	CARS	5	28	R/ELN	1	*Avoided the outside knowledge trap*
MCAT Demo Test	CARS	5	29	S	1	*Answered in own words first, kept track of Q type*
MCAT Demo Test	CARS	5	30	I	1	*Used passage actively*
MCAT Demo Test	CARS	5	31	R/ELN	2	*Eliminated all the answers at first*
MCAT Demo Test	CARS	6	32	I	1	*Went back to P1 to find the info-easy*
MCAT Demo Test	CARS	6	33	Ⓘ/ELN	⑤	*Forgot the EXCEPT!*
MCAT Demo Test	CARS	6	34	NI	2	*Didn't fully understand the question at first*
MCAT Demo Test	CARS	6	35	I	1	*Found it in P5, used major themes of passage*
MCAT Demo Test	CARS	6	36	I	1	*Hard question done well! :-) Used passage actively*
MCAT Demo Test	CARS	7	37	MI/PP	1	*Used Bottom Line*
MCAT Demo Test	CARS	7	38	NI	1	*Translated the question well*
MCAT Demo Test	CARS	7	39	I	1	*Used passage actively*
MCAT Demo Test	CARS	7	40	I	1	*Used passage actively*
MCAT Demo Test	CARS	7	41	S	1	*Paid close attention to wording in the passage, thought about how P4 relates to P3*
MCAT Demo Test	CARS	7	42	R	1	*Easy Retrieval from passage*

Test or Book/pg #	Section	P #	Q #	Q type	Result Code	Notes
MCAT Demo Test	CARS	7	43	I/ELN	1	*Kept track of the NOT!*
MCAT Demo Test	CARS	8	44	S/ELN	1	*Kept track of the "not" :-) and read choices word for word (caught "introduction" in A)*
MCAT Demo Test	CARS	8	45	I	1	*Used the passage actively, identified theme of the question*
MCAT Demo Test	CARS	8	46	S	1	*Kept track of Q type—needed <u>purpose</u> of reference*
MCAT Demo Test	CARS	8	47	Ⓘ	⑤	*Careless reading :-(*
MCAT Demo Test	CARS	8	48	I	1	*Stayed within scope of the passage, including author's tone*
MCAT Demo Test	CARS	9	49	I/RN	⑤	*Didn't do good RN POE*
MCAT Demo Test	CARS	9	50	S	1	*Could have been tough, but went back to passage to look for separate support for the quote (none)*
MCAT Demo Test	CARS	9	51	I	1	*Used careful reading, good POE, and tone*
MCAT Demo Test	CARS	9	52	I	2	*Almost fell for (incorrect) outside knowledge, but used passage and caught it*
MCAT Demo Test	CARS	9	53	MI/PP	1	*Used Bottom Line including tone*

Individual CARS Questions Analysis

Joe decided to consider his results passage by passage rather than result code category by category, so that he could more easily analyze how he moved through the CARS section from beginning to end. Joe reviewed the nine passages in the same order in which he completed them during the test.

Passage 1

Joe is taken aback when he sees that he missed three questions on this passage (Questions 3, 5, and 6). This passage seemed to be one of the easier ones (and still appears to be a Now passage, even though Joe didn't do well on it), and during the test he was happy because he thought he could move through it relatively quickly, banking time for other harder passages to come. In retrospect, however, he sees that he moved through it too quickly, answering many of the questions based on memory (which led to some right answers but to many wrong answers as well.) Given that his results are so unexpected, he decides to look closely at all seven questions for this passage in the order in which he completed them, so that he can identify exactly what went wrong.

- Question 7: Joe answered Question 7 first (and the rest in reverse order from there) since he previewed the questions from first to last, and then worked the passage from the screen containing Question 7. In reviewing it, he sees that he used good strategy here: He went back to the passage, identified the theme that required strengthening, and found the answer that was most consistent with that theme (while eliminating answers that contradicted the passage). As he remembers, he didn't spend a lot of time on that question, since he had a good guide based on the question task and on the passage to use as he went through POE.

- Question 6: Based on the work he had done for Question 7, he knew that item III was supported by paragraph 2. That eliminated choices A and B. Given that items I and III were included in both C and D, Joe decided he only needed to look at item II. He remembered seeing this statement in paragraph 3, so he went with 'I, II, and III" without going back to the passage. Looking at it now, however, he sees that this is not true about "writing in the modern tradition" as a whole, but rather just for novice writers. If he had gone back to the passage (which would have taken little time, since he knew based on his main points exactly where the statement was), he would have seen that item II was too broad when taken in the context of the question task. Joe realizes that he was getting overconfident at this point, and remembers telling himself that he should really pick up the pace so that he wouldn't run out of time later on in the section.

Use the passage actively: Don't rely only on memory.

- Question 5: Joe starts his review of this question by rereading the question stem. Choice D "Eliot" looks like the obvious choice now, given that paragraph 3 states that according to Eliot, literature should be an escape from one's personality, not an expression of it. Joe sees that two things happened when he was taking the test. First, he read the question stem too quickly and thought that it was asking what would be most *consistent*, not inconsistent with basing a work on one's own life. Second, although he sees now that the passage doesn't discuss whether or not Flaubert drew on his own life for his subject matter, Joe had taken a literature class and remembered from that class that Flaubert incorporated his own life experience into at least some of his works. If Joe had either read the question more carefully, or avoided using his own outside knowledge, he would have seen that choice C was incorrect and ended up with the correct answer, choice D.

Read the question stem word for word.

- Question 4: Joe got this question right for two reasons. First, he used his main points from the passage to eliminate one answer that was irrelevant to this question about Flaubert (choice A) and another that contradicted the passage (choice B). Second, when he was down to choices C and D, he went back to the passage and found that choice C is a point made about Mann in a different paragraph, while choice D matched up with the purpose and point of paragraph 3, where the author discusses Flaubert.

- Question 3: Joe realizes that he got this question wrong for the same reason as Question 5: he misread the question stem and missed that it asked about the author's current attitude toward writing. This was one question for this passage that he spent a fair amount of time on; he sees now that this was because he eliminated the correct answer (choice A) during his first cut through the choices, and then spent a lot of time debating between B and C. If he had either read the question more carefully up front, or re-read the question stem when he was down to two choices, he would have understood what the question was really asking (and wouldn't have wasted all that time deciding between two wrong answers).

  Re-read the questions when down to two choices.

- Question 2: Joe is happy with his efficient process on this question, in particular that he used tone to eliminate choices A, C, and D (which all in some way have a negative tone that doesn't match the attitude and purpose of the author in this part of the passage). The main point that he had already generated for paragraph 2 gave him enough basis on which to select choice B once he had eliminated the other three.

- Question 1: Joe is also pleased with his approach to this question. His Bottom Line made it clear that one problem with A, B, and D is that they are clearly too narrow to represent the primary purpose of the entire passage, while choice C nicely corresponded with that Bottom Line.

Joe learns a lot from analyzing his performance on this passage. First, he can't rush an easy passage too much. If he does, he will get easy questions wrong for silly and entirely avoidable reasons, such as not reading the question correctly. Second, while he can and should use his main points and Bottom Line actively, he still has to go back to the passage for anything that is more specific than a major theme in the passage. Plus, no outside knowledge allowed!

Passage 2

While Joe thought he had done badly on Passage 2, the results were actually pretty good. Joe is reasonably happy with his performance on this passage; he had settled down into a better pace, and was following his strategy more consistently, at least until the last two questions that he completed. So, he decides to just look at Question 11 (incorrect) and Question 12 (correct but the hard way) in more detail.

- Question 11: Joe did this question second-to-last, given that it is a Weaken question and he know he struggles with those. Joe sees that he did a good first cut through the answers, eliminating A, which would strengthen rather than weaken, and choice D, which was only mildly inconsistent with a minor point in the passage. However, once he was down to B and C which both sounded inconsistent with the passage, he bounced back and forth between them multiple times and then picked B because it sounded stronger. While he had one good impulse—to pick a strong answer on a weaken question—he neglected another important step, which was to make sure that the answer actually contradicts the author's own argument.

Now, going back to paragraph 3 (which he sees he should have done in the first place), Joe finds that the author himself says that coffee "has had to suffer from religious superstition." So, while choice B does express an anti-coffee point of view, it supports rather than weakens a claim the author has explicitly made. Choice C, on the other hand, directly undermines the author's central argument that coffee is a wonderful beverage. If Joe had gone back to the passage in the first place, he not only would have gotten the question right, but would have also saved all that time that he spent bouncing back and forth between choices B and C.

- Question 12: During the test, Joe skipped over Question 12 his first time through the questions and answered it last. While that was a good decision given the length of the question and the question type, he knows that he got impatient with it because he knew he had spent too much time on Question 11 (and he was still worried that he missed it, which distracted him). Reviewing his thought process in the moment, he remembers that the first time he read the question stem he basically skimmed it and went into his first POE cut just with "coffee is good" in mind for the theme of the new info. Furthermore, he wasn't really focused on the fact that all four choices were claims from the passage, and he needed to find the one that (1) had the same theme as the new info in the question, and (2) would be supported by it. Unfortunately all four claims from the passage cited in the answer choices, not surprisingly, were about benefits of coffee, so Joe hadn't made any progress at the end of his first cut. Then he went back and read the question stem more carefully and saw that it was about the nutritional value of coffee. At that point Joe saw that neither C nor D related to that, so he was down to A and B. Now, finally, Joe went back to the passage and saw that the word "democratic" in choice A was a trap. According to the passage, coffee is a "democratic beverage" because it is enjoyed by all classes of people, not because it contributed to the spread of democracy. (In fact, Joe already understood this, which is why he got Question 10 right, but in his flustered state he forgot.) In retrospect, Joe now sees how he could have avoided this convoluted path to the right answer, and it is so simple: Read the question carefully and translate it, identify the theme of the new information, define how it relates to the passage, and THEN go through POE. If he had followed that path, he most likely would have had the right answer by the end of his first cut through the choices.

What Joe learns from this passage is (1) do it right the first time (e.g., read and translate the question before anything else, go back to the passage as needed as soon as possible) and it will not only improve his accuracy but also save time, and (2) if he is feeling distracted or flustered, stop and take a few deep breaths and refocus before moving on to the next question or passage.

Joe did Passage 4 next; the cite for Passage 3 looked abstract and difficult, so he decided to leave it for later.

Passage 4

Joe knew before he looked at the score report that he didn't do as well as he would have liked on Passage 4. He was still flustered because of the last two questions he struggled through on Passage 2, and he had a hard time focusing as he read this passage. He decides to look at all the questions in more detail, since he was only confident of his answers on one or two of them as he did the passage. He completed all the questions in reverse order from last to first without skipping over any along the way, so he reviews them in that same order.

- Question 26: Joe felt at a loss on this question, and more or less guessed, but only after taking a fair amount of time to take multiple passes through the choices (he isn't sure how many—it's kind of a blur). He saw at the time that is was an Analogy question, but went straight into the choices without taking the time to define what he was finding an analogy to. All the choices included machines or technology of some kind, and Joe couldn't see any relevant differences between them. However, now he sees that he should have first gone back to paragraph 1 to find the punched cards and define their relationship to the Analytic Engine. The passage states that Babbage had a vision of the Analytic Engine as controlled through a program contained in punched cards, cards that would tell the Engine (just like the loom) what to do. So, the correct answer would need to first reference a thing that is constructed or created to direct the actions of something else in a particular way, and second, the thing being directed or controlled. Now that he has understood this, the right answer makes sense, and Joe sees the difference between his answer B and the right answer D (for one, a computer programmer is not *constructed* to direct the actions of something else). Joe realizes two things. First, he should have done this question last, not first. Second, it was absolutely necessary to go back to the passage before POE in order to have any idea of what he was looking for in the answers.

- Question 25: Joe had to read the question four times before he even began to understand it; he realizes that he should have read it more slowly and thoughtfully the first time (especially given the complexity of the question itself). However, his next step was appropriate; he went back to the passage and found the author's question in paragraph 3, and then thought through the main points of the following paragraphs. That took him down to A and C. But there he got stuck, feeing unsure of how he would know if something was directly or indirectly answered; it seemed at the time that you could define those terms in a lot of different ways. In the end, he guessed right between choices A and C, but it was more or less pure luck at that point. Now, however, he understands that he over-complicated it. If he had stuck to the passage and the exact wording of each choice, he could have seen that the author never states an answer you could actually point to or cite in those last three paragraphs, so A is definitively out. On the other hand, those final paragraphs do provide information that *suggests* the cause is the difficulty of programming flexibility into an inflexible machine.

- Question 24: Joe is seeing a pattern emerging not only within this passage but through all the passages from this test that he has reviewed so far: He is not using the passage actively enough, or soon enough. When he did this question during the test, he took multiple passes through the choices, all of which sounded like they would be true of computers, before he went back to the passage to find "unconsciousness" in paragraph 4. Once he glanced at that part of the passage, he was able to get it down to choices A and B. However, he couldn't decide between them and ended up on the wrong side of a 50/50 guess. Now that he reads that part of the passage more carefully, he sees that the right answer is more or less stated in the sentence that precedes the sentence with "unconsciousness" in it. If he had only read further above, and word for word, in the passage during the test, he would have had it down to that correct (in fact, obviously correct) answer.

- Question 23: Joe sees that yet again he didn't have a clear enough idea of what the question was asking, or what the relevant part of the passage was saying, before he started POE. He identified this as a Weaken question, but went into the choices without a clear idea of what he was supposed to weaken. He was looking for something that sounded inconsistent with the passage, but he didn't define ahead of time what the author's assertion in paragraph 5 was. After getting it down to B and D he more or less guessed between them, and guessed wrong. Now, however, he sees that the author asserts that AI research is all about creating strict rules that "tell inflexible machines how to flexible." With that in mind, it is clear that choice D—computers using rules to program themselves—isn't at all inconsistent, whereas choice B indicates that strict rules may not be necessary in the first place. Joe also realizes that he was biased against choice B because he thought it was impossible for computers to learn in this way; he should have taken the answer as a true statement, however, just like for any Weaken question.

★ Don't use outside knowledge or opinion!

- Question 22: This question took some effort to understand; Joe had to read it several times during the test (and again even now) to understand what it was asking. However, once he managed to translate it, he did take the appropriate next step: He paraphrased the relationship between reading and writing (you can't write unless you can read; therefore, if you can write, we know you must also be able to read) before he started in the answer choices. Joe wasn't 100% sure of C. However, he knew that (1) the passage indicates that flexibility may be necessary for intelligence, (2) C was the only answer among choices B, C, and D that had some aspect of one thing being necessary for another, and (3) choice A had to be wrong because unlike the punched card and the Analytic Engine, writing doesn't control reading. So, given all of that, Joe managed to pick C without too much debate or delay. Joe realizes that he made the question even harder by not reading the question stem more slowly and thoughtfully up front, but he congratulates himself for effective use of aggressive POE.

- Question 21: This question seemed easy during the test, for good reason. Joe identified the issue of the question, went back to the right part of the passage, found direct support for choice C in Paragraph 1, and moved through POE thoughtfully and efficiently. Joe gives himself a pat on the back for doing at least this one question with no wasted effort!

- Question 20: This question was much harder for Joe than Question 21, but he feels that he worked it as best he could. He was stuck for a moment between A and C, but then went back to the question and reminded himself that it was asking not just what the author said, but *why* the author included Lovelace's assertion. At that point, Joe's second cut decision became very clear: C described what, but not why, unlike choice A. Joe gives himself a mental round of applause.

Now that he is done reviewing the questions for this passage, Joe steps back and asks himself why he was so confused and unsure as he worked through them during the test. Yes, the passage was dense and complex (and he should probably have left it until later in the section), but it doesn't seem so bad now. He realizes that he paid way too much attention to all the details regarding the different types of rules in the last (very long) paragraph, details that ended up being irrelevant to answering the questions. That just fed into the frustration that was lingering from his experience with the last couple of questions from the previous passage. If he had simply stuck to the major themes and main points of the paragraphs, he would have gone into the questions with a clearer mind and would have been able to extract what he needed from the passage more efficiently as he attacked each question. Joe is disappointed that he didn't do as well as he could have, but sees that in a sense it was worth it, given that he has even more evidence now of what he needs to do differently in the future.

Joe did Passage 5 next during the test, so he takes another look at it now.

Passage 5
Joe got all the questions right on this passage! And fairly easily, except for Question 31, so he decides to take a closer look at that question.

- Question 31: Joe sees that it is the second half of choice A that makes it wrong; when he did the question during the test, he eliminated it in his first cut, and had to go through the choices a few times before he finally paid attention to "it is possible to derive truth from the natural world" (which contradicts Plato's thought as it is described in the passage). He also lost track of the EXCEPT the second time through the choices, which was another factor that necessitated a third cut. Joe knows that he sometimes gets turned around on questions formatted in this way; he commits to always use his scratch paper from now on to keep track of why he is keeping or eliminating answers on any Except/Least/Not question. He also further strengthens his resolve to read and consider every word of every answer choice the first time through, to avoid having to waste time by cycling back through the choices to find what he could have found the first time through.

✴ Take account of every word of every answer choice.

In thinking about how he worked through the passage text, Joe realizes that while the passage itself was long and often challenging to understand, unlike with Passage 4 he didn't get bogged down in details, or in trying to gain a deep understanding of every abstract idea. He also sees big blocks of green checks in the second half of the score report and for Passage 3 (which he went back to last). It seems that he was settling into his method and his pace (Joe was in the flow!) once he got past the first few passages he completed, in part because he was feeling more and more confident about his pacing. He reminds himself not to panic in the beginning of the section or rush the first few passages, trying to save time to use later (which as he had seen often led him to work inefficiently and go more slowly overall, as well as to miss questions that he could have/should have gotten right).

Passage 6
Overall, this passage went well. Joe is especially happy with how he worked the passage, not getting distracted by or tangled up in the abstract discussion in paragraph 5 (which ended up not being important for the questions, except on a superficial level). He is annoyed, however, that he missed another EXCEPT/LEAST/NOT (Q33) and he knows he struggled with New Info Question 34. So he decides to take a look at those two in more detail.

- Question 33: What happened here is what has happened to Joe on other EXCEPT/LEAST/NOT questions—he forgot the NOT. This is especially vexing, because Joe had been so proud of himself when he caught the tricky reason why choice D is NOT supported by the passage; he went back to the text and saw that pivotal phrase, "Yet here again we are disappointed…" At this point, Joe had eliminated all four choices and then took extra time to go back and talk himself into wrong answer (choice A), (thinking that maybe "departure" was too strong, even though Joe really knew that it wasn't). Joe resolves to track POE on his scratch paper for any and all EXCEPT/LEAST/NOT questions from now on.

✴ Use your scratch paper to track POE on Except/Least/Not and Roman numeral questions.

- Question 34: As with other New Information questions, Joe didn't read the question stem carefully enough or identify the theme of the new info up front. Instead, he had to read it over and over, going back and for the between the answer choices and the question stem, until he clarified the contrast: Beethoven (given in the passage as a composer ones listens to) is more popular than Schumann (a composer one plays) when listened to on the radio. Once Joe understood this, the rational for choice A became evident, but it took way too long to get there. Joe also realizes, however, that he also could have used more aggressive POE: B is a judgment not made by the author or supported by the new info, C even if true would not be inconsistent with the passage, and D is wacky, as in, completely out of scope. So, if Joe had (1) read and translated the question before anything else or (2) trusted his POE strategy or (3) both, he would have spent much less time on this question and saved time to use on harder questions later on.

Passage 7

Joe takes a moment to celebrate Passage 7: all code 1, and this was not the easiest passage to understand! Given that he did so well, he decides to take a look at what he did right on two question types that he tends to have trouble with: Question 38 (New Info) and Question 43 (NOT). Since that vexing NOT question from Passage 6 is still on his mind, Joe decides to look at Question 43 first.

- Question 43: First of all, even though he didn't use his scratch paper, Joe did keep close track of the NOT as he went through POE; as he read each choice, he said out loud in his head "If I find it in the passage, it's out." Secondly, he used the passage actively. Choice A looked good, given that he remembered it from the passage, but he went back to paragraph 3 to confirm that no, "They do not predict what is going to happen…". Joe then used his main point of paragraph 1 to efficiently go back to that paragraph where he found evidence supporting choices B and C. Choice D seemed trickier (it was a more minor point that Joe didn't remember), but he didn't panic and start searching through random parts of the passage; as he went back to paragraph 1 for B and C, reading above and below, he also came across the support for (as in, reason to eliminate) D. Once through the choices, with clear direction and focus, and Joe had his correct answer and was moving on.

- Question 38: Finally, Joe realizes, he took the time during the test to read the whole question word for word despite its length before he did anything else. He then paused and identified the theme of the new info: Humans manage to exterminate themselves at some point in the future. Joe then paused again and thought about how this might be relevant to the passage, considered his main points which led him back to paragraphs 3 and 4, and went back to the text to find that according to the author, the world of a future history "must be habitable [by humans or by creatures with humanity]" who "will be able to direct, predict, and shape history to bring about the least amount of suffering." With that in mind, Joe was able to easily see that choice A was the opposite (given that people have never before exterminated themselves) and choice B had the wrong tone (the passage indicates that future history is pretty optimistic). Joe then hesitated a moment on choice C, since the passage does not in fact directly discuss war, but then Joe reminded himself that New Information questions will, by their nature, bring in something that is not in fact already stated in the passage. The question to ask is, is it relevant? War *could* in fact be relevant to our expectations of the future, which eliminates choice C. This leaves Joe with choice D, which he recognizes with ease, given what he has already understood about the question task and the relevant part of the passage. Joe reaffirms his resolution to take New Information questions step by step from now on, always keeping the nature and requirements of the question task firmly in mind.

Passage 8

Joe felt good about this passage (about how he attacked it, not about the somewhat morbid subject matter!) during the test; he is a bit surprised, therefore, that he missed what seemed to be an easy Inference question. Joe investigates.

- Question 47: Joe sees that he missed this question because, yet again, he did not read the choices carefully enough. He missed "in general" in choice A (he picked it because he was thinking about the fact that *in one way* England was slow to change). He also didn't pay enough attention to "in certain capacities" in right choice C; he eliminated C because he thought it was too extreme. Now he sees that choices A and C are two sides of the same coin. The author uses the word "paradoxically" in paragraph 2 to suggest that it is surprising that England held on to the practice of public executions for so long; it would only be paradoxical or surprising if the English legal system was generally fairly progressive. This is not an easy concept to get from the passage, and it requires a close reading of the text and at least a bit of thought. Joe realizes that he underestimated the difficulty of the question and got a bit too careless in his approach. Finally, Joe sees in retrospect that if he had not so cavalierly eliminated A, it would have given him the chance to compare A and C in a second cut through the choices, which would have made it more clear that they went in opposite directions. That could have sent him back to the passage with a real focus, at which point he would have understood the author's somewhat subtle implication. In sum, there was a cascading effect, starting with a bit of overconfidence, leading to careless reading, from there to inadequate POE, and finally to a wrong answer.

Passage 9

Joe sees that he missed another Roman numeral question here. He also got hung up on Question 52 (which should have been an easy one); even though he got it right, taking a lot of time on that question made him rush a bit in the last passage, so he wants to go back through it to see exactly where he got off track.

- Question 49: Joe sees that he didn't read item I carefully enough; he assumed it was about "cultural formation" (which would be supported by paragraph 4) but it really says "political formation." But once he decided that item I was correct, he happily eliminated everything but C. This was fine strategy-wise (although not accuracy-wise) so far. At that moment, he thought he really should look at item II, since it is included in choice C, and he found good support for it in paragraph 1. Again, good decision. However, he should have taken it a step further; he picked C without reading item III. For CARS, not reading all the numerals is tantamount to not reading all the lettered choices. Now he sees that if he had read item III, he would have recognized that it is clearly supported by paragraph 3. Given that there was no "I, II, and III" option, that would have sent him back to item I to read it more carefully, at which point he would have caught his initial mistake. Joe reminds himself to always read all three numerals, no matter how sure he is of one or two of them.

- Question 52: Joe retraces his thought process. He went into the choices without going back to the passage first. Joe has taken literature classes, and he thought maybe he could recognize the right answer without taking extra time to use the passage. He read choice A and immediately selected it, thinking "of course Eliot and James are British—I read their stuff in my English lit class!" But he reminded himself that he needs to look at all the answers before making a final choice, so he went on to B. Choice B looked pretty good too, based on that same outside knowledge. Choice C didn't look so good (periphery?), but at this point Joe was feeling more and more unsure, so he left it in and went on to D. Choice D was clearly wrong; Joe knew from the main point of paragraph 4 that these authors were on board with, not in opposition to, the "study of English." But now Joe was left with three choices; he read all three a few more times, but made no progress (and was getting more and more exasperated). Time was ticking away, but, he took a deep breath, didn't panic, and finally went back to paragraph 3 to take a closer look. And voila, the passage presents Eliot and James as writers on the periphery who became "more English than the English" by inserting themselves into "the imported culture." And, *the passage* never indicates that they were "canonized." Joe finally saw that A and C are in a way opposites of each other, and that it is choice C, not choice A, that is supported by the passage.

Thinking back over these two questions, even though he got one right and the other wrong, Joe sees a common thread: He tried to cut corners and paid the price in both time and accuracy. He also decides to write "no outside knowledge!!!" down on his scratch paper when he starts the CARS section on the real MCAT. Not only might his own outside knowledge be inconsistent with, or out of the scope of, the passage or the question, but what Joe "knows" may not even be accurate.

Finally, Joe went back to the last passage he completed, Passage 3.

Passage 3

Looking at it now, Joe realizes that the passage was not as hard to understand as he expected or as the passage cite seemed to indicate. Joe doesn't think that hurt him much this time, but he reminds himself to rank passages based on the first few sentences of the text, not based on the source cite. He is also pleasantly surprised that he only missed one (Q18); he was really rushing to get through it. So, he decides to look at Question 18 first, but then also at two of the other questions that he is surprised he got right.

- Question 18: This was a pure guess between B and C—they both sounded fine based on his overall understanding of the passage, and he didn't feel as if he had time to do a second cut. Now that Joe goes back to the passage, however, it is clear that the authors never attribute any thoughts regarding subcultures to Veblen. Rather the authors use Veblen's ideas regarding class to develop their own argument about this particular subculture. The question looks doable in retrospect, and Joe realizes that another 15 seconds or so to go back to the passage would have given him this question.

- Question 15: This is the other question Joe guessed on once he got it down to two. It was the last question he did, and time was almost up, so a reasonable (in fact necessary) decision in the moment. But, if he had been a bit more efficient on a few questions earlier on, he would have had the 15–30 seconds to either find choice A in paragraph 1, or to have read C more carefully to discover that it is reversing the causal relationship described in the passage.

- Question 16: Actually, Joe could have saved those 15–30 seconds here. He got it down to A and B, but then bounced back and forth between them without either breaking them down piece by piece or directly comparing them to each other. Once he finally did that, he saw that choice A was mixing together two separate issues (guard dogs and status), while each part of B checks out.

All in all, not bad, given the circumstances. But, Joe appreciates the fact that if he had stuck even more closely to his strategy (in this passage, especially in the second cut of POE), he could have gathered up one more correct answer.

Summary of CARS Analysis

After Joe finished his analysis of all of these questions, clear patterns emerged that gave him very specific things to work on.

Joe noticed that for many of the questions he missed, he either rushed and didn't go back to the passage carefully enough, or he didn't read the question or the answer choices closely enough. When looking back at those questions on the test, most of the answers seemed pretty obvious in retrospect; he knew he could have gotten most of them right if he had been a little more careful. As he thought back to what was going on in his mind as he was working the first passage (one of the two where he missed three question), he remembered that he was very concerned that he would take too much time in the beginning of the section and run out of time at the end; because he understood the passage pretty well, he zoomed through the questions without thinking them through. He was also distracted as he moved into Passage 4 (where he also missed three questions), and he didn't take the time to stop and refocus until he was done with that passage. Once he did that, the rest of the section went much better, so he realized he needs to stop and take a few deep breaths whenever he is flustered or distracted.

The good news was that he had a solid grasp of the Bottom Line on all the passages, and he saw that he used it well on many of the questions (even the Specific ones) to answer those questions efficiently. Furthermore, he often used good POE technique to get the right answer when he was down to two: He now needs to do that even more consistently. And while he saw that he needed to slow down on some questions, he also realized that if he had approached those "Code 2" questions correctly, it would have saved him time that he could have used to work other questions more carefully.

When Joe looked at the New Information and Weaken questions that he missed, he saw that he didn't adapt well enough to the difficulty level of the question. He also didn't think through what the question was really asking and what the correct answer needed to do. He decided to work through a bunch of examples of those question types so that he can refine and improve his approach. As for the EXCEPT/LEAST/NOT questions he missed, he could have gotten them right fairly easily if he had just kept track of the format all the way through POE. He vowed to always use his scratch paper to keep track of EXCEPT/LEAST/NOT and Roman numeral questions from now on.

Overall, Joe saw that he needed to:

- not rush through easier passages,
- avoid getting bogged down in dense or abstract portions of the passage the first time through,
- read the question word for word and consciously translate it before doing anything else (especially on Application questions),
- read each answer choice word for word and with an open mind,
- compare choices to each other when he is down to two,
- go back to the passage more consistently,
- stop using outside knowledge or his own opinion!

After finishing his review of the CARS section, Joe was feeling optimistic. Almost all of his mistakes came not from an inability to understand the passage or the questions, but rather from not holding as tightly to his strategies as he could have. Joe now had some very concrete things to work on, and he was confident that he will be able to continue to improve in the future.

Remember to...

- fill out the Question Review Worksheet soon after taking your practice test or drill
- fill out a separate Question Review Worksheet for each section, and tackle each section one at a time
- circle the questions you got wrong in red; for the science sections, use colored pencils to shade in the different subjects and make them stand out
- spend whatever time you need (usually about 2–3 hours per section) reviewing your test

6.5 PRACTICE TEST ANALYSIS—BIOLOGICAL AND BIOCHEMICAL FOUNDATIONS OF LIVING SYSTEMS

As with the Chem/Phys and CARS sections, Joe reviewed each question in the Bio/Biochem section. As he reviewed the questions, he filled out his Question Review Worksheet, coloring the Biochemistry questions blue, and the General Chemistry questions and Organic Chemistry questions green. He circled anything he got wrong in red.

Joe did a quick scan of his Bio/Biochem QRW to see if he could identify any big patterns. He first noted that the majority of the questions he got wrong were in Biology; he missed seven Biology questions, but only three Biochemistry questions. Furthermore, of the seven Biology questions he got wrong, five of them were immunology questions. Joe decided he needed to take a little time to review immunology before his next practice test.

Joe also noticed that about half the questions he got wrong were Explicit questions, and that he had a similar problem with this section that he did in the Chem/Phys section—he wasn't reading the passage carefully enough. In Questions 2, 5, 13, 25, 37, and 40 he missed critical information from the passage that would have helped him find the right answer. This reinforced his notion of needing to slow down a bit when skimming the passages.

After filling out the Question Review Worksheet, Joe decided to review the Biology questions first, and then go back to review the Biochemistry questions in more detail. Also, as before, he did not spend a lot of time thinking about, or reviewing further, any question he coded as a "1." (Note: As you read through Joe's analysis of his questions, you should have the MCAT Demo Test open for viewing.)

Biological Sciences Question Review Worksheet

- **Test or Book/pg #:** This is the diagnostic exam you are reviewing or the passage you have completed.
- **Section:** CP (chem/phys), CARS (critical analysis), BB (bio/biochem) or PS (psych/soc)
- **P # and Q #:** Passage number and question number
- **Q type:** Question type; for the science sections this is either M (memory), E (explicit), or I (implicit). For the CARS section, this is R (Retrieval), I (Inference), MI/PP (Main Idea/ Primary Purpose), T (Tone or Attitude), S (Structure), E (Evaluate), ST (Strengthen), WK (Weaken), NI (New Information), A (Analogy), and when appropriate also ELN (Except/ Least/Not) or RN (Roman numeral).

Result Code:

Code	Question Result	Action
1	correct, easy	none
2	correct, the hard way	review for shortcuts—POE strategies, deductions, etc.
3	correct, got it down to two	review, look for WHY you picked the correct answer, compare remaining, decide why the correct answer was better, consider what you will do next time
4	wrong, got it down to two	review, look for WHY you picked the incorrect answer, compare remaining, decide why the correct answer was better, consider what you will do next time
5	wrong, eliminated the right answer	review for comprehension—did you ID the question correctly? Did you RTFQ (read the full question)? Misapply POE strategies?
6	guessed randomly (letter of the day)	review for difficulty—did you attempt the easiest questions and passages?

Since we are unable to depict the color highlighting in this book, a circled number or letter = red = wrong, grey shading = blue coloring = Biochemistry. An oval around the text = green = General or Organic Chemistry. No shading or ovals = Biology. The full color version of this worksheet can be seen in your Online Companion.

Test or Book/pg #	Section	P #	Q #	Q type	Result Code	Notes
MCAT Demo Test	BB	1	1	E	1	*Biology (resp system)*
MCAT Demo Test	BB	1	2	(E)	(4)	*Biology (resp system) - couldn't be normal and wouldn't be pus. Couldn't find the info in the passage about air trapping, guessed vol. would go down since bronchial tubes were constricted*
MCAT Demo Test	BB	1	3	(E)	(5)	*Biology (resp system) - didn't know role of mast cells in inflammation*
MCAT Demo Test	BB	2	4	S	1	*Biology (resp system)*
MCAT Demo Test	BB	2	5	(E)	(5)	*Biology (immuno) - didn't know IgM was first line antibody, struggled by reading the passage to determine would not make anti-core or anti-e*
MCAT Demo Test	BB	2	6	(E)	(4)	*Biology (immuno) - eliminated A and D w/passage info, but again could not remember that IgM is first line and IgG is for long term response*
MCAT Demo Test	BB	2	7	I	1	*Biochemistry (viruses)*
MCAT Demo Test	BB	2	8	I	1	*Biology (mol bio)*
MCAT Demo Test	BB	FSQ	9	I	1	*Biology (cardiac)*
MCAT Demo Test	BB	FSQ	10	M	2	*Biochemistry (thermo) - thought about question too much. Didn't find the common things to eliminate choices quickly. Got turned around a bit with the LEAST.*
MCAT Demo Test	BB	FSQ	11	M	1	*Biology (digestive)*
MCAT Demo Test	BB	FSQ	12	M	1	*O-chem (acid/base)*
MCAT Demo Test	BB	3	13	(E)	(5)	*Biochemistry (enzyme regulation) - missed passage info about UTP inhibiting carbamoyl phosphate synthase*
MCAT Demo Test	BB	3	14	M	1	*Biochemistry (PPP)*
MCAT Demo Test	BB	3	15	E	1	*Biochemistry (enzyme reg)*
MCAT Demo Test	BB	3	16	E	1	*Biochemistry (redox)*
MCAT Demo Test	BB	3	17	I	1	*Biochemistry (PPP)*
MCAT Demo Test	BB	3	18	E	1	*Biochemistry (figure analysis)*
MCAT Demo Test	BB	4	19	M	1	*Biology (mol bio)*

Test or Book/pg #	Section	P #	Q #	Q type	Result Code	Notes
MCAT Demo Test	BB	4	20	I	3	*Biology (genetics) - struggled with this one a bit, didn't realize that C meant termination of the pregnancy*
MCAT Demo Test	BB	4	21	M	1	*Biology (lab techniques)*
MCAT Demo Test	BB	4	22	I	2	*Biology (genetics) - passage said it was a 2% chance. Took a bit to figure out had to divide by 2.*
MCAT Demo Test	BB	5	23	E	1	*Biology (mol bio)*
MCAT Demo Test	BB	5	24	E	2	*Biology (mol bio/development) - need to remember to look for 2x2 questions to eliminate choices more easily*
MCAT Demo Test	BB	5	25	(E)	(6)	*Biology (development) couldn't figure this out easily, couldn't find passage info, finally just guessed B because vaguely remembered something about crawling and involuting cells*
MCAT Demo Test	BB	5	26	I	1	*Biology (devel/cancer)*
MCAT Demo Test	BB	FSQ	27	E	1	*Gen chem*
MCAT Demo Test	BB	FSQ	28	M	1	*Biochem (cell resp)*
MCAT Demo Test	BB	FSQ	29	(M)	(6)	*Biochem (amino acids) - did not know amino acid properties*
MCAT Demo Test	BB	FSQ	30	M	1	*O-chem (separation techniques)*
MCAT Demo Test	BB	6	31	E	3	*Biology (renal) - wasn't 100% sure about vitamin D production but guessed correctly*
MCAT Demo Test	BB	6	32	I	2	*Biology (gene regulation) got it right, but it was hard, had to read and analyze every choice*
MCAT Demo Test	BB	6	33	I	1	*Biology (hormones)*
MCAT Demo Test	BB	6	34	I	1	*Biology (cell bio)*
MCAT Demo Test	BB	7	35	E	1	*Biology (immuno)*
MCAT Demo Test	BB	7	36	M	1	*Biology (hormones)*
MCAT Demo Test	BB	7	37	(M)	(5)	*Biology (immuno) - used I-II-III correctly, forgot that APCs express both MHC I and II, missed part in passage about APCs having roles in all types of rejections*
MCAT Demo Test	BB	7	38	E	1	*Biology (immuno)*
MCAT Demo Test	BB	7	39	E	1	*Biology (gene regulation)*

SAMPLE MCAT PRACTICE TEST ANALYSIS

Test or Book/pg #	Section	P #	Q #	Q type	Result Code	Notes
MCAT Demo Test	BB	8	40	(I)	(5)	*Biology (ion channels) - missed passage info about CNG channels being specific for ions, only saw part where it says they were in collecting duct cells*
MCAT Demo Test	BB	8	41	E	3	*Biology (heart) - elim. C and D quickly, struggled a bit with A and B. Finally decided B was not supported by passage.*
MCAT Demo Test	BB	8	42	I	1	*Biology (ANS)*
MCAT Demo Test	BB	8	43	E	1	*Biology (figure analysis)*
MCAT Demo Test	BB	FSQ	44	M	1	*Biochem (cell resp)*
MCAT Demo Test	BB	FSQ	45	M	1	*Gen chem (oxidation potential)*
MCAT Demo Test	BB	FSQ	46	M	1	*O-chem (amino acids)*
MCAT Demo Test	BB	FSQ	47	(M)	(5)	*Biology (immuno) - forgot role of antibodies, thought they would destroy receptors directly*
MCAT Demo Test	BB	9	48	E	1	*Biology (taxonomy)*
MCAT Demo Test	BB	9	49	E	1	*Biology (neurobio)*
MCAT Demo Test	BB	9	50	I	1	*Biology (neurobio)*
MCAT Demo Test	BB	9	51	E	1	*Biology (neurobio)*
MCAT Demo Test	BB	9	52	M	1	*Biology (lab techniques)*
MCAT Demo Test	BB	10	53	(I)	(5)	*Biochem (cell resp) - very confused by this passage and questions, didn't understand what was going on, couldn't figure out yes or no, tried to eliminate based on falsehoods. Knew B was correct, even if NO was wrong.*
MCAT Demo Test	BB	10	54	M	1	*Biochem (fatty acid ox)*
MCAT Demo Test	BB	10	55	I	3	*Biochem (data analysis) - eliminated C and D easily, but struggled between A and B, guessed A lucky*
MCAT Demo Test	BB	FSQ	56	E	1	*Biology (passage analysis)*
MCAT Demo Test	BB	FSQ	57	M	1	*Biochem (enzyme inhib)*
MCAT Demo Test	BB	FSQ	58	M	1	*Biology (hormones)*
MCAT Demo Test	BB	FSQ	59	M	1	*Biology (muscles)*

Individual Biology Question Analysis

- Question 2: Joe was able to eliminate two of the answer choices reasonably easily because he knew that there was no infection (so no pus) and figured that the lung volumes would not be normal. However, he couldn't find any information in the passage about increased lung volumes, and he just guessed that volumes would go down (since the bronchial tubes were constricted). Joe was starting to get a little annoyed with himself for continually missing these important bits of information in the passage, so he vowed to read more carefully, and maybe a little more slowly in the future.

- For Question 3, Joe successfully identified Items I and II as being possible medications to treat asthma; the β agonist was mentioned in the passage and Joe knew that glucocorticoids could be used to treat inflammation. He also recognized that if Item I was true, then Item IV (the β antagonist) had to be false. However, he could not remember the role of mast cells in causing inflammation. This was one of the immunology questions that Joe got wrong.

- Questions 5 and 6 were two more missed immunology questions, and even more annoyingly for Joe, questions where he again missed critical passage information. He was able to find the information in the passage about filamentous bodies not having core or genetic components, and so he knew for Question 5 that anti-core and anti-e (part of the core) would not be made. However, he forgot whether IgM or IgG was the first antibody made, and he didn't realize this information was in the passage until he reviewed the question. He had the same problem on Question 6; he was able to eliminate choices with anti-s since the passage stated that chronic infection was a failed immune response against HBsAg, but when choosing between the remaining two, he couldn't remember that IgG was for long term responses, and he didn't see this info in the passage.

> ✦ Make sure to review the content for missed questions!

- Question 25: This was a very challenging question for Joe. When taking the test, he had a hard time grasping the experiments and spent a long time thinking about each answer choice, trying to understand them. Finally, he realized that he was spending too much time on this question and more or less randomly selected an answer choice. On review, he spent time reading the experiments thoroughly to comprehend them and finally could see why the right answer was right. He decided that if a difficult question came up like this on the real MCAT (and he was pretty sure he'd see at least one of them) that he would mark it, make a guess, and come back if there was time.

- Question 37 was a Roman numeral question, and Joe correctly applied technique here. He had taken a quick look at the answer choices to see which of the three items was found in two of them; he discovered that Item I was found in two of the choices, as was Item III, so he started with Item I. Unfortunately, Joe forgot that antigen-presenting cells express MHC I as well as MHC II, and he incorrectly identified Item I as true. This caused him to eliminate choices A and C, thus eliminating the correct answer. This was the fourth immunology-based question that he got wrong on this test. Joe decided he definitely needed to study his immunology more. Furthermore, Joe noted that Item II was contradicted by passage information and was not true; if he had realized this at the time, he might have caught his error. When answering this question he had not even looked at Item II, because after eliminating choices A and C, Item II was in both of the remaining answer choices, so he figured it must be true.

- Question 40 frustrated Joe, because while he pulled some information out of the passage, he clearly had not pulled enough. The passage stated that CNG channels were ion channels, but Joe had only seen the part where the channels were important in "visual and olfactory systems, nephron collecting duct cells, and pacemaker cells." He figured that since they were in the collecting duct, they must play a role in water retention, thus he marked Item I as true. Since only choice D included Item I, Joe figured he was done and moved on, never even looking at the items. This was the second Roman numeral question that Joe got wrong where he hadn't looked at one or more of the numbered items. He made a mental note to at least glance at the other items before making his final answer choice.

- Question 47 was another missed immunology question. Joe knew to eliminate choices A and C because he knew that a "downstream response" would mean muscle contraction, and these patients experience muscle weakness. He also knew that helper T-cells don't destroy anything; they secrete chemicals to help the other cells of the immune system. However, when deciding between choices B and D, Joe knew that ultimately these receptors get degraded and so he selected choice D, forgetting that antibodies do not play a direct role in destroying anything. Another reason to review immunology.

Lastly Joe took a quick look at some of the questions he got right, but worked too hard at.

- He got Question 20 right, but thought too much about it. He easily eliminated choices A and B as false, and figured that the age of the parents was irrelevant for this type of genetic error, so he eliminated choice D as well. However, he pondered the correctness of choice C for too long instead of just confidently selecting it and moving on to the next question. He reminded himself that he did not have to understand why the correct answer was correct, he only needed to eliminate the three wrong answers, click on what's left over, and move to the next question.

  Don't be afraid to use techniques!

- Joe also got Question 24 right, but spent too much time on each individual answer choice. This is a 2x2 question, where two answer choice can eliminated together quickly, since they contain much of the same information. If Joe had realized this, he could have quickly eliminated choices A and C together, since the embryo would have to be pre-gastrulation for these experiments. Instead, Joe laboriously thought out each answer choice and this cost him some time. He reminded himself to keep a lookout for places where he could use techniques to his advantage.

- Joe had indicated that Questions 22, 31, 32, and 41 also took a long time, but on looking at them, Joe did not discover and trick or technique he had missed. He decided that some questions are just going to be harder than others, and they will take more time to answer.

Individual Biochemistry Question Analysis

After reviewing the Biology questions, Joe went back through the QRW and looked at the Biochemistry questions. He got far fewer of these wrong, so was encouraged that his understanding of Biochemistry was solid.

- Joe got Question 10 right, but struggled with it. First, the "LEAST" got him turned around a bit. He decided that for LEAST/EXCEPT/NOT questions he would try to rewrite it so that it is easier to understand, for example, "LEAST likely to be spontaneous" could be "non-spontaneous," and that would make it easier to eliminate choices. Also, he felt he could have looked for similarities between the answer choices to help eliminate them more quickly. For example, all of the answer choices say "low temperature" except choice C, so he could ponder just the temperature aspect to see how that might affect the spontaneity. Then he could have pondered entropy alone to see how that might affect it, etc.

- Question 13 was the same old theme: Joe had missed some important information in the passage that would have helped him select the correct answer. He really had to be more careful in his reading.

- Question 29 was a little bit of a wake-up call. Joe knew he had to memorize his amino acids and had been putting it off. This question reminded him that he needed to dig out those flashcards and get the amino acids learned.

- Question 53 was the hardest of the Biochemistry questions. Joe had found this entire passage confusing; he tended to struggle a bit with gene regulation/expression passages, where the expression of one thing inhibited another thing, that normally stimulated yet another thing... he tended to get turned around in these and somewhat lost. As a result, he tried to tackle this question by eliminating things he knew were false, and ignoring the "yes" "no" parts of the answer choices. He could eliminate A because he knew PDH was not used in gluconeogenesis, and he could eliminate D because the passage stated that Pdk4 inhibited PDH, and this would decrease acetyl-CoA, not increase it. The other two answers were harder to understand, especially choice C. He thought they were both true statements (which they are), but without understanding the "yes" "no" parts, he was forced to guess, and guessed incorrectly. However, he didn't think there was any particular content topic he could study to help with this one; he guessed that perhaps slowing down a bit and trying to analyze the experiment more carefully would help him on these types of questions.

  Experiment and graph analysis is important on the MCAT.

- Question 55 was in the same confusing passage as Question 53, but Joe was at least able to eliminate choices C and D as wrong, and made a lucky guess to get choice A right. On review, he realized that he didn't read the data correctly and confused absolute rates of oxidation with relative rates of oxidation. He reminded himself to be careful with that when analyzing graphs.

Summary of Joe's Biology and Biochemistry Analysis

In taking a final look at his Question Review Worksheet, Joe realized that he answered almost all of the freestanding questions correctly, and most of the memory questions correctly. He felt pretty good about his content knowledge, with the exception of immunology (which he would definitely be reviewing) and amino acids (which he just had to buckle down and study). The errors he made in this section reinforced what he had already learned from the Chem/Phys section: he needs to slow down just a little bit and read the passage more carefully. He also needs to look for information in the passage before just making assumptions about the answer choices.

Remember to...

- fill out the Question Review Worksheet soon after taking your practice test or drill
- fill out a separate Question Review Worksheet for each section, and tackle each section one at a time
- circle the questions you got wrong in red; for the science sections, use colored pencils to shade in the different subjects and make them stand out
- spend whatever time you need (usually about 2–3 hours per section) reviewing your test

6.6 PRACTICE TEST ANALYSIS—PSYCHOLOGICAL, SOCIOLOGICAL, AND BIOLOGICAL FOUNDATIONS OF BEHAVIOR

As with all of the other test sections, Joe reviewed each question in the Psych/Soc section. As he reviewed the questions, he filled out his Question Review Worksheet, coloring the Sociology questions blue, the Stats and Design questions in green, and circling anything he got wrong in red.

Joe did a quick scan of his Psych/Soc QRW to see if he could identify any big patterns. He noted that he did not get any Stats/Design questions wrong, so he was happy about that and felt confident in his knowledge. He missed approximately the same number of Psychology questions (five wrong) as Sociology questions (six wrong), and approximately the same number of Memory questions (five wrong) as Implicit questions (six wrong). He did not miss any Explicit questions, and at first was pleased, but on reviewing the notes he made about each question (in particular, Questions 6, 9, 20, 21, 22, 36, 40, 54, and 56), Joe realized that he was having a similar problem with this section as he did with the Chem/Phys and Bio/Biochem sections. He was just not pulling information out of the passage as well as he could be. Although he got a number of those questions right, he took too long and was inefficient; this caused him to run out of time on the passages.

After filling out the Question Review Worksheet, Joe decided to pay more attention to the Psychology questions this first time through, and then go back to review the Sociology questions in more detail. Also, as before, he did not spend a lot of time thinking about, or reviewing further, any question he coded as a "1." (Note: As you read through Joe's analysis of his questions, you should have the MCAT Demo Test open for viewing.)

Psychology and Sociology Question Review Worksheet

- **Test or Book/pg #**: This is the diagnostic exam you are reviewing or the passage you have completed.
- **Section**: CP (chem/phys), CARS (critical analysis), BB (bio/biochem) or PS (psych/soc)
- **P # and Q #**: Passage number and question number
- **Q type**: Question type; for the science sections this is either M (memory), E (explicit), or I (implicit). For the CARS section, this is R (Retrieval), I (Inference), MI/PP (Main Idea/ Primary Purpose), T (Tone or Attitude), S (Structure), E (Evaluate), ST (Strengthen), WK (Weaken), NI (New Information), A (Analogy), and when appropriate also ELN (Except/ Least/Not) or RN (Roman numeral).

Result Code:

Code	Question Result	Action
1	correct, easy	none
2	correct, the hard way	review for shortcuts—POE strategies, deductions, etc.
3	correct, got it down to two	review, look for WHY you picked the correct answer, compare remaining, decide why the correct answer was better, consider what you will do next time
4	wrong, got it down to two	review, look for WHY you picked the incorrect answer, compare remaining, decide why the correct answer was better, consider what you will do next time
5	wrong, eliminated the right answer	review for comprehension—did you ID the question correctly? Did you RTFQ (read the full question)? Misapply POE strategies?
6	guessed randomly (letter of the day)	review for difficulty—did you attempt the easiest questions and passages?

Since we are unable to depict the color highlighting in this book, a circled number or letter = red = wrong, grey shading = blue coloring = Sociology, boxed text = green coloring = Stats and Design. The full color version of this worksheet can be seen in your Online Companion.

Test or Book/pg #	Section	P #	Q #	Q type	Result Code	Notes
MCAT Demo Test	PS	1	1	(I)	(4)	*Psych - Had a difficult time understanding the question.*
MCAT Demo Test	PS	1	2	I	1	*Soc*
MCAT Demo Test	PS	1	3	I	1	*Psych*
MCAT Demo Test	PS	1	4	I	1	*Soc*
MCAT Demo Test	PS	1	5	E	2	*Stats/Design - Took longer than necessary; roman numeral question, use POE*
MCAT Demo Test	PS	2	6	(I)	(4)	*Stats/Design - Misread information in the passage, could not to eliminate the incorrect response*
MCAT Demo Test	PS	2	7	E	1	*Psych*
MCAT Demo Test	PS	2	8	I	3	*Psych - Got it down to two but had to guess, was shaky on Piaget*
MCAT Demo Test	PS	2	9	E	3	*Psych - Got it down to two but had to guess, did not highlight key words to see connection between object permanence and working memory*
MCAT Demo Test	PS	2	10	I	1	*Psych*
MCAT Demo Test	PS	FSQ	11	M	1	*Soc*
MCAT Demo Test	PS	FSQ	12	M	1	*Soc*
MCAT Demo Test	PS	FSQ	13	M	1	*Psych*
MCAT Demo Test	PS	FSQ	14	I	3	*Psych - Confused self-serving bias with self fulfilling prophecy, had to guess*
MCAT Demo Test	PS	3	15	E	1	*Stats/Design*
MCAT Demo Test	PS	3	16	(M)	(4)	*Psych - Had to guess between Huntington's and Parkinson's*
MCAT Demo Test	PS	3	17	I	1	*Stats/Design*
MCAT Demo Test	PS	3	18	M	1	*Psych*
MCAT Demo Test	PS	4	19	I	1	*Soc*
MCAT Demo Test	PS	4	20	E	2	*Psych - Did not map the passage effectively and spent more time than necessary*

SAMPLE MCAT PRACTICE TEST ANALYSIS

Test or Book/pg #	Section	P #	Q #	Q type	Result Code	Notes
MCAT Demo Test	PS	4	21	(I)	(4)	*Psych - Did not read carefully; missed subtle differences between answer choices*
MCAT Demo Test	PS	4	22	E	2	*Stats/Design - Misused highlighting techniques, took too long to go back and find information*
MCAT Demo Test	PS	5	23	I	2	*Stats/Design - Took too long going back and forth between passage and question*
MCAT Demo Test	PS	5	24	(M)	(6)	*Soc/Stats/Design - Guessed randomly, didn't know any of the classic experiments in psychology*
MCAT Demo Test	PS	5	25	(M)	(4)	*Soc - Misread the answer choices*
MCAT Demo Test	PS	5	26	E	2	*Soc - Roman Numeral POE*
MCAT Demo Test	PS	FSQ	27	M	1	*Psych*
MCAT Demo Test	PS	FSQ	28	M	1	*Psych*
MCAT Demo Test	PS	FSQ	29	M	1	*Psych*
MCAT Demo Test	PS	FSQ	30	(M)	(6)	*Soc - Review social influences*
MCAT Demo Test	PS	6	31	M	3	*Psych - Got it down to punishment causes misbehavior and only effective when present*
MCAT Demo Test	PS	6	32	M	1	*Psych*
MCAT Demo Test	PS	6	33	I	1	*Psych*
MCAT Demo Test	PS	6	34	(M)	(5)	*Psych - Eliminated the correct answer because ideal answer "conditioned response" was not there, did not use POE*
MCAT Demo Test	PS	6	35	M	1	*Psych*
MCAT Demo Test	PS	7	36	I	2	*Psych - Spent a lot of time looking for information, misused passage highlighting*
MCAT Demo Test	PS	7	37	I	1	*Psych*
MCAT Demo Test	PS	7	38	E	1	*Stats/Design*
MCAT Demo Test	PS	7	39	M	1	*Psych*
MCAT Demo Test	PS	8	40	I	2	*Stats/Design - Spent a long time, misused highlighting techniques and passage analysis strategies*

Test or Book/pg #	Section	P #	Q #	Q type	Result Code	Notes
MCAT Demo Test	PS	8	41	I	2	*Stats/Design - Spent a long time because of lots of text in question, long passage*
MCAT Demo Test	PS	8	42	I	4	*Soc/Stats/Design - Spent a long time, got it down to two, waited too long to guess*
MCAT Demo Test	PS	8	43	I	2	*Psych - Spent a long time*
MCAT Demo Test	PS	FSQ	44	M	1	*Soc*
MCAT Demo Test	PS	FSQ	45	M	1	*Soc*
MCAT Demo Test	PS	FSQ	46	M	1	*Psych*
MCAT Demo Test	PS	FSQ	47	M	2	*Psych - Did not correctly analyze the question although it was 2x2*
MCAT Demo Test	PS	9	48	M	1	*Psych*
MCAT Demo Test	PS	9	49	E	1	*Stats/Design*
MCAT Demo Test	PS	9	50	I	3	*Psych - Knew it had to be monozygotic so got it down to A and C quickly, guessed correctly*
MCAT Demo Test	PS	9	51	M	1	*Psych*
MCAT Demo Test	PS	10	52	M	1	*Soc*
MCAT Demo Test	PS	10	53	E	2	*Soc - Spent a lot of time looking for information*
MCAT Demo Test	PS	10	54	I	5	*Soc - Misread the passage, led to incorrect inference*
MCAT Demo Test	PS	10	55	M	1	*Soc*
MCAT Demo Test	PS	10	56	I	3	*Stats/Design - Read the passage too quickly*
MCAT Demo Test	PS	FSQ	57	I	6	*Soc - Left until end of test, ran out of time*
MCAT Demo Test	PS	FSQ	58	I	1	*Stats/Design*
MCAT Demo Test	PS	FSQ	59	I	1	*Psych*

Individual Sociology Question Analysis

Since Joe missed more questions in Sociology than in Psychology, he decided to start his analysis with the Sociology questions he got wrong.

- Joe had to guess randomly on Question 24 and answered wrong. He simply did not memorize the classic experiments in social psychology that he needed to be able to answer the question. He made a note to find each of the experiments in The Princeton Review's *MCAT Psychology and Sociology Review* text and learn them.

- Question 25: Joe answered narrowed it down to two but did not guess correctly. Choices B and D were inconsistent with what Joe expected to happen with in group identification. He thought there would either be more in group bias or people would be less likely to seek other in groups. He could not decide which was more likely so he guessed. However, individuals with strong in group identification can still seek many other in groups, and there is no evidence that they are less likely to seek out other in groups. Joe could have used this line of reasoning to select the correct answer choice.

- On Question 30, Joe guessed randomly because he did not review normative social influences. He made a note to focus on that topic while he looked over Sociology in greater depth.

- Joe used figure analysis on Question 42 to eliminate choices A and C, but he did not select the correct answer. He knew that taking care of children was unlikely to account for the vast difference between immigrant and non-immigrant women in cortisol levels expressed in Figure 1. Immigrant women reported slightly higher stress about children, but both immigrant and non-immigrant women were close to an average score of 3 and the difference was minor. English fluency was not directly mentioned, and non-immigrant women actually worried slightly more about racial discrimination. Now Joe spent a lot of time clicking between the figures and re-reading the passage to try to eliminate choices B or D. He did not see any direct evidence for either better coping mechanisms among non-immigrants or that immigrants were more likely to take care of their parents. He ended up guessing between these two and choosing the incorrect answer. Joe's takeaway from this problem was that he spent too much time on a problem that he had narrowed down to a 50/50 chance. He could have used this time more efficiently on other problems, especially Free Standing Questions.

  Skip questions that take a long time to analyze to save time for easier questions.

- Joe misread Passage 10 and he made an incorrect inference on Question 54 that led him to eliminate the correct answer. Joe was coming to the end of the test and fatigue was setting in. Joe made a note to allocate his time better on the test so that he did not rush on any questions that were within his ability. With more careful analysis, he could have gone back to the passage and seen that the hypothesis predicts that individuals from individualist cultures are more likely to practice individualist values, and therefore less likely to practice collectivist values.

  When taking practice tests, experiment with different foods during your breaks to see which one best sustains your energy until the end of the test.

- Question 57 was another question where Joe could have benefited from leaving more time at the end of test. He had to guess randomly and did not select the correct answer. Joe left this question until the end of the test, however, it is a Free Standing Question, and Joe knew from his analysis that he did extremely well on this type. If he would have left more time, this is likely a question that Joe would have answered correctly. Again, Joe noted to allocate his time better and make sure he had enough time to work on all the questions within his ability.

Individual Psychology Question Analysis

Joe continued his analysis with Psychology, starting with the questions he got wrong.

- Joe got Question 1 wrong because he did not understand what it was asking. The question was long, with complex language. He correctly left this question until the end of the passage, but he allowed himself to get bogged down in the details of the question. Joe was able to eliminate choice B because he remembered that catecholamine acts on the sympathetic, not the parasympathetic nervous system. He also knew that high catecholamine levels are associated with more stress, not less, and would probably lead to increased cortisol levels. Joe was able to use POE in this way to get it down to two. This gave Joe a 50/50 chance to select the correct choice, but when he reviewed the test he realized he could have also eliminated choice C because it is unlikely that muscle contractions would burn enough calories to lead to weight loss.

- On Question 6, Joe got the wrong answer because he was uncertain about the information in the passage and became confused between choices B and D. Both emotional regulation and orientation and engagement were associated with high scores on object permanence, however, a link between the two was not expressed in the passage. Joe made a note to read the results more carefully and look for links that are explicitly stated. Joe remembered that the MCAT will often set traps that draw extraneous links; Joe noted afterwards that the passage states that "object permanence tasks can also be used as memory assessments for younger children." He made a note also that high emotional regulation is correlated with high performance on object permanence task and that the correct response is choice D.

- Joe got Question 16 wrong after getting it down to two. He remembered that like Alzheimer's Disease, both Huntington's Disease and Parkinson's Disease are late onset neuro-degenerative disorders. However, he had to guess between the two because he could not remember which was more similar to Alzheimer's. He made a note to review all his disorders in more detail and make sure that he knew how to identify the most important ones by symptoms. He realized from reviewing the explanation for Question 16 that he also missed the first sentence of paragraph 3, where the passage states that Alzheimer's is an "autosomal dominant mutation," just like Parkinson's. Joe's takeaway was to review this specific area of content in depth and improve his passage mapping.

Pull important information out of the passage!

- Joe got Question 21 wrong because he rushed through the answer choices and didn't see that choice A stated presentation of a media problem and choice C stated presentation of a life problem. He was left to guess between the two answer choices. Joe remembered to read the answer choices more carefully and look for subtle differences between answer choices. He was able to get it down to two because he knew that analysis of text would yield the best memory improvements in the depth of processing model. This brought the choices down to two, and with more careful reading, Joe could have eliminated the other incorrect choice. Joe got the answer wrong and his takeaway was that Question 21 was a question he could have answered correctly if he had more time, and that he should allocate more time for questions like this and spend less time on low yield, very difficult questions like several of the questions in Passage 8.

- Joe eliminated the correct answer on Question 34. He thought classical conditioning was too broad to be the correct answer and eliminated choice C. He knew the correct choice was a type of response so he selected choice D. However, the response is a conditioned, not an unconditioned response, so Joe should have eliminated choice D. Since "conditioned response" is not a choice but is a part of classical conditioning, choice C is correct. The MCAT will often leave out information or omit the best possible answer, leaving test takers to choose among other less ideal choices. Joe made a note that it is better to eliminate only if he is certain an answer is wrong since he can always do more in depth POE when he is down to two.

Joe next looked at Psychology questions he got right, but took a long time on or was otherwise inefficient.

- Question 8: Joe answered this question correctly but guessed between two. He remembered that before children learn conservation in the concrete operational phase, they think that water poured into a glass with a different shape will actually change in content. He therefore knew that the child would think that one of the two glasses contained more water, but he did not remember which. Since it was a memory question, he knew he simply made a note to review Piaget's stages in greater detail.

- Joe also answered Question 9 correctly after using POE to get it down to two. This was the second question on this passage that Joe struggled with because he did not notice the connection between working memory and object permanence. Joe concluded that he made a mistake in the way he mapped the passage. Object permanence is a key word, so he should have highlighted any instance of it in the passage. If he had done so, he would have seen that it was related to working memory and he could have more certainly selected choice A, since the hippocampus is the most prominent brain region in memory formation.

- Joe answered Question 14 correctly but he had to guess because he confused self-serving bias with self-fulfilling prophecy. As a result, he did not eliminate choice D and had to guess between choices C and D. He was lucky to chose the right answer, but he made a note to review attribution in more detail to avoid such mistakes in the future. He also noted that even between self-serving bias and learned helplessness, learned helplessness is still the better choice since it fits the situation almost perfectly, so Joe could have used his techniques to get the correct answer with more confidence.

- On Question 31, Joe got it down to two by eliminating implausible answers, then guessed correctly. He knew punishment is not the single most effective form of behavior modification. Also, administering any form of behavior modification in an inconsistent manner seemed unlikely to lead to better outcomes. This left choices A and D. Joe wasn't sure which of these was better, because he remembered reading that

Review topics that you are unsure about.

punishment did lead to some unintended consequences. Joe made a note to review the effects of punishment in behavior modification since he was somewhat unsure.

- Joe got Question 50 down to the last two and was lucky to guess correctly. When Joe saw heritability, he knew that the best way to show heritability is with research methods that incorporate monozygotic twins, since they are genetically identical. Joe guessed correctly among the monozygotic choices. However, when he reviewed the test, he realized he should not have had to guess on this problem. He knew in retrospect that heritability should isolate genetic factors, and therefore twins reared apart would be the best choice. However, since he was pressed for time on the end of the test he began to rush. He did not make the differentiation between the two choices to be able to select the correct answer. Joe's takeaway was to manage time better and guess more quickly between two on questions like 42 where he cannot narrow it down more quickly.

Keep an eye on the timer to manage your pacing; know how many minutes each passage should get.

Summary of Joe's Psychology Sociology Section Analysis

Joe combined his Question Review Analysis with a final look at the score report for the Psychology and Sociology section. He went to the category view and reminded himself that in Sociology, he missed 2 out of 5 questions about Groups, and 3 out of 5 questions about Socialization. He made a mental note to review those topics before his next practice test.

Joe also decided to review the rules for pacing and to practice this in his homework and practice passages as well as on his full-length tests. He felt like he made some mistakes that could have been prevented by not rushing and feeling fatigued.

Remember to...

- fill out the Question Review Worksheet soon after taking your practice test or drill
- fill out a separate Question Review Worksheet for each section, and tackle each section one at a time
- circle the questions you got wrong in red; for the science sections, use colored pencils to shade in the different subjects and make them stand out
- spend whatever time you need (usually about 2–3 hours per section) reviewing your test

Part II

The Critical Analysis and Reasoning Skills (CARS) Section

Chapter 7
Critical Analysis and
Reasoning Skills
on the MCAT

7.1 OVERVIEW

The Critical Analysis and Reasoning Skills (CARS) section can be intimidating for many test takers, and this is why, even though it is the second section of the test, we are addressing it before the science sections. You've been studying hard for many years, packing your brain with lots of science knowledge and refining your memorization skills. But now, as you confront the CARS section, all those facts and mnemonics are useless; you have to employ an entirely different approach. Even if you have taken lots of Humanities and Social Science classes and have been speaking and reading English for many years, you may find that you aren't doing as well as you expected on CARS. This is because you haven't yet learned to adapt to the specific nature and requirements of the MCAT.

There are many false beliefs out there regarding CARS, one of which is "either you get the passage or you don't." According to this myth, your CARS score depends on luck; if you get "good" passages, all is well, but if you don't, you're in trouble. However, this is in fact completely untrue; there are ways any test taker can improve his or her CARS score and get points on even the most difficult passages.

Many of you reading this chapter will fall into one of two categories:

1. your science scores are high on practice tests or past real MCATs, but your CARS score is hovering at or below average; or,
2. your CARS score is above average, but now your goal is to move it even higher.

Regardless of which category you are in, you can boost your score in two ways. First, you must follow a methodical and consistent approach. Many people who are already good at CARS rely on their existing reading comprehension skills: They just "read the passage and pick the answer that sounds right." However, no matter how good of a reader you already are, you need to employ analytical methods specific to the unique nature of this section of the test. Second, you must also do consistent and detailed self-analysis to figure out the types of mistakes you are making and develop a strategy to avoid those mistakes in the future. While the same fundamental plan of attack works for everyone, different people think and read differently, and you have to adapt the basic tactics that we will be discussing in this chapter to your own needs.

MCAT CARS is very different from the reading you're used to.

Change is scary, especially if you are already doing fairly well in CARS. However, in order to improve, you will have to do something different. Simply taking test after test or working passage after passage won't do it; you need to refine your strategy in order to increase your score. In the rest of this chapter, we'll look at the skills you need and review the basics; even high scorers can benefit from solidifying their basic approach. We will also discuss advanced methods for refining your skills and pushing your score even higher.

7.2 MCAT CRITICAL ANALYSIS AND REASONING SKILLS[1]

The following is a general list of the skills tested in the CARS section.

Reading Comprehension—you will need to:
- recognize the main theme or purpose of a passage
- recognize the purpose of different parts of the passage
- recognize explicit and implicit claims contained in the passage
- identify a correct paraphrase of complex details and information
- ascertain the meaning of important terms used in the passage
- draw inferences from passage information
- identify different points of view presented within the passage
- identify the passage author's tone or attitude
- recognize relationships between different parts or aspects of the passage

Reasoning Within the Text—you will need to:
- determine how solid a particular argument or reasoning step is
- decide on the relevance of facts or data to an argument or claim
- decide whether a source of information is reliable or plausible
- decide whether or not a claim is well supported within the passage
- evaluate the evidence for a conclusion to determine its validity

Reasoning Beyond the Text: Applying Passage Information to New Situations—you will need to:
- identify what situation or idea would be most analogous to a situation or idea in the passage.
- recognize the most likely reason for a specific occurrence or outcome based on passage information
- use information from the passage to solve a particular issue or problem, and recognize the range of application of theories, reasons, and conclusions
- predict the result of a theoretical situation based on new information as well as information in the passage
- ascertain the implications for the real world of particular assumptions or outcomes

Reasoning Beyond the Text: Applying New Information to the Passage—you will need to:
- identify processes or outcomes that would contest theories given in the passage
- identify reasonable competing conclusions or theories that could be drawn from passage information
- decide on the influence of new facts and data on arguments presented in the passage
- figure out how a conclusion from the passage can be altered to make it more consistent with new data
- decide what new information is most consistent with the information or argument presented in the passage

---

[1] Adapted from *The Official Guide to the MCAT® Exam (MCAT 2015)*, 2014 ed. Association of American Medical Colleges.

7.3   BASIC PREPARATION

Before we get into the specific CARS Techniques, let's talk about other ways to build up your skills.

Outside Reading

Many MCAT students feel uncomfortable with the CARS passages because they are more used to reading science texts than material from the Social Sciences or Humanities. If this is true for you, build up your reading comprehension and active reading skills using material similar to that which you will encounter on the test. Find a text written at a fairly high level (that is, not a simple news article) and treat it like a passage: highlight it, summarize the main point of each paragraph, define how the paragraphs relate to each other and what the author's overall argument is in each chunk of paragraphs. If you are using printed material, make a Xerox copy (never highlight a library book!). Even better, find material online and work with it on the screen rather than printing it out. Remember that you are not reading it to learn the content but rather to practice your CARS skills, so don't get caught up in the subject; focus on analyzing the structure of the material.

Some useful sources:

- Periodicals: *The New Yorker, Atlantic Monthly, The Economist, Legal Affairs, Foreign Affairs, Harper's.*
- Authors: Here are some authors whose work is similar to the material you will find in CARS passages (in fact, work by many of these authors has been used in the past by the real MCAT writers):
    - René Wellek
    - Austin Warren
    - Joseph Campbell
    - Will Durant
    - Walter Jackson Bate
    - Henry Giroux
    - Donna Haraway
    - George Lakoff
    - Erwin Panofsky
- Gutenberg.org and Authorama.com
    - These are sites where you can download material that is not copyrighted or whose copyright has expired. This is a good source for MCAT-like material that you can practice reading and working on a computer. Go through their catalogs and find material that looks unfamiliar and difficult to understand (just like the hardest CARS passages).

Build Endurance

If you are just beginning to study for MCAT CARS, start by doing one or two passages at a time. In this initial stage, check your answers immediately after completing those passages so that you can remember your thought process and see where you may have failed to apply the correct method (as well as where you succeeded). Gradually build up to the point where you are doing at least three passages, and ideally seven to nine passages, at a stretch. At this stage, do not check your answers after every passage or two. You want to get used to working through a new passage without the reassurance of knowing how you did on the previous passage. Also, practice dealing with distraction. Do some timed work in less than ideal conditions (a library where people are moving around, a calm but not dead-silent coffee house, etc.). Practice tuning out your surroundings and keeping your energy focused on the test.

Timing

Start by doing passages untimed. Whenever you learn a new skill, you need to practice it slowly until you learn to do it right. Once you've become comfortable with the basic steps and techniques, start keeping track of the time you spend per passage or on a chunk of passages. Eventually work up to doing timed CARS sections and full-timed practice tests. Keep in mind that you should be working up to your ultimate test pace, rather than going as fast as possible from the beginning of your prep. If you've been studying for a while but have never done much untimed work, this might be a good time to go back and work a series of passages without timing yourself. In particular, list the mistakes you tend to make on timed passages, and then work through a series of passages untimed, focusing on avoiding those same mistakes.

Self-Evaluation

As you saw in the Test Analysis section, self-evaluation is a necessary component of the quest to maximize your score. This is especially true of CARS, since only your logical and analytical skills, not your factual knowledge, is being tested. You will see in the rest of this chapter that whenever we discuss advanced methods and ways in which to refine your skills, they will always tie back to self-evaluation.

Implementing Your Skills

Using whatever resources are available to you, take as many full timed practice tests as you can. Don't wait to start taking practice tests until a few weeks before the real exam. Taking full tests and evaluating your performance is an essential part of your preparation. Test takers may make different kinds of mistakes on timed passages than on untimed passages, on timed CARS sections than on individual timed CARS passages, and during full-timed MCATs than during isolated timed sections.

Stress Management

Most test takers feel a certain level of stress on and before the big day. A certain level of anxiety can be useful; it motivates you, keeps you alert, and sharpens your focus. However, if you find that your stress levels get so high that they interfere with your studying or with your concentration during a test, find ways to alleviate your stress and bring it down to manageable levels. Here are some suggestions:

- **Deep breathing.** When you realize that your focus is fading or your muscles are tensing up during a test, sit back from the screen (or the book), close your eyes, and take three slow, deep breaths. It can be hard to look away from the screen during a timed test, but if those 10–15 seconds of relaxation help you concentrate and work productively for the rest of the time, it is the best investment of time that you can make.
- **Positive reinforcement.** It's easy to fall into negative thinking during moments of frustration, and this can push you into an overly self-critical mindset. It doesn't help to beat yourself up over mistakes you have made. Instead, think about (1) what you can learn from those mistakes, and (2) all the questions you got right and how you did it.
- **Reward yourself.** Studying for this test should be a high priority for you over the next few weeks or months. However, there is no point in burning yourself out physically or emotionally. If you go into the test in a state of exhaustion, you will not be able to put all that time and effort to good use. Build time for enjoyable activities into your studying schedule. This is especially important during the week leading up to the day of the real test. Taper off in your studying in those last few days, and do little if any MCAT work the day before test day (basic review at the most, but no timed practice tests or timed sections).

Now let's go through each of the steps of doing CARS in more detail, discussing the basic approach and how to further refine your skills. Included within these steps are instructions on how to navigate most efficiently through a passage when doing a computer-based MCAT.

7.4 THE SIX STEPS TO CARS

First, we'll go through an outline of the Six Steps you will take to approach every CARS section and passage. Then we'll break down each step in more detail, using a sample passage.

▬ STEP 1: RANK AND ORDER THE PASSAGES

Decide if the passage is a relatively easy "Now" passage, a more difficult "Later," or a "Killer" (an especially difficult passage that you will do last or on which you will randomly guess).

▬ STEP 2: PREVIEW THE QUESTIONS

After writing down a heading for that passage on your scratch paper, quickly read through the question stems for that passage from first to last, looking for and highlighting references to passage content. The purpose is to get an idea of what will be important in the passage and to help you annotate the passage text more effectively.

▬ STEP 3: WORK THE PASSAGE

Read through the passage relatively quickly, but with enough attention that you can track its logical structure and the main points of each paragraph. Highlight key words and phrases within the passage text, using your scratch paper to take notes as needed. Work the passage from the screen containing the last question for that passage.

STEP 4: DEFINE THE BOTTOM LINE

Define the main idea, purpose, and tone of the entire passage.

STEP 5: ATTACK THE QUESTIONS

Translate and define the question task. When the question gives you a reference to the passage, go back to the passage text first, read above and below that reference, paraphrase what you just read, and generate an answer in your own words. Go through the choices using POE; look for what is wrong with each answer and eliminate down to the "least wrong" choice. Attack the questions from last to first for that passage. Save particularly hard questions for last; do them as you click forward toward the next passage.

STEP 6: INSPECT THE SECTION

Use the Review screen to make sure that you haven't left anything blank; if you have, go back and fill in random guesses. Get this done at least by the 5-minute warning, but ideally before you start your last passage.

STEP 1: RANKING AND ORDERING THE PASSAGES

In the CARS section, some passages will be significantly harder than others. However, you don't get any more credit for correctly answering the hardest question in the section than for correctly answering the easiest question. And the passages are rarely presented in order of difficulty from easiest to hardest (that would be too easy). Often, the most difficult passage or passages are buried in the middle of the section. Therefore, if you just plug away at the passages from first to last, you will likely spend lots of time struggling with the hardest passage in the section, perhaps getting a high percentage of those questions wrong and spending a lot of time doing it. Or, you will run out of time and have to randomly guess on, or rush through, one of the easier passages, missing questions that you could have gotten right. Maximizing your CARS score is all about taking control over the section, and one way to do this is to attack the passages in the order that works best for you. You need to make well-founded decisions about which passages to complete and when.

Do the passages in the order that works best for you—start with the easy ones!

Ranking

Here's how to predict the overall difficulty level of a passage:

- Skim the first two or three sentences of a paragraph.
- Try to paraphrase what you have just read.
- If you can paraphrase easily, the passage is likely to be fairly easy to read and understand. If all you can do is repeat the words you have just read because the meaning is difficult to extract, the passage text is likely to be difficult as a whole.
- Give the passage a ranking of NOW (one you will complete early on in the section), LATER (a passage you will come back to and complete after the easier ones), or KILLER (a passage you will do last or randomly guess on).

Note: Given that the questions are delivered on separate screens, it is too cumbersome to take the apparent difficulty of the questions into account when ranking. However, as you attack the questions you may decide to temporarily skip over some questions as you go backwards through the set, and leave them to do last as you click forward to the next passage.

So, let's look at passage and question difficulty in a little more detail.

Evaluating the Passage Text

Read through each of the following paragraphs quickly, and write a paraphrase in the space provided below.

1. In his consideration of the meaning of the evolution of forms of punishment and imprisonment in different societies over time, Foucault shows that the way in which punishment is inscribed upon the body, or rather, the way in which it may be sequestered from public view and carried out behind the walls of institutional constructs, indicates the meaning of crime within that society and the ramifications of trespassing against accepted modes of behavior within different cultural nets of significance. Ontological considerations necessarily follow from identification of different disciplinary modes: Meaning is fluid.

    _____

    _____

    _____

2. Prison overcrowding is a serious problem in modern society. When prisons are filled beyond their capacity, it is difficult or impossible to carry out necessary rehabilitation programs. This failing contributes to recidivism and future crime rates.

    _____

    _____

    _____

Did you find the first paragraph to be much more of a challenge? If so, why? Beyond having vocabulary that may have been unfamiliar, it is highly abstract. The complicated sentence structure adds insult to injury; when sentences are constructed out of several parts cobbled together with commas and colons and semicolons, you will have to put a lot of effort into untangling them in order to get any understanding of the author's meaning. The second paragraph, while on the same overall topic (prisons and punishment), is concrete, descriptive, and written in a straightforward manner. The rest of the passage is likely to continue along the same lines. If these were two passages on a real exam, you'd want to do the second first and the first later (or never).

Evaluating the Questions

As we mentioned above, your passage ranking should be based on the passage text alone. However, you may improve your performance on the set of questions attached to that passage by leaving the hardest questions for last (but before you move on to the next passage). So, being able to quickly judge the likely difficulty level of a question is a useful skill to develop. Questions that ask you to extract information from the passage, or to summarize the main theme of the passage as a whole, tend to be faster and easier to answer. On the other hand, complex questions that ask you to apply new information to the passage text, or to evaluate the strength of the author's argument, will tend to be more difficult. And all other things being equal, longer questions and answer choices tend to be harder to manage than shorter question stems and choices.

Take a look at the following questions and decide if they are likely to be easy or hard to answer. Circle your choice (Easy or Hard) for each of the five, and then read through the explanations below.

1. Which of the following statements, if true, most *undermines* the author's contention regarding the debate between Reynolds and Adams?
    Easy or Hard?

2. Which of the following statements regarding Impressionism is best supported by the passage?
    Easy or Hard?

3. Assume that it was shown that the political goals of the Surrealists were in direct conflict with their artistic mission. What impact would this have on the author's argument regarding Louis Aragon, as that argument is presented in the passage?
    Easy or Hard?

4. By "recidivism," the author most likely means:
    Easy or Hard?

5. Which of the following statements best captures an accurate evaluation of the strength of the author's argument regarding the impact of the growth of coffee sales on Central American economies in the absence of a stable infrastructure?
    Easy or Hard?

Evaluation

Question 1: Hard. This question asks you to take new information in the answer choices and apply it to the passage. It also requires you to pick an answer that goes against the author's argument, making it easy to get turned around.

Question 2: Easy. This question essentially asks you to locate what the author says about Impressionism, and to find the choice that is best supported by that part of the passage.

Question 3: Hard. This question gives you new information in the question stem, and requires you to decide how it would apply to the author's argument.

Question 4: Easy. Questions that ask for definitions tend not to be that challenging, especially if the passage text is reasonably comprehensible. Even if you are unfamiliar with the word being defined, if you can understand that part of the passage you will get the question right.

<u>Question 5: Hard</u>. To answer this question, you will not only have to understand what the author has to say on this issue, but to take another step and decide whether or not it is well founded or well supported.

Summary of Ranking

Even though ranking takes a bit of time up front, it will pay off in the section as a whole by helping you to avoid getting stuck in a hard passage early on, and to as well to avoid choosing an easy rather than a hard passage to guess on if you are not completing all nine.

Spend 15–20 seconds per passage making your ranking decisions.

Overall, you should be spending about two to three minutes, spread out throughout the 90 minutes you have on the section, making your ranking decisions.

Ordering the Passages Based on Ranking

The ordering system that works best for most test takers is the Two-Pass System.

First Pass

If a passage is a NOW, go ahead and complete it once you have identified it (before you rank the next passage). Do your scratch paper work under the heading (e.g., "Passage 1 Q 1–5") you have just written down. If it is a LATER or KILLER, skip over it in your first pass. (You might wait until you have done all the NOW passages to make the final distinction between LATER and KILLER passages.) If you are skipping over a passage, write a big "SKIPPED" under your scratch paper heading, and leave room beneath in case you decide to come back and do this passage later. Also, go ahead and mark and randomly guess on all the questions for that passage. If you decide never to come back to them, you will have already made your guesses, and there will be no risk of leaving questions blank. If you decide to return and do it as a LATER passage, it takes little or no time to change your answers as you work through the questions. (Note: Since you should rarely, if ever, come back to rework CARS questions once you have finished a passage and moved on, this is most likely the only time you will be marking questions within the CARS section.)

Mark passages you are skipping and fill in guesses just in case you don't have time to come back.

Second Pass

Once you have completed the easier passages, come back through the section a second time, completing the LATER passages. At or by the 5-minutes-left warning (ideally, before you start your last passage), check the Review screen to make sure that you haven't left anything blank.

Advanced Ranking and Ordering: Refining Your Skills

Improving your score by working on these skills requires taking your current pacing into account (how many questions and passages you are completing). Take a look at the following two categories. If your pacing changes in the future, you may move into a new category; at that time, reconsider your ordering strategy.

Finishing All Nine Passages

If you are currently working at this pace and scoring a 128 or above, passage choice is still important. (If you are completing all nine and not yet scoring at this level, you may need to slow down your pace to eight passages, at least for now.) Skip over at least one, ideally at least two, during your first pass. Many who are planning to finish all the passages feel that there is no need to rank them, since they will be working them all at some point. However, getting stuck on a hard passage early on in the section can throw off the rest of your timing, causing you to become frustrated and lose your cool, rush through other easier passages and make unnecessary mistakes, and lose concentration and work less efficiently.

As you work through the passages, when you come across one that looks more difficult than the others (in particular, if the passage text is highly abstract and difficult to understand), skip over it in your first pass. This way, you can make sure that if you do run short on time and have to guess on a few questions, it will be on the hardest passage. And you don't risk hitting a bump early on that throws you off your game for the rest of the section. If you are going to lose your form, better that it happens in the last 10 minutes than in the first half of your time, when you could be scoring easy points.

Finishing Eight or Fewer Passages

If the pacing that is currently working best for you is randomly guessing on one or more passages, skip over two to four LATER/KILLER passages during your first pass. Since you will not be completing all the passages, it is important that you make well-considered choices and avoid wasting your time on the hardest one. You want to be able to compare several passages with each other toward the end and make the best choice.

You may even find that effective passage ordering helps you speed up and get to more questions in the end, especially if you usually tend to waste time struggling with one hard passage.

7.5 READING AND MAPPING THE PASSAGE (STEPS 2, 3, AND 4)

Students who are already scoring above average in CARS often get blasé about how they are working the passage. They tend to rely on their natural reading skills without thinking very much about how they are working through the passage text. It certainly all comes down to the questions in the end, but to answer the questions as accurately and efficiently as possible, you need to have an appropriate foundation in the passage. If you aren't working the passage to the best of your abilities, you will not get the highest possible score. So let's review the basic process of passage reading and mapping. There are three phases in this process: Previewing the Questions, Working the Passage, and Defining the Bottom Line. Let's take a look at each, using a sample passage. After we get through the basics for each phase in the process, we will discuss ways in which you can refine your skills within each stage.

STEP 2: PREVIEWING THE QUESTIONS

Why preview the question stems before reading the passage text? After all, you will be reading them again to answer the questions. However, there are several advantages to this step.

First, there are no line references in the questions (and sometimes only a few paragraph references) to help you locate the information in the passage that you need. Test takers who don't preview the questions often find themselves on long meandering searches through the passage trying to find specific topics. This eats up a lot of your precious time. If you know the question topics ahead of time, you can locate and highlight them as you read, setting up a map for yourself to follow once you hit the questions. **Important:** At this stage, ignore words indicating the question type (e.g., "According to the passage," "What can be inferred," "What would most strengthen," "What would be most analogous," etc.). While knowing the question type is crucial when you enter into the process of answering the question, it won't help you work the passage any better.

Second, not everything in the passage is important for answering the questions. If you know what at least some of the key issues are ahead of time, you can maximize your efficiency in working the passage, paying attention to what is most important and reading more quickly through what is less crucial.

Third, reading a passage without previewing is like jumping into the middle of a discussion and trying to figure out what's going on with no context to guide you. Knowing something about the overall passage topic before you begin to read gives you a base to which you can connect all the new information; it helps you make sense of the passage more quickly. It also improves your focus. If you have found yourself realizing halfway through a passage that you have no idea what you are reading, previewing can go a long way toward helping you keep your concentration.

After a bit of practice, previewing the questions should take you 15–30 seconds. This is generally *not* a time to use your scratch paper; don't take notes as you preview, but rather focus your mind on each issue as it arises. Think about how the different topics you are discovering might relate to each other. If your mind is staying active and engaged, you will naturally find yourself generating questions about those relationships. This also helps you maintain focus and interest in the passage text.

To see how this works in practice, let's take a look at a set of sample questions. (These are the questions attached to the sample passage we will be working through later in the section.)

Below are the questions attached to the sample passage. **Important:** On the MCAT, there will be 5–7 questions for each CARS passage. For the purposes of talking through each of the ten question types later in this chapter, there will be 10 questions attached to this passage, which is why we have 10 questions to Preview here. In the Preview stage you should *not* be looking at the answer choices, so only the question stems are provided for now. You can highlight within the question stems (but not the answer choices or Roman numerals), so highlight the lead words referencing passage content as you go. Preview them from first to last for about 20 seconds, looking only for references to passage content and not worrying at this stage about the question type. Then, for the purposes of this drill, answer the Preview Question that follows the list of questions before reading through the explanation.

Sample Passage: Question Stems

1. According to the passage, anthropologists can still gain understanding of the meaning and function of early human myth by:

2. The author implies that the need ancient peoples had for myth's clarity and reassurance came mainly from:

3. The author's primary purpose in the passage is to:

4. In this passage, the author's tone is one of:

5. In the passage, the author draws an analogy between:

6. The author's assertion that science plays the same role today as myth played in ancient societies is supported:

7. Which of the following statements, if true, would most strengthen the author's claim that most modern people see myth as little more than superstition or fantasy?

8. Which of the following statements, if true, would most *weaken* the author's argument that Malinowski's work in the Trobriands does justice to the true function of myth in that culture?

9. Suppose an original poetic text from the first century B.C. celebrating the heroic deeds of the god Apollo were discovered in an archeological dig. How would this discovery affect the author's claim that we in modern society find it difficult to comprehend the meaning of myth in ancient societies?

10. Which of the following would be most analogous to the relationship between the role of myth in ancient societies and the role of medicine and astrophysics today, as those roles are described in the passage?

Preview Question: What will be important in the passage text? _____

_____

_____

_____

_____

_____

_____

_____

Before answering that question together, let's see what you could have gotten out of each question stem.

- Question 1 asks about the meaning of early myths. This also appears to relate closely to what you saw in Question 9: understanding the meaning of ancient myths
- Question 2 alerts you to the fact that the author will be discussing why ancient people needed clarity and reassurance from myths.
- Question 3 is a generic Main Idea/Primary Purpose question. You will quickly learn to recognize these generic questions and to immediately move on to the next question. You are always defining the Bottom Line of the passage (main point, purpose, and tone of the passage as a whole), regardless of whether or not there is a General question attached to it.
- Question 4 asks for the author's tone. Like Question 3, this is a generic general question; you should always be tracking the author's tone in the passage, even if there is no question explicitly asking about it.
- Question 5 asks about an analogy used by the author. Now you know to be on the lookout for where this kind of logic appears in the passage
- Question 6 asks what the author says about the role of science today as compared with the role of myth in ancient society. Given the previous questions, you now know to be alert to comparisons or contrasts between modern and ancient peoples.
- Question 7 focuses on the modern view of myth as superstition and fantasy. Note that just like Question 6, this question indicates that the passage will compare and/or contrast ancient and modern peoples.
- From Question 8, you know that you need to find and understand what the author has to say about Malinowski's work as it relates to the function of myth.
- Question 9 contains new information. Once you recognize this in the preview, it is reasonable to move on; it may take too much time to separate the new information from the passage reference. However, you might have seen that this question refers to an ancient text and to the author's argument about what myths meant to ancient societies. You might also be thinking about how this relates to Question 1, which asks about the meaning of early myths.
- Finally, Question 10 will require you to find what the author says about the relationship between the role of myth in ancient societies and the role of medicine and astrophysics today, which sounds very similar to Question 6.

Based on all this, you might have answered the Preview Question as follows:

The importance and function of myth in ancient societies and how we might understand it, especially through Malinowski's work.

Advanced Previewing: Refining Your Skills

Ask yourself if you are getting what you need out of this step. If not, here are some things to consider.

- Do you find that once you start reading the passage, you can't remember anything that you previewed? If so, you may be previewing too quickly. If you are simply running your eyes over the questions without pulling out (and highlighting) the content, you probably aren't getting enough of a sense of the passage, or remembering enough of the question topics, to make it worthwhile. In this situation, try spending an extra 10–15 seconds to see if they stick better. Or, it may be an issue of focus rather than time. Imagine that you are imprinting each topic on your brain as you read. With a half-second pause after each question, the topics are more likely to make it into your memory bank and to stick around for the passage.

- Are you spending too much time previewing (more than a minute)? If so, you are likely reading for too much detail, including the question type (which is irrelevant at this stage). Practice running your eyes over the question stem until you hit true content, and only then slowing down to read more carefully. Familiarizing yourself further with the common ways in which question tasks are worded will help you focus on the passage content in the question stem (or to recognize and skip over a generic question) and to tighten up the process as a whole.

- Do you become distracted by your memory of the question topics, to the extent that you find yourself just searching for certain words in the passage rather than understanding the author's main points? If so, think of the question topics as clues, not the whole story. You are a detective gathering those clues, and once you read the passage, you are building the story around them. Also, once you improve your skills in working the passage, previewing will contribute to, rather than detract from, your understanding of the key themes in the passage text.

STEP 3: WORKING THE PASSAGE

There are two tasks to accomplish as you work through each paragraph of the passage: highlight the important parts of the passage text and summarize the main point of each paragraph or chunk. Let's talk about each in turn.

Highlighting

Passages are made up of parts that work together to communicate the author's argument. Some of these parts are more critical than others, however. Obviously, anything related to the question topics will be important to understand. However, to get the correct answers to the questions as efficiently as possible, you also need to have an understanding of the logic of the passage. Highlighting allows you to both maintain your focus on those logical aspects and to leave a trail of breadcrumbs behind so that you can follow it back to the information you need when answering the questions. If you think of yourself as a "good reader," meaning that you read relatively quickly with good comprehension, you may feel that you don't need to highlight at all. However, unless you have a photographic memory and can remember every detail and the major themes with perfect accuracy after a 2–4 minute reading of the passage, you will do better if you use some highlighting.

As you read, highlight key words and phrases that (1) relate to question topics you saw in your preview, and (2) tell you about the logical structure of the passage. Authors use words to communicate clearly. Take advantage of this by noticing and highlighting these "indicator words."

The key to effective highlighting is to avoid the extremes of highlighting too little or too much. On one hand, highlighting everything that "sounds important" will cause you to highlight a large portion of the text. This does not help you focus on, or understand, the major themes as you read, and it doesn't provide you with a useful map to rely on as you answer the questions. On the other hand, if you do little or no highlighting, you are wasting a handy tool kindly provided to you by the test makers. While some people will legitimately highlight less or more than others, there are basic categories of things that should always be highlighted.

1. **Question topics.** You will not only have to find these references again as you answer the questions, but you will need at least a basic understanding of the surrounding text. Highlight a few key words as a marker, not multiple sentences.
2. **Author's opinion.** Knowing the author's tone is crucial; many wrong answers are wrong because they misrepresent the author's opinion. If the author says good or bad things about anything, highlight the words that indicate attitude. Make sure to separate the author's opinion from the opinions of others cited by the author, and to define whether or not the author expresses agreement or disagreement with those other opinions.
3. **Transitions.**
    *   **Pivotal words:** Words like "however," "but," and "although" tell you something very important about the logical structure of the author's point. Tricky wrong answers often *appear* to be supported by the text, but once you take a logical pivot or shift into account, end up being the opposite of what the author is really trying to say. By highlighting these words (or phrases), you plant a signal for yourself to pay attention to that shift.
    *   **Continuations:** Authors use words such as "furthermore," "additionally," and "also" to show that two or more ideas are connected to each other and that the latter idea is some kind of extension of the first. As with pivotal words, the test writers will give you wrong answers that look good if you haven't taken those connections into account.

4. **Conclusion indicators.** Authors use words like "therefore" or "thus" to tell you, "Here's what everything I just told you was leading up to," or, "Here is the most important thing to get out of all of this information." Conclusions are inherently important to the logic of the author's argument, and by marking them and focusing on them, you will much more easily distinguish the details from the main points.

5. **Comparisons and contrasts.** A common passage structure is one that discusses similarities and/or distinctions between different things. Use your highlighting to delineate what is being compared or contrasted and how. As you highlight the indicator words, ask yourself what the *purpose* of the comparison or contrast is: What role does it play within the author's argument? Wrong answers will often mix up the two, suggesting that things compared are instead contrasted, or vice versa, or that two or more things mentioned in the passage are compared/contrasted when in fact they are not.

6. **Different points of view.** When an author quotes or cites someone else, highlight the name or marker for the other point of view. Also ask yourself as you read *why* the author is citing someone else's ideas. Is it to agree? To disagree? To add support to the author's own claims? To contrast different points of view?

7. **Emphasis words.** When an author says something like "most importantly," "primarily," or "key," take him or her at his or her word. The point that follows is more or less guaranteed to be important to the author, and it is often "crucial" to answering the questions as well.

These first seven categories are important for understanding the big picture: the author's main point, tone, and purpose. In addition, there are a few other categories of words and phrases that should be highlighted for location purposes. That is, highlight them so that you can find them again if and when you need to as you answer the questions, but don't spend a lot of time mulling them over, memorizing them, or trying to gain some deep understanding of the details in that section of the passage.

8. **Example indicators.** When you see "for example," "in illustration," or "in this instance," your main focus should be on figuring out what this is an example of (that is, the larger claim being supported) rather than on the details of the example itself. However, by highlighting the indicator words, you leave yourself a sign to guide you back to the details of the example if you need them to answer a question.

9. **Lists.** If you see a list strung together with words like "first," "second," and "third," as with examples (and lists are often lists of examples), ask yourself what this is a list of and what purpose it serves within the passage. However, highlight just the list markers to help you locate any of those items on the list if they become important to the questions.

10. **Names.** It is very annoying to spend large amounts of time hunting down a name to answer a question when you can't remember where it showed up. If you find that by skimming through a text, you easily locate names (which, like numbers, tend to stand out from the surrounding text), you might decide not to highlight them. However, if this is not the case, highlight names wherever they appear. If you do this consistently, you have a guarantee that by skimming through your highlights you will quickly locate them when needed.

This may seem like a lot to keep track of. However, once you practice highlighting for a while you will find yourself doing it automatically; it becomes a natural part of how you read. Furthermore, elements from all the categories of indicator words will not appear within a single paragraph. Even if you highlight all these things consistently, it will only add up to a relatively small percentage of the text.

Advanced Highlighting: Refining Your Skills

Developing your highlighting skills, like all other things CARS, requires careful self-evaluation. As you review completed passages, ask yourself: "Did I highlight too much? Too little? Did I fail to highlight parts of the text that would have helped me answer the questions more accurately or efficiently? Did I neglect to use my highlighting at times when it would have led me to the correct answer? Did I highlight so much that I couldn't sort through it all?"

- **Highlighting too much and/or highlighting the wrong things:** This often occurs when students treat a passage like a Science textbook. When you are studying for a class, you are often most focused on the details and facts, and your highlighting reflects this. In the CARS section, however, the details are least important during your first reading of the passage. Save your highlighting for select words and phrases: those clusters of words that tell you something about the main theme of the paragraph and of the passage as a whole. Think of it as signposting; you don't need in most cases to highlight entire sentences or blocks of text, but rather just the signposts that tell you what important things happen within those blocks of text. Additionally, given the challenge of doing large amounts of reading on a computer screen, sometimes students overhighlight just to keep their eyes moving and to track their progress through the passage. However, while this may seem useful at the time, it does you little or no good once you are answering the questions. Practice questioning why you are about to highlight something. If there is no defined reason, leave it clean. After a while, you will find yourself highlighting less, and only those things that serve a logical or location purpose.

- **Highlighting too little:** Ironically, the cause of highlighting too little can be the same as a cause of highlighting too much: thinking of the passage as an undifferentiated series of facts to be learned and memorized, rather than as an argument made up of different parts to be mapped and analyzed. Or, you may feel that there just isn't enough time to highlight effectively. However, highlighting is one of those small investments of time that pays off in the long run. If you tend to highlight too little, review the list in the previous section. Then do some practice passages untimed, consciously looking for and highlighting the indicator words. As you answer the questions, pay attention to how useful those highlighted chunks are in finding the correct choice and in defining what is wrong with the bad choices. Once you train yourself to highlight as a natural part of reading, and once you can see how it contributes to your speed and accuracy, it gets easier and easier to do it effectively and quickly under timed conditions.

- **Not using your highlighting:** One of the more frustrating experiences is to look back at a question that you have missed, or a question that took you too long to get right, and see that you had the relevant part of the passage highlighted but never looked at it as you were answering the question. This usually happens partway through the learning curve: You are now highlighting well, but working the questions as if you hadn't highlighted at all. It seems simple, but all you need to do in this situation is remind yourself to look at your highlighting. You may even want to write "Look at highlighting!!!" on the top of your scratch paper. A basic reminder may be all it takes for you to remember to take advantage of that effort you put into mapping the passage.

Don't let your good highlighting go to waste—use it!

Summarizing the Main Point of Each Paragraph

Paragraphs (or different chunks within long paragraphs) are generally made up of claims and evidence: There is some central claim being made, and evidence is provided in support of that claim. Or an entire paragraph may consist of evidence intended to support a claim made elsewhere in the passage. Either way, your goal is to separate the claims from the evidence and to keep your focus on the author's central points (and to skim over the details that may or may not be needed to answer the questions). Sometimes an author will do the work for you by giving you a topic sentence at the beginning or end of the paragraph. At other times the burden is placed on you to imagine what that topic sentence would be, given the information presented in the paragraph. Regardless, after you read each paragraph, pause and ask yourself, What is the one central idea to which this chunk of information relates? Why did the author write this paragraph in the first place? What function does it serve within the passage as a whole?

Knowing the main point of each paragraph or chunk not only keeps you focused on the main themes of the passage, it also gives you a label for that chunk that you can use to locate information later on as you answer the questions. This is the main use to which you will put your scratch paper in the CARS section: writing down a very brief summary (say, 5–10 words) of each main point as you read. Some test takers will write more or less than others (you may find, for example, that you only need to physically write down the main points during more challenging passages), but every student will benefit from using his or her scratch paper actively (to some extent). Whenever you use your scratch paper, do so in an organized fashion: Write down the passage number on the top of the space you are using for that passage and label each paragraph as you go.

Aside from helping you analyze the author's logic and locate information for the questions, defining the main points serves an even more basic function: It keeps you awake. If you are passively reading through 600–700 words of (often not so fascinating) text, it can be a challenge to keep your mind engaged. However, if you give yourself this task to perform after each paragraph, it keeps you alert and focused.

Advanced Summarization: Refining Your Skills

- **Getting the main point wrong:** If you find that you often misidentify the main point, ask yourself if you focused too much on one part of the paragraph to the exclusion of the rest. In particular, did one subsidiary detail stand out and stick in your mind, distracting you from the larger purpose of the paragraph? Also, while topic sentences often come at the beginning or end of a paragraph, there is no guarantee that the first or last sentence will in fact sum up the purpose of the paragraph as a whole. Did you miss some key indicator words (for example, a conclusion indicator or a pivotal word) that would have pointed you toward the true central theme of the paragraph?

  If any of this sounds familiar, put yourself through a series of main point drills: Do a set of passages untimed, requiring yourself to write down the main point of each paragraph on scratch paper. While doing this, concentrate on the highlighting skills we discussed above, paying close attention to indicator words, especially conclusions, pivotal words, and expressions of the author's opinion. Even if this entails more writing than you think you will need to do for the actual test, the act of putting it into words and writing it down (for each and every paragraph) will force you to engage with the logic of the material. This is the way to learn how to avoid mistaking the author's real argument, or to keep yourself from passively identifying things that "sound important" in the paragraph as the main point. You may find that writing more doesn't actually take up too much of your time and that it contributes significantly to your accuracy. Or, you might go back to only using your scratch paper for harder paragraphs or harder passages, but with an improved ability to mentally articulate the major themes.

- **Writing too much:** If you find yourself essentially rewriting each paragraph on your scratch paper, you may be writing an outline of that chunk of passage rather than distilling the information down to one central theme. Keep your focus on the overall purpose of the paragraph rather than on all the facts and details within it. Limit yourself to eight words at most, and think of the main point as a label rather than as an outline. Sometimes writing too much comes from thinking too little; it is easier (but more time consuming and less useful) to regurgitate every detail of the paragraph than to stop and ask: What theme do all those details relate back to? If this sounds familiar, take a distinct pause after you finish each paragraph to ask yourself what that overall theme is before you take the next step of jotting down the main point.

Keep your main points short and sweet.

STEP 4: DEFINING THE BOTTOM LINE

The Bottom Line of the passage is the main point, purpose, and tone of the passage as a whole. While you don't necessarily need to define each of those three aspects separately, thinking of them as facets of the Bottom Line can help you put it into words. If you have worked the passage effectively as we have discussed above, defining the Bottom Line should come fairly easily. Essentially, it is the connecting thread that ties all the paragraphs together. And nicely enough, the Bottom Line is one of the most powerful tools you have in hand when answering the questions. Many answers even on Specific questions are wrong because they violate or are inconsistent in some way with the Bottom Line, and recognizing this is often the fastest way to eliminate those choices. You may find it useful to jot down a concise expression of the Bottom Line on your scratch paper for every passage or at least for the most difficult passages. Make sure that you have a clear idea of the point and purpose of the passage before you start on the questions.

Advanced Bottom Lining: Refining Your Skills

As we suggested above, problems defining the Bottom Line often track back to troubles with mapping the passage. If you find that you often just flat out get it wrong, ask yourself if you paid enough attention to key indicator words as you were reading the passage. If, for example, you thought the Bottom Line was the opposite of what it really was, did you miss an opinion/tone indicator? Did you overlook a pivotal word or phrase that sent the passage in a different direction from where it first appeared to be going? If you find that your Bottom Line was too narrow (and you got General questions wrong because of this), did you focus too much on one paragraph to the exclusion of the others? In particular, did you incorrectly assume that the main point of the last (or the first) paragraph was the main point of the whole passage? Sometimes the first or last paragraph will sum it all up for you, but not always. Think of the passage as a puzzle, with the paragraphs as the pieces. The Bottom Line is the picture made by fitting all the pieces together.

Putting it All Together

Let's practice your passage mapping and Bottom Line skills on a passage. This is the text that goes with the questions you have already previewed. We will use this same passage later in our discussion of question types and strategies; for now, however, we are just focusing on working the passage itself. First, go back to the discussion of previewing the questions and remind yourself of the topics that appeared in the question stems. Then, read and highlight the passage below, and jot down the main point of each paragraph in the spaces provided. Finally, define the Bottom Line and write it down as well. Then, read through the explanations that follow and see if you worked the passage effectively, and how you could have worked it even better. These explanations, in addition to providing a statement of the main points and the Bottom Line, will walk you through an analysis of the thought process you want to follow as you work the passage yourself.

Whenever you are working a passage on paper, use a highlighting pen to map the passage.

For the purposes of this drill, there are spaces provided under each paragraph for notes. When doing passages on your own, however, use scratch paper, just as you will when taking a test on a computer.

Sample Passage: Passage Text

In our contemporary world so obsessed and controlled by science and technology, the idea of myth has fallen into disrepute. For most people, if one were to ask them, "myth" amounts to little more than superstition, wives' tales, illusion, fantasy, or false conception. But the great ancient civilizations from which our own society evolved cherished fabulous tales of gods and heroes.

Main Point of paragraph 1: _____

_____

For the civilizations that produced them, myth occupied a place and served a function within the social fabric reserved today for medicine, astrophysics, and cybernetics. Myth blazed like a beacon of clarity and reassurance in an uncertain and terrifying universe. Myth gave people a finite idea of their place in the scheme of things, taught them how to see themselves in relation to forces beyond their control and how to survive and relate within a human society built on hierarchical power and often ruthless savagery.

Main Point of paragraph 2: _____

_____

The chasm of experience and time separating our lives at the third millennium from those who created the classical myths in antiquity makes it difficult for us to comprehend the feelings of those to whom myth represented a living reality. We lack the testimony of the committed believers, who knew Athena's power as we know the atom's, who consulted the Delphic oracle as we do the Hubble telescope, who deciphered the Muses' secret whispers as we decode the chromosomal helices. (For that matter, even the texts that have come down to us across the epochs are suspect, rescripted along the way by thousands of oral poets, censors, translators, and politically correct intelligentsia of every stripe.)

Main Point of paragraph 3: _____

_____

Nevertheless, in certain far-flung corners of the globe, more or less impervious to the glitter, flash, and buzz of this Early Electronic Age, communities of humans who maintain their people's ancient knowledge still practice the traditional rituals, still follow the folkloric customs. Anthropologists willing to shed their cosmetics of doctrine and costumes of theory might thus still gain a firsthand understanding of essential myth. For just as astronomers study astroradial photographs of exploding supernovas to learn about the evolution of planets and the origins of organic life, so might we study modern aborigines to discover the strategies and insights of human consciousness in its primal attempts to process perceptual reality into cultural rules.

Main Point of paragraph 4: _____

_____

Prior to the work of Sir James Frazer, mythologists for the most part lined themselves up in one of two opposing camps. On one side were the naturalists, who believed that aboriginal peoples limited themselves to an elegiac worship of cosmology, investing the sun, moon, stars, and climate with anthropomorphic identities. On the other side, the historicists argued that aboriginal myth amounted to nothing more than historical chronicle, a fact-based record of past events. Yet neither of these approaches does adequate justice to the fundamental power and function of myth in aboriginal societies.

Main Point of paragraph 5: _____

_____

By venturing into the field to live within aboriginal society, however, Bronislaw Malinowski, one of Frazer's disciples, penetrated the core of the matter. His pioneering work in the Trobriand Islands led him to a comprehensive view of myth as a "vital ingredient of human civilization; not an idle tale, but a hard-worked active force; not an intellectual explanation or an artistic imagery, but a pragmatic charter of faith and moral wisdom."

Main Point of paragraph 6: _____

_____

Bottom Line of the passage as a whole: _____

_____

Sample Highlighting and Analysis

In our contemporary world so obsessed and controlled by science and technology, the idea of myth has fallen into disrepute. For most people, if one were to ask them, "myth" amounts to little more than superstition, wives' tales, illusion, fantasy, or false conception. But the great ancient civilizations from which our own society evolved cherished fabulous tales of gods and heroes.

Analysis: The first appearance of the word "myth" is highlighted. As long as the passage continues to discuss myth, you don't need to highlight every recurrence of the word. The pivotal word "But" marks a contrast between how most people today think of myth and the importance it had for ancient civilizations. When you come across phrases like "for most people," or "many people claim," or "in the past it was believed," look out for the pivotal word that often follows to suggest a contrast or some other kind of shift.

Main Point of paragraph 1:   Unlike today, myth important in past.

For the civilizations that produced them, myth occupied a place and served a function within the social fabric reserved today for medicine, astrophysics, and cybernetics. Myth blazed like a beacon of clarity and reassurance in an uncertain and terrifying universe. Myth gave people a finite idea of their place in the scheme of things, taught them how to see themselves in relation to forces beyond their control and how to survive and relate within a human society built on hierarchical power and often ruthless savagery.

Analysis: "Function," "clarity and reassurance," "medicine," and "astrophysics" showed up in our preview of the questions. Both the word "function" and the phrase "reserved today" relate to the continuation of the contrast the author began to draw in the first paragraph: the difference between ancient and modern societies in relationship to myth. This part of the passage tells us that myth served the same function for ancient societies that medicine and science serve for us today, and it describes that function in more detail. This analogy is something we were on the lookout for, based on our preview of the questions.

Main Point of paragraph 2:   Myth in past same function as science today.

The chasm of experience and time separating our lives at the third millennium from those who created the classical myths in antiquity makes it difficult for us to comprehend the feelings of those to whom myth represented a living reality. We lack the testimony of the committed believers, who knew Athena's power as we know the atom's, who consulted the Delphic oracle as we do the Hubble telescope, who deciphered the Muses' secret whispers as we decode the chromosomal helices. (For that matter, even the texts that have come down to us across the epochs are suspect, rescripted along the way by thousands of oral poets, censors, translators, and politically correct intelligentsia of every stripe.)

Analysis: Most of the highlighting in this paragraph relates to both the continuation of the author's contrast between past and present ("chasm of experience and time"), and a series of comparisons between how knowledge was gained in the past versus in the present. Notice that a new idea has been introduced: the difference between ancient and modern society and the lack of reliable evidence makes it difficult for us to understand the true meaning of myth for those who lived in the distant past. The word "suspect" relates to this problem of evidence and carries a negative tone.

Main Point of paragraph 3: Understanding of ancient meaning of myth limited by lack of evidence.

Nevertheless, in certain far-flung corners of the globe, more
or less impervious to the glitter, flash, and buzz of this Early
Electronic Age, communities of humans who maintain their
people's ancient knowledge still practice the traditional rituals,
still follow the folkloric customs. Anthropologists willing to
shed their cosmetics of doctrine and costumes of theory
might thus still gain a firsthand understanding of essential myth.
For just as astronomers study astroradial photographs of
exploding supernovas to learn about the evolution of planets
and the origins of organic life, so might we study modern
aborigines to discover the strategies and insights of human
consciousness in its primal attempts to process perceptual
reality into cultural rules.

Analysis: The pivotal word "Nevertheless" sends the passage off in a different direction at this point. However, this is not entirely unexpected; we saw a question about ways in which we may be able to gain an understanding of the meaning and function of early myths. The phrase "thus still gain a firsthand understanding" continues this shift into a discussion of how we may in fact be able to gain firsthand evidence of the ancient or essential role of myth. This phrase is highlighted because it performs a variety of roles: It relates to a question topic, it introduces a conclusion, and it presents a contrast with the theme of the previous paragraph. In the second half of the paragraph, the author introduces another analogy, indicated by the words "just as" and "so might."

Main Point of paragraph 4: Might study aboriginal myths to understand ancient myths.

Prior to the work of Sir James Frazer, mythologists for
the most part lined themselves up in one of two opposing
camps. On one side were the naturalists, who believed that
aboriginal peoples limited themselves to an elegiac worship
of cosmology, investing the sun, moon, stars, and climate with
anthropomorphic identities. On the other side, the historicists
argued that aboriginal myth amounted to nothing more than
historical chronicle, a fact-based record of past events. Yet
neither of these approaches does adequate justice to the
fundamental power and function of myth in aboriginal societies.

Analysis: This paragraph has a fairly complicated structure. The word "Prior" at the beginning of the paragraph introduces a new contrast: mythologists before and after Frazer. Within this contrast is embedded a further distinction, that between the naturalists and the historicists. Then the phrase "Yet neither of these approaches does adequate justice" indicates the author's negative opinion about both of these schools of thought. At this point you would want to be on the lookout for the other side of the suggested contrast in time. This was true of mythologists before Frazer, so what was different about those that came after?

✴ If there is a "before," look for what the "after" might be.

Main Point of paragraph 5:   Two types of mythologists before Frazer—both inadequate.

By venturing into the field to live within aboriginal society, however, Bronislaw Malinowski, one of Frazer's disciples, penetrated the core of the matter. His pioneering work in the Trobriand Islands led him to a comprehensive view of myth as a "vital ingredient of human civilization; not an idle tale, but a hard-worked active force; not an intellectual explanation or an artistic imagery, but a pragmatic charter of faith and moral wisdom."

Analysis: This paragraph answers the question we just posed, beginning with the word "however." Malinowski, in following Frazer, was "pioneering" and came up with a "comprehensive view." Both of these phrases indicate a contrast between Malinowski and the mythologists mentioned in the previous paragraph; both also have a positive tone within the context of the author's discussion. The repeated pairing of "not" and "but" in the rest of the paragraph continues the contrast between the naturalists and historicists on one hand, and Malinowski on the other. Note that this paragraph is also a continuation of the idea introduced in paragraph 4, where the author indicates how we may actually be able to find evidence to help us understand the essential function of myth.

Main Point of paragraph 6:   Malinowski, studying aboriginal people, able to develop better understanding of myth.

Bottom Line of the Passage: Myth played an important role in ancient society, and we may come to better understand it through studying aboriginal societies today.

STEP 5: ATTACKING THE QUESTIONS

Now it comes down to the heart of your CARS score: answering the questions as quickly and accurately as possible. A common reason even high-scoring students miss questions is that they approach them too "intuitively." That is, they quickly read the question, go though the answer choices, and look for something that seems like a reasonable answer. If something jumps out at them, they pick it and move on. If not, they reluctantly go back to the passage to look for something that appears to support one of the answer choices. If you are already scoring at or above average, this process is often leading you quickly to the right answer. However, unless you are already getting the score you want, sometimes it isn't. So, let's go though the basic approach to answering the questions, the different question types and strategies, and ways in which to refine your skills.

Basic Approach

1. **Read the question stem word for word.**

   You will have already skimmed through the question stems during the previewing process. However, if you previewed effectively, you were not paying attention to the question type at that stage. Now, every word in that question is potentially important. If you misread the question at this point in the process, it is difficult to recover.

2. **Identify the question type and format, and translate the question task.**

   Ask yourself, "What is this question asking me to do?" This defines your strategy from that point on.

3. **Go back to the passage to find the relevant information.**

   This applies to all questions that include some reference to a defined area of the passage. (If the question is asking about an issue that appears in multiple paragraphs, or if it has no reference to particular passage content, go directly to the answer choices.) Read at least five lines above and below the reference in the passage; pay attention to indicator words that may tell you that you need to read even more of the text. Paraphrase what the author had to say.

4. **Generate an answer in your own words.**

   Based on the question task and your paraphrase of the passage text, come up with a guide to what the correct answer needs to do or say.

5. **Use Process of Elimination (POE) to choose an answer.**

   Read all four answer choices word for word. Paraphrase complicated wording to make sure that you understand the meaning of each choice. Strike out choices that are clearly wrong; don't, however, select an answer until you have read all four carefully and thoughtfully. Often, you will need to take two passes or "cuts" through the choices before you make a final selection. Even though you may have a good idea of what the answer should be, don't just look for the closest match. Instead, approach the choices negatively: Look for what is *wrong* with each choice, and eliminate down to the "least wrong" answer.

   Even test takers who have followed good form up to this point (both in how they worked the passage and interpreted the question) can still get the question wrong if they don't use good POE. The test writers purposefully construct certain wrong answers to be "Attractors." That is, they are written to sound even better than the credited response, and to distract you away from it. Those writers may even take into account what someone who has understood the passage and the question task will be looking for, in order to tempt that person into picking the Attractor without reading the rest of the choices carefully (or at all). Stay on your toes: Often the answer that looks good at first glance turns out to have something wrong with it. However, don't fall into paranoia, striking out an answer just because it looks too obvious.

   > Answering in your own words before looking at answer choices makes you less likely to fall for Attractors.

   POE is so fundamental to improving your score that it is worth further discussion here, before we get into the details of the different question types and formats. Let's go through the different types of tricky wrong answers that most commonly appear in the CARS section and discuss ways to identify and avoid them.

Advanced POE: Attractor Types

- **Out of scope:** These are choices that bring in issues not discussed in the passage. They are often the most clearly wrong answers and therefore usually the easiest ones to eliminate. Do be careful, however, not to overuse this rationale: Just because something isn't directly stated by the author doesn't necessarily mean that it is irrelevant to what the author does have to say.

- **Too extreme/too absolute:** This is a common Attractor for questions that ask you in some form what the author or the passage would support. These answers take information from the passage but take it too far beyond what the question is asking and what the author is claiming. They may include strong words like "all," "none," "most," "rarely," "should," or "must." However, a statement doesn't have to explicitly include these words in order to be too strong to be supported by the passage; the test writers know that students often have learned to look out for these words. Think about the meaning of the statement, not just the individual words that it includes. Also keep in mind that a strongly worded passage can support a strongly worded answer choice. This is why you should think of this Attractor not as "extreme" or "absolute" but *too* extreme and *too* absolute. That is, *too* strong for what the question is asking and for what the passage will support.

> ✳ Pay attention not only to the content of the answer choice but also to the strength of its language and of its claim.

- **Half right/half wrong:** These choices are partially but not fully supported by the passage; even one word is enough to make an answer wrong. In fact, the "good" part of this Attractor may sound even better than the whole of the correct answer. The test writers dangle the good part in front of you like a lure, testing to see if you can look past it to discern that there is something else in that statement that invalidates the whole choice.

> ✳ Part wrong means all wrong.

To avoid this trap, always read the answer choices word for word the first time through the choices, and take every word into account. It can be tempting to try to rehabilitate these choices by talking yourself into ignoring the bad parts (and to take up a lot of time doing so); remind yourself instead that part wrong means *all* wrong.

- **Words out of context:** These are traps set for students who are not going back to the passage, or not going back carefully enough. They have words or phrases lifted directly from the passage text, but the meaning of the statement is not supported by the passage.

To avoid this trap, use the passage actively rather than relying on your memory. Also, don't choose answers based on "word matching"; that is, don't choose an answer only because it includes a certain number of words that match back to the passage. Instead, paraphrase the answer choices to see their true meaning. It is the meaning, not the words themselves, that must match. However, don't get paranoid and eliminate an answer only because it reproduces wording from the passage; it might just be an easy question (such things do in fact exist!).

- **Outside knowledge:** These are statements that are either true in the real world or consist of claims with which any reasonable person would agree. However, they are not supported by the passage text. If you are working too quickly and carelessly, these will seem like super-easy questions; the answer looks so obvious that you feel like it would only be wasting time to go back to the passage. However, the CARS section never tests outside knowledge (and the correct answer doesn't have to correspond to common sense). It's all about whether or not the answer is supported by the passage in some form.

  To avoid this trap, use the passage more actively. Go back to the passage before reading the choices whenever possible; if you already have found what the author actually had to say on the issue, you will be much less tempted by these Attractors.

- **Opposites:** These choices state the exact opposite of what the passage says, or of what the question requires. The test writers may accomplish this by using a negation. That is, they take what would be a correct answer and drop a negative word like "not" into it (or, take out a negative word that should be included). Don't feel stupid if you discover that you have fallen for this trap; sometimes everything in them is good except for that one word that switches the direction. However, people often fall for this because they are not reading carefully enough, or because they are looking for an answer that sounds most like what they think it should say, rather than using careful POE.

  To avoid this trap, read word for word but also pay close attention to: 1) the direction in which the right answer needs to go, and 2) the direction in which each choice actually goes.

- **Right answer/wrong question:** Unlike the previous Attractors, these choices *are* in fact supported by the passage text. However, they don't address the question. These are traps intended for students who fail to pay sufficient attention to the question itself, or who lose track of it as they get caught up in evaluating the choices.

  To avoid this trap, read the question word for word and translate it before you look at any of the choices. If you have narrowed it down to two answers, re-read the question before making your final decision.

Summary: Refining your POE skills

These are not the only ways in which choices can be wrong, and we will discuss some more Attractors in the next section that are specific to certain question types. However, if you find that you often waste all the good work you put into working the passage by falling for a trap answer at the last minute, learn these common types and use that knowledge actively to ask questions of the choices (especially when you are down to two). That is, ask questions such as: "Are you too extreme? Do you have one word that makes you wrong? Are you the exact opposite of what you should say?" Asking these questions keeps your mind focused on POE and often alerts you to a problem that you may have overlooked the first time through the answers.

Read the question and answers carefully and remember to go back to the passage.

7.6   QUESTION TYPES AND STRATEGIES

There are ten different question types, and three formats in which they can appear. The ten types can also be grouped into four categories: **Specific** questions that ask about a particular issue within the passage, **General** questions that ask about the passage as a whole, Reasoning questions that ask you to describe or evaluate how the author constructs his or her argument, and Application questions that require you to apply new information from the question stem or the choices to the passage. Here are the ten types by category.

Specific Questions
1. Retrieval
2. Inference

General Questions
3. Main Idea/Primary Purpose
4. Overall Tone/Attitude

Reasoning Questions
5. Structure
6. Evaluate

Application Questions
7. Strengthen
8. Weaken
9. New Information
10. Analogy

These ten types appear in three different formats:

1. Standard
2. Except/Least/Not
3. Roman numeral

These labels will make much more sense if we examine what the questions look like in action. Let's go over each type and format using the sample passage that we have already highlighted. Remember that MCAT CARS passages will have five to seven questions attached; there are ten questions on this passage only for the purposes of this exercise. As we go through the steps for each question type and format, we'll group steps 1 and 2 under "Reading and translating the question task," steps three and four under "Going back to the passage and generating an answer," and then go through step five, POE.

Sample Passage

Here is the set of questions you already previewed, now with the lead words highlighted. We have also provided the passage text below to make it easier to reference; this is the same passage you just read and highlighted, and the main points and Bottom Line are included as well.

Question stems:

1. According to the passage, anthropologists can still gain understanding of the meaning and function of early human myth by:

2. The author implies that the need ancient peoples had for myth's clarity and reassurance came mainly from:

3. The author's primary purpose in the passage is to:

   ☀ If there are no lead words referencing content, skip over the question in the Preview stage.

4. In this passage, the author's tone is one of:

5. In the passage, the author draws an analogy between:

6. The author's assertion that science plays the same role today as myth played in ancient societies is supported:

7. Which of the following statements, if true, would most strengthen the author's claim that most modern people see myth as little more than superstition or fantasy?

8. Which of the following statements, if true, would most weaken the author's argument that Malinowski's work in the Trobriands does justice to the true function of myth in that culture?

9. Suppose an original poetic text from the first century B.C. celebrating the heroic deeds of the god Apollo were discovered in an archeological dig. How would this discovery affect the author's claim that we in modern society find it difficult to comprehend the meaning of myth in ancient societies?

   ☀ You may decide to skip over long New Information questions in the Preview stage.

10. Which of the following would be most analogous to the relationship between the role of myth in ancient societies and the role of medicine and astrophysics today, as those roles are described in the passage?

Passage Text

In our contemporary world so obsessed and controlled by science and technology, the idea of myth has fallen into disrepute. For most people, if one were to ask them, "myth" amounts to little more than superstition, wives' tales, illusion, fantasy, or false conception. But the great ancient civilizations from which our own society evolved cherished fabulous tales of gods and heroes.

For the civilizations that produced them, myth occupied a place and served a function within the social fabric reserved today for medicine, astrophysics, and cybernetics. Myth blazed like a beacon of clarity and reassurance in an uncertain and terrifying universe. Myth gave people a finite idea of their place in the scheme of things, taught them how to see themselves in relation to forces beyond their control and how to survive and relate within a human society built on hierarchical power and often ruthless savagery.

The chasm of experience and time separating our lives at the third millennium from those who created the classical myths in antiquity makes it difficult for us to comprehend the feelings of those to whom myth represented a living reality. We lack the testimony of the committed believers, who knew Athena's power as we know the atom's, who consulted the Delphic oracle as we do the Hubble telescope, who deciphered the Muses' secret whispers as we decode the chromosomal helices. (For that matter, even the texts that have come down to us across the epochs are suspect, rescripted along the way by thousands of oral poets, censors, translators, and politically correct intelligentsia of every stripe.)

Nevertheless, in certain far-flung corners of the globe, more or less impervious to the glitter, flash, and buzz of this Early Electronic Age, communities of humans who maintain their people's ancient knowledge still practice the traditional rituals, still follow the folkloric customs. Anthropologists willing to shed their cosmetics of doctrine and costumes of theory might thus still gain a firsthand understanding of essential myth. For just as astronomers study astroradial photographs of exploding supernovas to learn about the evolution of planets and the origins of organic life, so might we study modern aborigines to discover the strategies and insights of human consciousness in its primal attempts to process perceptual reality into cultural rules.

Prior to the work of Sir James Frazer, mythologists for the most part lined themselves up in one of two opposing camps. On one side were the naturalists, who believed that aboriginal peoples limited themselves to an elegiac worship of cosmology, investing the sun, moon, stars, and climate with anthropomorphic identities. On the other side, the historicists argued that aboriginal myth amounted to nothing more than historical chronicle, a fact-based record of past events. Yet neither of these approaches does adequate justice to the fundamental power and function of myth in aboriginal societies.

By venturing into the field to live within aboriginal society, however, Bronislaw Malinowski, one of Frazer's disciples, penetrated the core of the matter. His pioneering work in the Trobriand Islands led him to a comprehensive view of myth as a "vital ingredient of human civilization; not an idle tale, but a hard-worked active force; not an intellectual explanation or an artistic imagery, but a pragmatic charter of faith and moral wisdom."

Scratch Paper Notes

1: *Unlike today, myth important in past.*
2: *Myth in past same function as science today.*
3: *Understanding of ancient meaning of myth limited by lack of evidence.*
4: *Might study aboriginal myths to understand ancient myths.*
5: *Two types of mythologists before Frazer—both inadequate.*
6: *Malinowski, studying aboriginal people, able to develop better understanding of myth.*

Bottom Line of the Passage: Myth played an important role in ancient society, and we may come to better understand it through studying aboriginal societies today.

Question Types

1. Retrieval Questions

Reading and Translating the Question Task   These questions are usually phrased "According to the passage..." or "As stated by the author...". They will also usually give you some fairly specific reference to the passage. These are essentially "go fetch" questions; they usually give you a specific issue and send you back to the passage to find what the author says about it.

Here is our sample Retrieval question for this passage:

1. According to the passage, anthropologists can still gain understanding of the meaning and function of early human myth by:

Going Back to the Passage and Generating an Answer   Once you have read the question word for word and identified the question type, the next step is to go back to the passage and find where the author discusses the cited issue. Our main point of paragraph 4 is, "Might study aboriginal myths to understand ancient myths." This sends us back to that paragraph for the answer. The author states (with our original highlighting):

> Anthropologists willing to shed their cosmetics of doctrine and costumes of theory might thus still gain a firsthand understanding of essential myth. For just as astronomers study astroradial photographs of exploding supernovas to learn about the evolution of planets and the origins of organic life, so might we study modern aborigines to discover the strategies and insights of human consciousness in its primal attempts to process perceptual reality into cultural rules.

So, your answer in your own words might be: "studying modern aborigines." Once you have an answer in your own words, compare it to the answer choices. Remember, however, that you are still using POE, looking for what is wrong with each choice.

POE   Here are the answers that go along with our sample Retrieval question:

A) developing computer models based on modern aboriginal communities.

B) applying contemporary theories and doctrines to interpret aboriginal social structures.

C) learning about the role played by myth in the lives of aborigines today.

D) adopting aboriginal traditions and truths as guiding moral precepts and analytical tools.

Taking each choice in turn, choice A is half right, half wrong: The author never discusses computer models. This is an excellent reason to strike it out. Choice B is going in the opposite direction. The author suggests that we should get a "firsthand understanding of essential myth" by observing it in as pure a state as possible in aboriginal cultures, not that we should apply our own modern ideas to aboriginal social structure. So, choice B is out. Choice C is more or less exactly what we had in mind, so we will keep it in. Choice D goes too far. The author states that we should study aboriginal myths and traditions, but not that we should follow them ourselves. This leaves you with choice C as correct.

Advanced "Retrieval": Refining Your Skills   Retrieval questions tend to be the easiest ones, so if you are missing a significant percentage of them, you definitely need to figure out why, and to make corrections in your approach. When high-scoring students miss these questions, it is often due to overthinking. Answers that are more or less straight from the passage can seem too obvious, leading you to think that there must be something wrong with them. This in turn leads you to talk yourself into some other answer. Keep it simple: You want the answer that is closest to what the passage says (and relevant to the question).

High-scoring students (or even those who are not yet high-scoring) may also miss these questions because they rely too heavily on memory, or on a cursory glance back at the passage. If you commonly fall for the "words out of context" Attractor for this question type, this is a clear sign that you need to use the passage more consistently and carefully.

2. Inference Questions

Reading and Translating the Question Task   Inference questions can be worded in a variety of ways, such as, "It can be inferred that…," "The author implies/suggest/assumes that…," "With which of the following statements would the author be most likely to agree?," or "Which of the following statements is best supported by the passage?" Here is our Inference question for this passage:

> **2.** The author implies that the need ancient peoples had for myth's clarity and reassurance came mainly from:

Going Back to the Passage and Generating an Answer   These questions may or may not give you a specific reference to the passage within the question stem. If it does, approach it in the same way as a Retrieval question by going back to the passage and locating the relevant information. For this question, we had already highlighted the key words in the second paragraph based on our preview of the questions. The second paragraph states:

> Myth blazed like a beacon of clarity and reassurance in an uncertain and terrifying universe. Myth gave people a finite idea of their place in the scheme of things, taught them how to see themselves in relation to forces beyond their control and how to survive and relate within a human society built on hierarchical power and often ruthless savagery.

Your answer in your own words therefore might be, "People's sense of insecurity and lack of control."

POE   As you use POE, ask yourself which choice is best supported by the passage. Although Inference answers tend to be less directly stated in the passage than Retrieval answers, your logical process on both types is essentially the same.

Now let's take a look at the choices:

> A)   feelings of powerlessness and vulnerability.
> B)   an unstable social fabric.
> C)   ineffective medical techniques.
> D)   a finite sense of themselves.

Choice A appears to be closely related to, and consistent with, the author's description of myth helping people to deal with the existence of "forces beyond their control" and with the challenges of survival in a sometimes "savage" society. Choice A is also a close paraphrase of our own answer. But since we haven't read all the choices yet, we will just keep it in contention for now. Choice B sounds good at first glance because the author does mention an "uncertain" universe. However, the passage does not describe the "social fabric" itself as uncertain or unstable. This is a "Words Out of Context" trap, and we can strike out choice B.

Choice C is out of scope; you might also think of it as words (or word) out of context. The author does mention that today's medicine performs the same function that myth did in the past. However, there is no mention or suggestion of medicine being ineffective in the past. Also be careful not to use outside knowledge or to overthink it. Medicine may well have been relatively ineffective in the ancient past, and we might be tempted to speculate that this would make people feel powerless, which for all we know might have caused them to turn to myths for reassurance or guidance. However, none of this would be supported by the passage, and thinking this way would be a big waste of your time.

Finally, choice D is an example of a combination of two different Attractors: "Opposite" and "Right Answer/Wrong Question." Looking back at the passage, the author says that "Myth gave people a finite sense of themselves," not that myths were *created because* of people's finite sense of themselves. Choice D would be a great answer for a question that asked what myth provided or resulted in, rather than for this question, which asks where it came from. This answer would also be perfect if it said the opposite of what it actually says: that is, "the *lack* of a finite sense of themselves."

In the end, therefore, we are left with choice A as the credited response.

Advanced "Inference": Refining Your Skills

It is important to keep in mind that this is not a test of your real inferring skills. People sometimes get into trouble with Inference questions because they overinterpret or misunderstand what these questions are really asking. In the real world, "inference" is most often used to indicate "conclusion" or "deduction." However, while some answer choices in the CARS section will fit this definition, others will not. Defining it this way can lead you to overlook the easiest Inference answers: those that closely paraphrase the passage. On the other hand, we also sometimes think of inferences (or suggestions or implications) as insinuations or speculation. This can cause you to pick incorrect answers that "might be true" or "could be true," rather than relying only on what is already stated in the passage.

What it all comes down to is: an inference (or assumption, or suggestion, or implication, or what the author would most likely agree is true) is defined as "the answer choice that is *best supported* by the passage, compared to the other three." Correct inferences appear in a variety of guises. They may be more or less restatements of passage information or directly supported by a particular paragraph within the passage. Additionally, an Inference question stem that includes a reference to something within one paragraph may require you to take evidence from two or more paragraphs into account in order to locate the correct answer. The correct answer is always the one that is closer to the passage and better supported than the other three choices. As you can see, comparing choices to each other is an especially important part of your Inference strategy.

Now we are back to self-evaluation. You will probably discover that a high proportion of the questions you miss are Inference questions; this may be in part because Inference questions are one of the most common question types. Ask yourself if you tend to eliminate choices that seem too obvious. If so, you may be taking the definition too narrowly, as a deduction and not potentially as a paraphrase. Or, do you only look for choices that are in fact essentially stated in the passage? If so, remind yourself that an answer can be directly supported by the passage without being directly stated in the text. Do you miss correct answers because they required combining information from two or more paragraphs or chunks of the passage? If so, remember to look at all areas where the issue of the question appears in the passage. Finally, do you pick incorrect answers because you add in too much of your own information or speculation? If so, remind yourself to stick as closely as possible to the passage text. If you hear yourself thinking, "Well, if X were also true, and if Y and Z also happened, then this would be a pretty good answer," you are probably straying too far afield.

3. Main Idea/Primary Purpose

Reading and Translating the Question Task   These questions ask you for a summary of the central point or purpose of the passage. They are most commonly phrased like this: "The main idea/central thesis of the passage is…" or "The author's primary purpose is…". Here is our sample question:

> **3.** The author's primary purpose in the passage is to:

Although the wording of the two subtypes is different, they are really asking for the same thing: The Main Idea is the central claim or overall theme of the passage, while the Primary Purpose is what the author does in order to communicate that claim or theme.

Going Back to the Passage and Generating an Answer   To answer these questions, you generally will not need to go back to the passage before you start evaluating the answer choices. You have already answered in your own words when you defined the Bottom Line. Our Bottom Line for this passage was, "Myth played an important role in ancient society, and we may come to better understand it through studying aboriginal societies today."

POE   As you go through the answer choices, make sure that you keep the scope of the question (the entire passage) and the tone of the passage in mind. Here are the answer choices:

A) demonstrate the impossibility of understanding the function of myth in ancient society.

B) criticize the naturalist and historicist schools of thought for presenting inadequate visions of the place and power of myth.

C) explain the role of myth in ancient society and suggest ways of overcoming the problems involved in understanding that role.

D) explain why, given advances in science and technology, we no longer need myths to represent the roles we play in society and nature.

Choice A is too strong. While the author says that it is difficult to understand, the last paragraph tells us that Malinowski was able to express "a comprehensive view of myth." Be on the lookout for choices that take a theme or idea expressed in the passage too far. Choice B represents one theme in the passage (from paragraph 5), but it is only one part of the author's overall argument. This is an Attractor specific to General questions: answers that are too narrow for the scope of the question task. Choice C is similar to our own Bottom Line and doesn't appear to have anything wrong with it, so we will keep it in contention. Choice D is something the author suggests to be true in the second paragraph. However, while D could be a correct answer for an Inference question, it is too narrow to be the primary purpose of the passage as a whole. This leaves us with choice C as the correct answer.

Advanced Main Idea/Primary Purpose: Refining Your Skills   The most important thing to keep in mind when answering these questions is scope. An answer that captures the main point of a paragraph, or even of multiple paragraphs, will be incorrect if it leaves out some major theme in the passage. On the other hand, an answer that is too broad in scope is incorrect as well. The Goldilocks approach that we discussed for highlighting applies here as well: not too big or too small, but just right.

If you consistently miss Main Idea or Primary Purpose questions, ask yourself if it may be due to problems you are having working the passage in the first place. Are you explicitly defining the Bottom Line before you attack the questions? If not, the "too narrow" choices that are only the main point of a paragraph or two will be especially tempting. In particular, look to see if you have picked wrong answers that are the main point of the last paragraph but not of the passage as a whole. Also check to see if you are missing these questions because you got the tone of the passage wrong. If this is the case, focus on looking for attitude and opinion indicators as you work the passage the first time through. Overall, a low level of accuracy with this question type may be a symptom of a larger problem, and an indication that you would benefit from refining your strategy in the passage-working phase.

4. Overall Tone/Attitude

Reading and Translating the Question Task   In their General form, these questions will be phrased fairly simply: "Which of the following statements best describes the author's tone in the passage…" or "The author's attitude can best be described as…". (Be on the lookout for the occasional Specific Tone/Attitude questions, which ask for the author's attitude toward a particular issue within the passage, rather than about the passage as a whole.) Let's work through our sample question:

> **4.** In this passage, the author's tone is one of:

Going Back to the Passage and Generating an Answer   As with Main Idea/ Primary Purpose questions, there is usually no need to go back to the passage before you start on the answer choices. Tone and attitude are parts of the Bottom Line, and you have already defined this once you finished working the passage. Here, given our Bottom Line, we could answer in our own words: "admiration for the function of myth in ancient society, and for Malinowski's work."

POE   As you go through the choices, look out for two basic things: answers with the wrong tone (e.g., positive when it should be negative), and answers that are too extreme (e.g., "dismay" when it should be "disappointment"). Here is a set of choices for our sample question:

> A)   disappointment.
> B)   dismay.
> C)   appreciation.
> D)   excitement.

Although the author does express some level of disappointment with the naturalists and historicists in paragraph 5, this does not capture the overall tone of the passage, which leads up to a positive evaluation by the end. Dismay goes even further in the wrong direction. So, choices A and B are out. Choice C goes in a positive direction, which is promising, and it could apply to both the role of myth and Malinowski's work. So, we keep it in. Finally, "excitement." It's tempting because it also has a positive tone, and because perhaps we can imagine the author being excited when he heard of Malinowski's work, or speaking in an excited way when discussing the role of myth. However, that's too much from our imagination, with not enough direct support from the passage. This leaves us with choice C as the correct answer.

Advanced "Tone/Attitude": Refining Your Skills

The first thing to keep in mind when answering these questions is the scope of the question task. If it is a General question, you need a general answer that captures the author's tone in the passage as a whole, not just in one part of the passage to the exclusion of others. Be on the lookout for choices that are too narrow.

> Make sure the scope of the answer matches the scope of the question and passage.

As you are doing these questions, it can help to visualize the tone of the passage and the tone of the choices you are considering. Imagine a spectrum, from totally negative on the left (say, "severe condemnation") to strongly positive on the right (such as "joyful advocacy") and with "neutral description" in the middle.

(–)_____neutral_____(+)

When you are answering tone questions in your own words, visualize where along this line the passage would fall. As you go through the choices, do the same (especially if you are down to two). For our question above, we might have visualized something like this:

B   A   C   D
(–)_____ passage _____ (+)

If you are down to two on opposite sides of the spectrum, or between "neutral description/analysis" and something with an either positive or negative tone, you need to go back to the passage and look for more evidence. However, if you are down to two answers on the same side of the spectrum, the answer is usually the more moderate of the two.

Also be suspicious of descriptors that suggest uncertainty, such as "ambivalent" or "reluctant." Authors may express both positive and negative evaluations within a passage, but they are usually pretty firm and decisive about those opinions. Finally, correct answers are rarely emotional or personal. In the question above, "excitement" would be a bit strange to see in a passage; the kind of writing you usually find on the MCAT is not the kind of writing that usually expresses excitement, or fear, or sadness, or joy. Don't eliminate these choices thoughtlessly (sometimes things outside of the norm do show up), but if you are stuck between two, it is safest to go with the more "normal" choice.

If you tend to miss Tone/Attitude questions, or if you often miss other question types because you mistook the author's tone, you need to consider how you are working the passage in the first place. Are you consciously looking out for words that indicate attitude? If so, are you consistently highlighting them? Are you taking them into account when you define the Bottom Line (and are you defining the Bottom Line in the first place)? Issues with tone are usually a symptom of larger problems with how you are working the passage, problems that will affect other question types as well.

5. Structure

Reading and Translating the Question Task   Structure questions ask you to describe, in some form, the logical structure of the passage. This often involves describing the relationship between different parts of the passage. The most common phrasing uses the words "in order to," as in, "The author mentions Frazer in order to…". But, let's take a look at a more challenging version of a Structure question:

> **5.** In the passage, the author draws an analogy between:

The correct answer will describe or match a part of the passage where the author compares two things in this way.

Going Back to the Passage and Generating an Answer   We have a few possibilities already highlighted in the passage, based on our preview of the questions. In paragraph 2 we saw:

> For the civilizations that produced them, myth occupied a place and served a function within the social fabric reserved today for medicine, astrophysics, and cybernetics.

In paragraph 4, we saw another analogy:

> For just as astronomers study astroradial photographs of exploding supernovas to learn about the evolution of planets and the origins of organic life, so might we study modern aborigines to discover the strategies and insights of human consciousness in its primal attempts to process perceptual reality into cultural rules.

If we hadn't already found and highlighted these analogies based on either our preview or on the fact that they are comparisons, we would skip this step and go directly to the choices. Keeping these two analogies in mind, let's take a look at the choices.

POE   Here are the answer choices:

> A) naturalist and historicist approaches to understanding the role of myth in aboriginal society.
> B) the role of science in the modern world and the place of myth in antiquity.
> C) ancient gods and heroes and anthropomorphized cosmological entities in today's aboriginal cultures.
> D) science and anthropology.

Looking at choice A, and going back to paragraph 5, we see that this is the opposite. These two schools of thought are contrasted, while analogies are based on similarities. Choice B is the first of the two analogies we already pulled out of the passage, so we'll hang on to it. Choice C is tempting because these things were in fact mentioned in the passage (paragraph 1 and paragraph 5), and it seems reasonable that they might play analogous roles in myth. So, let's say we hold on to choice C for now. Choice D is half right, half wrong. The analogy is between science and myth, not science and anthropology.

Now that we are down to two, it's time to go back to the exact wording of the question stem. It asks what the *author* draws an analogy between, not what *we* might see as analogous. This takes it down to choice B as the correct answer.

Advanced "Structure": Refining Your Skills

When answering these questions, make sure that you take indicator words into account. If the phrase "for example" appears in front of something, you know that thing is an example of a larger point made previously in the passage. If the word "therefore" shows up, it indicates that what follows is a conclusion based on evidence or an explanation that most likely immediately preceded it.

Sometimes Structure questions ask you to see the connection between things that sit in different parts of the passage. Don't assume that everything you need to take into account for a single Structure question will be within a single paragraph.

If you consistently struggle with these questions, it may be because you are not paying enough attention to the logical structure of the author's argument when you work the passage. If this is the case, review the list of indicator words given earlier in this chapter, and practice your highlighting.

6. Evaluate

Reading and Translating the Question Task

Evaluate questions will ask *how well* a claim made in the passage is supported. For example, here is our sample question:

> **6.** The author's assertion that science plays the same role today as myth played in ancient societies is supported:

The answer choices then might be variations on "strongly" and "weakly" with explanations why.

Going Back to the Passage and Generating an Answer

This question sends us back to paragraph 2, where the author writes:

> For the civilizations that produced them, myth occupied a place and served a function within the social fabric reserved today for medicine, astrophysics, and cybernetics. Myth blazed like a beacon of clarity and reassurance in an uncertain and terrifying universe. Myth gave people a finite idea of their place in the scheme of things, taught them how to see themselves in relation to forces beyond their control and how to survive and relate within a human society built on hierarchical power and often ruthless savagery.

Looking back at this paragraph, we see that the role of myth is explained in a fair amount of detail. However, although the author claims that science (that is, medicine, astrophysics, and cybernetics) plays the same role today, there is no evidence given for that claim. How do we know that science provides clarity and reassurance? The author appears to assume that we will agree with this statement, and so no evidence is given. Thus, our answer is "weakly, because of the lack of evidence or examples."

POE   Here is a set of choices to go with our sample question:

A)   strongly: The analogy between astroradial photographs and the study of modern aborigines supports the claim.

B)   strongly: Evidence is provided of the role science plays to reassure us of our finite place in the world.

C)   weakly: This claim contradicts the author's statement that it is difficult to understand the role of myth in ancient society.

D)   weakly: No description or evidence of the role of science today is provided.

Choice A heads off in the wrong direction from the first word, "strongly." However, you should always read every word of every answer. In this case, though, choice A just gets worse. Yes, there is such an analogy made in paragraph 4, but on a different issue (how studying current evidence can teach us about the past). Choice A is out. Choice B also begins with the opposite word "strongly," and the description that follows is inaccurate. There is in fact no such evidence provided. Choice C is more promising, but the second half of it is wrong. The author claims in paragraph 3 that it is difficult to understand the feelings of those for whom myth played an essential role, not that we have little understanding of the function that myth served. Finally, both parts of Choice D match up. The claim is weakly supported, and the explanation of why is accurate. Choice D therefore is correct.

Advanced "Evaluate": Refining Your Skills   Just as for Structure questions, Evaluate questions require you to take into account the logical structure of the passage: how the author constructs his or her argument, and additionally how good a job he or she does. Use your highlighting actively as you attack these questions, especially indicator words that mark conclusions, examples, and pivotal words.

If you are down to two choices that are opposites of each other (e.g., "strongly" vs. "weakly"), there is likely to be something important about the passage that you haven't understood. Go back to the relevant paragraph or paragraphs and re-read carefully. If you are down to two choices on the same side of the fence (e.g., both "strongly" or "weakly"), it is likely that the description that follows one or the other doesn't match the logic of the passage. Compare the two choices to each other, look for differences in the descriptions, and go back to the passage to find out which one does not fully match up.

If you tend to miss these questions, this may mean that you are not reading critically enough. Normally you take the passage as true (except for Weaken questions) and only treat the answer choices skeptically. For these questions, however, you need to shift gears and approach the passage skeptically as well, looking for flaws in logic. The most common flaw you will see is lack of examples or evidence supporting a claim. Again, this goes back to highlighting effectively and using your highlighting actively while answering the questions.

7. Strengthen

Reading and Translating the Question Task Strengthen questions give you new information in the answer choices, and they ask you to find the statement that does what it needs to do to the passage. A Strengthen question can be worded, "Which of the following claims, if valid, would most strengthen the author's argument in the passage?" or "Which of the following, if true, would most support the author's conclusion in the last paragraph?" Here is our sample Strengthen question:

> **7.** Which of the following statements, if true, would most support the author's claim that most modern people see myth as simply superstition or fantasy?

Going Back to the Passage and Generating an Answer To answer Strengthen questions, first find the relevant part of the passage if you are being asked to strengthen a particular part of it. Paraphrase what the author has to say on that issue. You can't literally answer these questions in your own words, because the answers will bring in new information that wasn't in the passage. Your goal at this stage, then, is to come up with a guide to the correct answer: What does it need to do or say to accomplish the strengthen task? If the question stem doesn't specify a particular issue within the passage, use your Bottom Line as a guide to the choices. Regardless, you need to find an answer that is not only consistent with the passage, but that adds something new that makes the author's argument or claim even more compelling than it already was, and that goes the furthest of all the choices in accomplishing this.

For Question 7, the relevant part of the passage is in the first paragraph:

> In our contemporary world so obsessed and controlled by science and technology, the idea of myth has fallen into disrepute. For most people, if one were to ask them, "myth" amounts to little more than superstition, wives' tales, illusion, fantasy, or false conception. But the great ancient civilizations from which our own society evolved cherished fabulous tales of gods and heroes.

So, we need an answer choice that goes as far as possible to indicate that this is in fact the view of myth taken by most modern people.

POE Here are the answer choices:

> A) Most people today believe that myths, like fairy tales, are appropriately used only to entertain children with wild stories that have little to do with everyday life.
> B) Many people in contemporary society learn very little about ancient myths in the course of their primary or secondary education.
> C) Myths tend to take very different forms within different cultures.
> D) Most people believe that modern life is much less uncertain and terrifying than life in ancient times.

Choice A may initially seem out of scope, given that it brings in fairy tales and the entertainment of children, which are never mentioned in the passage. But for Strengthen questions, you need to take each choice as a true statement, and to remember that the right answer will bring in new information. This choice may also sound extreme, but for a Strengthen question, you want the answer that gives the strongest possible support to the passage. So, you would want to keep choice A in contention; it does add additional evidence for the author's claim. Choice B, on the other hand, may look good at first glance. However, it doesn't go far enough. "Many" doesn't mean "most," and this choice doesn't indicate anything about how people actually view the nature of myth. So, choice B is out.

Choice C doesn't address the issue; the fact that myths take on different forms in different cultures doesn't tell us anything about how myth is viewed in those different cultures. Therefore, choice C is out. Finally, choice D may also be very tempting, as it indicates that people view modern life as different than life in ancient times. But, the question is about a contrast between how people see the role or nature of myth now versus in the past not how people view the nature of life now versus in the past. Choice D leaves open the possibility that most modern people could still perceive myth to be relevant to their own experience, even if the character of that experience has changed over time. That leaves us with choice A as the correct answer.

Since the approach to Strengthen and Weaken questions is quite similar (even though the answers will go in opposite directions), let's go over Weaken questions first, and then advanced strategy for both.

8. Weaken

Reading and Translating the Question Task   Like Strengthen questions, Weaken questions give you new information in the answer choices, and they ask you to find the statement that does what it needs to do to the passage. In this case, however, you will be looking for the answer that goes the furthest to cast doubt on the author's argument. Weaken questions that don't actually include the word "weaken" might be phrased, "Which of the following statements, if true, would most *undermine* the author's claims?" or "Which of the following, if proven, would go farthest to *call the author's argument into question?*" Generally, the words that indicate "weaken" are italicized within the question stem (however, words that indicate a Strengthen question are not). Here is our sample Weaken question:

> **8.** Which of the following statements, if true, would most *weaken* the author's argument that Malinowski's work in the Trobriands does justice to the true function of myth in that culture?

Going Back to the Passage and Generating an Answer   To answer Weaken questions, just as with Strengthen questions, first find the relevant part of the passage if you are being asked to weaken a particular part of it. Read it carefully and then paraphrase the author's argument. If the questions asks you to weaken the author's overall argument in the passage, remind yourself of the Bottom Line. Don't try to come up with an actual answer; the correct choice will bring in something new, and perhaps something unpredictable. However, do create a guide to the correct answer. What does it need to do or say to accomplish the task of weakening? To weaken, you need something that contradicts the passage as much as possible; put the opposite of the author's argument into your own words as a guide to the choices. If the question stem doesn't specify a particular issue within the passage, use the opposite of the Bottom Line as your guide. The correct answer doesn't need to disprove the author's claim or claims, but it does need to be the one of the four choices that goes the furthest in that direction.

For our sample Weaken question, the relevant part of the passage is the last paragraph, where the author writes:

> His pioneering work in the Trobriand Islands led him to a comprehensive view of myth as a "vital ingredient of human civilization; not an idle tale, but a hard-worked active force; not an intellectual explanation or an artistic imagery, but a pragmatic charter of faith and moral wisdom.

Therefore, we need an answer choice that indicates a reason why Malinowski's work in the Trobriands may NOT provide an accurate picture of the real function of myth in that culture.

POE   Here are the answer choices:

A) Sir James Frazer had as a primary goal the reconciliation of the naturalist and historicist schools.
B) The specific myths that define Trobriand society contain some images and themes found in no other ancient or modern cultures.
C) The presence of outside anthropological observers significantly changes the speech and behaviors of the members of the culture being observed.
D) Many well-respected anthropologists have rejected Malinowski's conclusions.

Choice A is out of scope for two different reasons. First, the question is about Malinowski; even though Malinowski was Frazer's disciple, we don't know that what was true of Frazer was necessarily true of Malinowski. Second, there is no reason to think that an attempt to reconcile the two schools of thought would inherently fail to capture the true function of myth; even if this were true of Malinowski as well as of Frazer, it would not by itself weaken the author's argument. Therefore, we can strike out choice A. To evaluate choice B, we need to check back to the passage: does the author ever suggest that Malinowski's conclusions were based on an assumption that the Trobriand myths themselves were identical to myths in other cultures? Looking back at paragraphs 3–6, we can see that it is the function of myth that the author claims to be the same, not the specific myths themselves. Therefore, choice B does not weaken the passage.

Choice C, at first glance, looks irrelevant. The author never talked about the effect of observers on the observed. However, since the right answer will bring in new information, we can't eliminate it on that basis alone. And, if the presence of an outsider would change how people act, it is possible that Malinowski did not in fact get a true picture of how myth functioned in Trobriand society; his data or observations may have been inaccurate. So, we will keep choice C in for now. Choice D is momentarily attractive because it sounds like a negative judgment of Malinowski. However, the question we need to ask of this choice is, "Is the opinion of some anthropologists, no matter how well-respected, enough to cast significant doubt on Malinowski's claims?" The answer is no. By whom.

Now let's go through advanced strategy for improving on both Strengthen and Weaken questions.

Advanced "Strengthen" and "Weaken": Refining Your Skills   In general, a correct Weaken answer will provide empirical evidence against the claim being weakened. It may also suggest an alternate cause or explanation, or question the methodology used to support the claim. Often a correct Strengthen answer will give empirical evidence in support of the claim. It may also fill in a logical gap in the argument, state that an assumption made in the passage is in fact true, or rule out possible objections to, or problems with, the claim being strengthened.

There are a couple of things about Strengthen and Weaken questions that distinguish them from other question types. First, the correct answer will have new information in it that you must apply to the passage. If you treat these too much like Inference questions (especially easy to slip into on the Strengthen version), you will eliminate the correct answer, thinking that it is out of scope. In fact, the wording of some Strengthen questions sounds a lot like Inference questions. If the question asks "what is supported by the passage," this is an Inference. If it asks "what supports the passage," it is a Strengthen. If you tend to miss Strengthen questions, use your Question Review Worksheet and self-evaluation to figure out if you are mistaking them for Inference questions.

Pay attention to the direction of the author's argument in the passage.

The second aspect of Strengthen and Weaken questions to keep in mind is that you want a strong answer rather than a wishy-washy one. If you are doing any other question type (except for Except questions), strong language is suspicious, and choices are often wrong because they are too extreme or absolute. However, for a Strengthen or Weaken question, the stronger the language is in the answer choice, the better that choice is, all other things being equal. If you tend to eliminate the right answer the first time through the choices, look to see if you eliminated it because you thought it was too strong.

A third aspect, this time of Weaken questions in particular, is that they require keeping close track of the direction of the passage, the direction required by the question task, and the direction of each answer choice. Given that you are more used to picking answers that go along with the passage than choices that go against it, it can be a challenge to keep your wits about you and keep headed in the right direction on Weaken questions. If you find that you tend to get turned around and pick an answer that is the opposite of what it should be, or that you waste a lot of time having to backtrack and start all over because you get confused, this is a good time to use your scratch paper. Write down a paraphrase of the argument from the passage that you are weakening, jot down a guide to the correct answer (the opposite of what the passage said), and refer to that guide as you make your way through the choices.

9. New Information

Reading and Translating the Question Task   All New Information questions have one thing in common: They give you a new fact or scenario in the question stem and ask you to apply it in some form to the passage. New Information questions have become quite common in the CARS section, to the extent that they now rival Inference questions as one of the most commonly seen question types.

There are two types of these questions: New Information/Inference and New Information/Strengthen/Weaken. New Information/Inference might be phrased something like: "If X were shown to be true, what, based on information in the passage, would also be true?" For these, you take the new information, combine it with existing passage information, and find the answer choice that is best supported by that combination.

New Information/Strengthen/Weaken questions ask you what effect the new information in the question stem would have on the author's argument in the passage. For example, the question might ask, "Which of the following claims made in the passage would be most weakened by data showing X?" or "Suppose X were proven to be true. This finding would offer the most support to the author's claim that…".

Regardless of which type it is, the key to answering these questions is to paraphrase the new information in the question stem (treat it like a chunk of passage and figure out its theme or main point), and then decide on its relationship to information provided in the passage.

Since the New Information/Strengthen/Weaken variation tends to be especially challenging, we took our sample question from that category:

> **9.** Suppose an original poetic text from the first century
> B.C. celebrating the heroic deeds of the god Apollo were
> discovered in an archeological dig. How would this
> discovery affect the author's claim that we in modern
> society find it difficult to comprehend the meaning of
> myth in ancient societies?

The theme of this scenario is, "We found new primary evidence of an ancient myth."

Going Back to the Passage and Generating an Answer   The relationship of this evidence to the passage is, "This appears to be less 'suspect' than the evidence discussed in paragraph 3. However, it doesn't seem to be enough to represent a 'living reality.' So, it doesn't appear to either significantly weaken or strengthen the author's argument."

POE   Here are the choices:

> A) It would refute the claim by indicating that data from
>   living cultures can give us some insight into the role and
>   power of myth.
> B) It would support the claim, because rescripted texts are
>   inadequate indicators of what myth meant to the people
>   of that time.
> C) It would be irrelevant to the claim, which is about
>   mythological stories, not poetry.
> D) It would not fully refute the claim, because even an
>   original text does not recreate the living reality essential
>   to cultural meaning.

Choice A is, first of all, too strong. As we already decided, the new evidence is not enough to significantly undermine the passage. If we weren't sure about it on that basis, there is something else wrong with this choice: This is an ancient text, not one from a "living culture." Choice B also begins in a dubious manner; the new information doesn't directly support the author's claim. And, as in choice A, choice B makes another mistake: There is no indication that this is a "rescripted" (rather than original) text. Choice C isn't clearly wrong from the very beginning. Having no significant impact could perhaps be described as "irrelevant." However, the author's argument is not limited to *nonpoetic* mythological stories. Therefore, this choice is incorrect. Finally, choice D matches our own answer and does not misrepresent either the passage information or the new information in the question stem. This leaves us with choice D as the correct answer.

Advanced "New Information": Refining Your Skills   For both types of New Information questions, if you are down to two answers, compare them on the basis of the following: Which one of the two is most relevant to both the question stem and the passage information? If one of them relates to both the passage and the question, while the other is supported by the passage but has no direct connection to the new information, the first of the two is a more likely choice.

For New Information/Inference questions (just as on Specific Inference questions), beware of choices that are too extreme to be supported by the passage and/or the new information. Beware of choices that go in the opposite direction or that focus on the wrong issue in the passage. Additionally, extreme language can in fact be a problem for New Information/Strengthen/Weaken questions (unlike for regular Strengthen/Weaken), if the language of the answer goes too far past the actual impact of the new information on the passage.

10. Analogy

Reading and Translating the Question Task   These questions ask you to take something described in the passage, logically abstract it, and then compare that abstracted logic to new situations in the choices, looking for the best match. Like Strengthen and Weaken questions, the new information will be in the answer choices. Unlike those questions, however, the answer choice will match the logic of what is stated in the passage, rather than make it better or worse. Here is our sample Analogy question:

> **10.** Which of the following would be most analogous to the relationship between the role of myth in ancient societies and the role of medicine and astrophysics today, as those roles are described in the passage?

Going Back to the Passage and Generating an Answer   In paragraph 2, the author states:

> For the civilizations that produced them, myth occupied a place and served a function within the social fabric reserved today for medicine, astrophysics, and cybernetics. Myth blazed like a beacon of clarity and reassurance in an uncertain and terrifying universe. Myth gave people a finite idea of their place in the scheme of things, taught them how to see themselves in relation to forces beyond their control and how to survive and relate within a human society built on hierarchical power and often ruthless savagery.

The relationship between myth on one hand, and medicine and astrophysics on the other, is that they perform the same function ("clarity and reassurance") in different societies. So, in the choices we are looking for something like different things, same function.

POE   Here are the choices for our Analogy question:

A)   Eyes and ears
B)   Teeth and fur
C)   Wings and fins
D)   Teeth and tongue

Choice A gives us two different structures with different functions (seeing and hearing), which eliminates choice A. Choice B has a similar problem: Perhaps teeth and fur both perform a protective function, but we need a tighter analogy. Choice C is the best so far: Wings and fins are both forms of locomotion (and are generally used by, or attached to, different kinds of animals). Choice D doesn't match the relationship in the passage in a different way than choices A and B fail to match. Teeth and tongue usually work together in the mouth. So, while they may perform the same (or a related) function, it isn't in two different contexts. This leaves us with choice C as the best match.

Advanced "Analogy": Refining Your Skills   Don't panic! While the answer choices may all seem out of scope at first glance, this is because you need to match the logic, not the content, of the passage. But, this makes it especially important that you go back to the passage first. And, once you have read the relevant part and paraphrased it, take one more step and identify the more abstract theme or logic of that part of the passage. That is, generalize it before you start POE, to prime yourself to identify that "different content but same logic" correct answer. Expect to take two passes through the choices for most of these questions. On your second pass, compare the pieces of the remaining choices to each other (within the choice and between different choices) in order to eliminate "half right/half wrong" answers. Also beware of wrong answers that match or connect to the content in the passage, but not the logic of it.

Question Formats

Before we wrap up our discussion of question strategies, let's take a look at the three formats in which these ten question types can appear.

1. **Standard**
    This essentially means not Roman numeral and not Except/Least/Not. That is, you have one of the ten question types in its pure form.
2. **Roman numeral**
    These questions give you three statements labeled with numerals, and the choices present you with different combinations of those numerals. An example of how one of these questions might be structured is:

    With which of the following statements would the author
    be likely to agree?

    I.   blah blah blah
    II.   blah blah blah
    III. blah blah blah

    A)   I only
    B)   III only
    C)   I and II only
    D)   I, II, and III

The most efficient strategy in approaching these questions is to work with the combinations in the choices as you evaluate the statements in the numerals, and to eliminate choices as you go. You can't strike out numerals on the screen, only the lettered choices, so this is also a good time to use your scratch paper. Let's say you were unsure of I and II, but you have a solid reason to eliminate III. Cross off III on your scratch paper, and strike out choices B and D on the screen, since they include III. Now compare what you have left, choices A and C. You see that I is in both of the possible answers. Now, you don't have to worry about I anymore: It all comes down to whether or not II is sufficiently supported.

3. **Except/Least/Not**

These questions try to confuse you by asking, for example, what is NOT supported by the passage rather than what IS supported. Or, what LEAST Weakens rather than what most Weakens. The key to these questions is to not let yourself get turned around. Use your scratch paper to keep track of POE. Quickly jot down A–D vertically on your paper. As you strike out each choice on the screen, jot down a note next to the letter on your scratch paper indicating WHY you crossed it off. For example, if it is a Strengthen Except question, write an "S" next to each choice that you eliminate because it does in fact Strengthen. This will keep you focused on eliminating answers for the right reasons and will alert you to what has gone wrong if you get confused.

The most challenging Except/Least/Not questions tend to come in combination with Strengthen and Weaken questions. Do not translate "Weaken Except" as "Strengthen" or "Least Strengthen" as "Weaken." A choice that does go to the opposite extreme (for example, it weakens on a "Strengthen Except") may in fact be the right answer, but the right answer doesn't *have* to go to the opposite extreme. It may instead have no impact on the passage. For example, if three of the choices do significantly strengthen the passage, and one of them does nothing (or strengthens less than the other three), that "does nothing" or "barely strengthens" answer is the correct choice. As you can see, keeping track of your direction and comparing remaining choices to each other is crucial for doing these questions as quickly and accurately as possible. It can help keep your focus on what you are eliminating rather than on what you are choosing. For example, if you have a "Weaken Except" question, write down on your scratch paper "cross off what weakens" and keep track of POE accordingly.

7.7 SELF-EVALUATION

We've been discussing the specifics of self-evaluation throughout this chapter and the previous one as well. Here, then, let's summarize the big categories in which to look for additional room for improvement.

Overall Pacing

The first step is to diagnose if you are going too fast or too slow, and then to decide the best way to adjust.

Too Fast

- You are completing 8 or 9 passages but missing on average three or more per passage, or you tend to crash and burn on one passage that you are rushing through at the end of the hour.
- You often miss easy questions.
- You are completing all 9 passages and not scoring a 129 or above.

Strategy Adjustments

- Slow down from 9 to 8, or from 8 to 7 passages, and work on improving your accuracy. If your accuracy improves, you may then be able to bring the pace back up. If you are scoring well (but not as well as you would like) and completing all 9 passages, try randomly guessing on 1–3 questions and saving that time for getting the rest of the questions right.
- Read the question stems and answer choices more carefully the first time through.
- Go back to the passage more carefully and consistently.

Too Slow

- You consistently get all or most of the questions that you answer correct, but you are completing 7 or fewer passages.
- You spend a disproportionate amount of time on one passage, or on one or two questions within a passage.
- You spend 6 or more minutes reading the passage the first time through.

Strategy Adjustments

- Force yourself to spend less time on your first read-through of the passage. Remember that you don't have to memorize it, or even fully understand every aspect of it, on your first reading; you can always go back to find what you need.
- If you often have to read the question stem or choices multiple times, read it more slowly and translate/paraphrase it the first time. Better to read it once well than to get stuck reading it five times over.
- Use aggressive POE. You don't always have to know exactly why the right answer is right as long as you know why the other three are wrong. Compare choices to each other when you are down to two, keeping the focus on finding what is more wrong with one of them.
- Pick your passages more carefully, especially if you tend to waste a high percentage of your time bogged down in a Killer passage.

Working the Passage and Bottom Line

Do your mistakes in the questions tend to track back to mistakes you made when reading the passage the first time through? If so, focus on:

- Mapping and highlighting for logical structure and tone,
- Defining the main point of each paragraph based on that structure: jot it down on your scratch paper,
- And defining the Bottom Line as a distinct step before you attack the questions. Ask yourself, Does my Bottom Line include all the major themes of the passage? Does it take into account any major shifts in the passage? Does it match the author's tone?

Attacking the Questions

Do you find that you had a beautifully mapped and understood passage, and yet something went wrong in the questions? If so, diagnose exactly where you strayed from the path leading toward the correct choice, and come up with a strategy to stay on that path next time. Ask yourself:

- Did you misread or misidentify the question? If so, read word for word and paraphrase the question task. Also, review the ten question types in the previous section.
- Did you understand the question, but misunderstand the relevant part of the passage? If so, read the passage text closely at this stage, read farther above and below, and pay attention to indicator words. Make yourself paraphrase the author's argument before taking the next step.
- Did you understand the question task and the relevant part of the passage, but got turned around in the answer choices? If so, focus on answering in your own words, keeping both the question task and passage information in mind.
- Did all of that go great, up to and including having a perfect answer in your own words, and yet you still picked the wrong answer? If so, focus on reading each choice word for word the first time through, looking for what's wrong rather than for what "sounds right." Review the types of Attractors discussed earlier in this chapter, and look for patterns in the types of Attractors that you tend to fall for.
- Did you in fact select the right answer and then change it to a wrong answer? If so, live by the following rule: Never change an answer unless you can define exactly what was wrong with your first choice. If the other answer just "sounds better," leave it be.

Final Note

To improve your score, you have to do something different, even something radically different, perhaps even something you would never had done on your own unless someone had (strongly) suggested it. As we have discussed, simply doing test after test or passage after passage will get you nowhere. Don't be afraid to experiment in order to find what works best for you. Nothing is set in stone until test day (or perhaps a few days before). You may be surprised at the good results you get once you step out of your strategy comfort zone and try something new!

Chapter 8
Critical Analysis and Reasoning Skills Practice Section

PRACTICE PASSAGE 1

Anyone who has had the misfortune to go to the emergency room of a modern hospital will be familiar with the ugly face that high-technology medicine presents to the patient. The long wait before anything happens, the filling out of forms, the repetitive answering of questions, the battery of routine chemical and physical tests carried out by masked technicians, and finally the abbreviated contact with the physician. The thing the patient needs the most, and the thing hardest to find, is personal attention.

Since personal attention has become the scarcest resource in high-tech medicine, it is inevitable that it should be distributed unequally. The majority of advanced countries have national health services that attempt to distribute medical attention fairly. But the escalating costs of medical attention make social justice more difficult to achieve. One way or another, as personal attention becomes scarcer, people of status tend to receive more of it. In the United States, which has never had a national health service and does not pretend to distribute medical resources equally, the prospects for achieving social justice are far worse. In the United States, a medical system based on the ethic of the free market inevitably favors the rich over the poor, and the inequalities of medical treatment grow sharper as the costs increase.

Similar dilemmas exist in the world of high-technology computing and communications. Here too, there is a clash between the economic forces driving the technology and the needs of poor people. Access to personal computers and the Internet is like medical insurance. Almost everybody needs it, but most poor people don't have it. Increasingly jobs and business opportunities are offered through the Internet. People who are not wired are in danger of becoming the new servant class.

The computer and software industries are driven by two contradictory impulses. On the one hand, they sincerely wish to broaden their market by making computers accessible to everyone. On the other hand, they are forced by competitive pressures to upgrade their products constantly, increasing their power and speed, adding new features and new complications. In the tug-of-war between broadening the market and pampering the top-end customer, the top-end customer usually wins.

The problem of unequal access to computers is only a small part of the problem of unequal opportunity in our society. Until the society is willing to attack the larger problems of inequality in housing and education and health care, attempts to provide equal access to computers cannot be totally successful. Nevertheless, in attacking the general problems of unequal opportunity, computer access may be a good place to start. The Internet easily infiltrates through barriers of language, custom, and culture. No technical barrier stops it from becoming universally accessible. The Internet could then become an important tool for alleviating other kinds of inequality.

Adapted from: F. Dyson, "The Sun, The Genome, and The Internet," *New York Public Library Lectures in Humanities.* © 1999 by New York Public Library.

1. The relationship between the two market impulses described in paragraph 4 would be most similar to which of the following?

    A) A medical school committed to providing both top-notch laboratory facilities for profitable research and a high quality education for practicing doctors seeks to accomplish both through integrating more medical students in ongoing research projects.
    B) A public school serving a community with a wide range of socio-economic levels seeks to equalize certain educational outcomes by instituting a program to make sure that all of the students have access to good quality computers.
    C) A state university, which has committed to lowering tuition for all students, offers a special zero-tuition scholarship program and newly upgraded facilities to the top performing academic students in the state, in order to lure more high performing students away from competing private colleges.
    D) A private school, which has been seeking to expand enrollment over the last decade, raises tuition to cover the costs of a several new athletic programs that will distinguish it from other high-end private schools.

2. Which of the following, if true, would most *undermine* the author's position concerning the relationship of computer access to contemporary manifestations of social inequality?

    A) Hospitals with the most up-to-date technology can often make use of the resulting efficiencies to provide services and personal attention to patients of all socio-economic backgrounds.
    B) Many Western markets have seen a significant overall decline in computer sales as cell-phones, almost universally available, become more capable of performing the same functions.
    C) No compelling documentation exists linking the availability of computers within elementary schools to improved academic performance or higher eventual economic potential.
    D) Although the price of new computers continues to decline overall in the United States, the cost of high-speed Internet services have remained high and, in some cases, risen over the last 5 years.

3. The author of the passage would likely expect each of the following to be a typical experience in an emergency room in the United States, EXCEPT:

A) a patient has blood drawn twice for reasons that are never explained to the patient.

B) a patient is misdiagnosed, in part because certain presenting symptoms were never discussed with the doctor.

C) the doctor reviews all the questions the patient previously answered with the nurse practitioner.

D) a patient with high-end insurance waits much less time before receiving medical treatment than does a patient who lacks insurance.

4. Which of the following claims about health care in the United States would constitute the most effective support for the author's position regarding the likelihood of achieving social justice within United States health services?

A) Despite various attempts to control costs of medical care, the pressure of the marketplace and the aging population all but guarantee that medical costs will continue to rise and outpace inflation for the foreseeable future.

B) Studies indicate that those patients who receive a larger share of direct attention from treating physicians, regardless of income level, experience improved health outcomes.

C) As improved medical technology becomes more widely available and easier to manufacture, it is very likely that some medical costs will decline.

D) As more individuals gain access to the Internet, overall knowledge about health and wellness will be more consistently spread through the population.

5. Which of the following outcomes does the passage suggest is/are likely to be correlated with wealth in the modern world?

    I. Better outcomes from medical treatment
    II. Feeling pressure to adopt new technologies that enter the marketplace
    III. Access to better quality education

A) I and II only
B) I and III only
C) II and III only
D) I, II, and III

6. A recent international report shows that within local communities whose access to the Internet has increased significantly over the past 10 years, there has also been an increase in the number of those seeking treatment for certain serious conditions such as cancer and heart disease. What effect would this data have on the author's overall argument?

A) If the increased access to the Internet is due largely to more affordable providers, then the report would weaken the author's overall argument.

B) If the increase in those seeking treatment corresponds to better health outcomes for those people, then the report would strengthen the author's overall argument.

C) If the increase in those seeking treatment only coincidentally relates to increases in Internet usage, then the report would weaken the author's argument.

D) If increases in those seeking treatment also have occurred in wealthy communities in which high-speed Internet was already readily available, then this report would weaken the author's overall argument.

7. Which of the following scenarios would most nearly parallel the author's description of the intersection between providing equal access to computers and addressing broader issues of social equality?

A) The consensus among economists is that the economy will not be able to support a minimum wage that would constitute a true living income unless other changes occur within the larger economy. On the other hand, an immediate moderate increase in the minimum wage may pave the way to some of those other economic transformations.

B) Most physicians agree that exercise will contribute significantly to weight loss, although if performed incorrectly exercise can be dangerous and contribute to various injuries. Still, most physicians do recommend exercise to patients who desire to lose weight.

C) It is clear that the introduction of police cameras will not, by themselves, alleviate problems of police brutality and the pervasive societal distrust of the nation's police personnel. Still, installing cameras would be a beneficial first step toward repairing some of these systemic problems.

D) It seems certain that the widespread problem of homelessness will not be fully addressed without also successfully addressing broader issues around poverty. In particular, as long as new housing is primarily oriented toward wealthier consumers instead of serving as many as possible, it is unlikely that sufficient low-income housing will be available.

PRACTICE PASSAGE 2

Language takes on for Chomsky the role of reason in Descartes' philosophy; that is, language becomes the essence that defines what it is to be human. Language is also universal and innate, an autonomous capacity of mind, independent of any connection to things in the external world. Language must also have an essence, something that makes language what it is and inheres in all language. Language does not arise from anything bodily. Studying the brain and the body can give us no insight into language.

There is an intimate link between the philosophy underlying Chomsky's linguistics and his political philosophy. As a [follower of Descartes's ideas], Chomsky believes there is a single universal human nature, that the mind is separate from and independent of the body, and that what makes us distinctively human is our mental capacities, not our bodies. We can think freely, free of any physical constraints. This gives us free will. Thus, by human nature, all people require maximum freedom. Being ruled by a government is inherently oppressive and an ideal political system is maximally anarchic.

Since what makes us human is our minds, not our bodies, what makes us essentially human is not material. It follows from this philosophical perspective that universal human nature does not include a need to acquire material possessions (beyond what is required to live). Capitalism is thus a perversion of universal human nature and nonstate socialism is in accord with universal human nature. From this perspective, the major sins against universal human nature are oppression and greed on the part of capitalistic governments and large corporations. Much of Chomsky's political writings focus on uncovering instances of governmental oppression and corporate greed and on seeing world politics and history from this perspective.

In Chomsky's philosophy, rationality and freedom take center stage, while culture, aesthetics, and pleasure (e.g., religion, ritual, business, music, art, poetry, and sensuality) play no essential role in human nature; for Chomsky, these things simply get in the way of proper politics and have nothing to do with reason and language. The same is true of one's bodily relation to the physical environment or to "lower" animals, which Chomsky sees as devoid of language and reason and lacking in free will.

One reason for including this excursion into Chomsky's political philosophy is simply to demonstrate the coherence of his overall philosophical views. His political philosophy derives from the same source as his linguistic philosophy. There is a reason why "language" for Chomsky does not include poetic language. It is also why one finds in his work no serious discussion of the role of culture in language. In both Chomsky's linguistics and his politics, one finds the systematic

Cartesian denial of the role of the body and of our animal nature in human nature.

Adapted from G. Lakoff and M. Johnson, *Philosophy in the Flesh.* ©1999 by Basic Books.

1. Which of the following claims, if true, would most *undermine* Chomsky's conclusion that capitalism is a perversion of human nature?

A) It is possible to maintain a capitalist economy while still largely minimizing the influence of corporate greed and corruption.

B) The essence of capitalism has less to do with material possessions than with freedom from restraint in pursuing one's own economic interests.

C) Within a socialist economy, it can still be difficult to ensure that all people are provided with those basic possessions necessary for living.

D) Most individuals raised in capitalist cultures experience the acquisition of material possessions as a basic human good.

2. Which of the following would be most analogous to the relationship between reason and the body as presented in Chomsky's philosophy?

A) Mathematical truths are fundamentally independent of the calculations produced by some calculator or even by a human brain, since human brains and so the calculators they construct are always limited by their capacity for error.

B) Music, as an abstraction, can be thought of as independent of any instrument, but of course without instruments (including the human voice) we would have no conception of music.

C) The promise of artificial intelligence now makes it reasonable to suppose that computers will achieve modes of thinking not directly linked to any specific human-made program, since computers may, as they experience new situations, program themselves in ways human cannot currently imagine.

D) Beauty represents the highest achievement of art. Although art often falls short and can be marred by ideology or the simple physical limitations of artist or artistic medium, still art allows us to conceive of true beauty.

3. The author most likely mentions Descartes in order to:

A) establish a link between language and reason that will be explored throughout the passage.

B) demonstrate that philosophy can be applicable to politics, since both relate to the relationship of mind and body.

C) support Chomsky's argument that studying the brain and body do not give insight into language.

D) introduce an analogy that will help to clarify Chomsky's position and identify one influence on Chomsky's thinking.

4. Which of the following statements, if true, would most strengthen Chomsky's argument that the ideal political system is maximally anarchic?

A) Free will, according to Chomsky, allows human beings to make decisions that cannot directly be attributed to biological states, such as certain neural processes.

B) Government intervention is not needed in order to keep some from illegitimately intruding on the rights and freedoms of others.

C) In the absence of government rule and controls, the wealthy and strong within a given society control the poor and weak.

D) Governments, by their very nature, do not exercise free will, and in fact act in ways more similar to "lower" animals than to human beings.

5. Elsewhere the author of this passage challenges Chomsky's claim that studying the brain gives no insight into language; the passage author argues that understanding brain function in fact constitutes a critical component of an adequate scientific account of the function and structure of all types of verbal communication. This argument would most *undermine* which other position in the passage attributed to Chomsky?

A) Human beings are essentially different from lower animals and our "animal nature" does not crucially influence our rational behavior.

B) Capitalism is a perversion of human nature and corporate greed should be actively resisted.

C) Chomsky's political philosophy is coherent with his philosophy of language, in that both rely on a systematic denial of the role of the body.

D) All languages that human beings use to communicate with each other must share a basic essence.

6. Which of the following, given the descriptions in the passage, would most reasonably be expected as the title of an article published by Chomsky?

A) "Enjoying the fruits of one's labor: the fundamental human right of economic freedom from constraint"

B) "Free will as a neurological epiphenomenon: the gaps between the synapses"

C) "Man vs. Corporate Machine: Separating the good from the goods"

D) "Language without limits: Free verse and expanded consciousness"

PRACTICE PASSAGE 3

Those afflicted or affected by psychosis have put up in its place the image of the Mother: for women, a paradise lost but seemingly close at hand, for men, a hidden god but constantly present through occult fantasy. And even psychoanalysts believe in it.

Yet, swaying between these two positions can only mean, for the woman involved, that she is within an "enceinte" separating her from the world of everyone else. Enclosed in this "elsewhere," an "enceinte" woman loses communital meaning, which suddenly appears to her as worthless, absurd, or at best, comic—a surface agitation severed from its impossible foundations. Oriental nothingness probably better sums up what, in the eyes of a Westerner, can only be regression. And yet it is jouissance, but like a negative of the one, tied to an object, that is borne by the unfailingly masculine libido. Here, alterity becomes nuance, contradiction becomes variant, tension becomes passage, and discharge becomes peace. This tendency towards equalization, which is seen as a regressive extinction of symbolic capabilities, does not, however, reduce differences; it resides within the smallest, most archaic, and most uncertain of difficulties. It is powerful sublimation and indwelling of the symbolic within instinctual drives. It affects this series of "little differences-resemblances" (as the Chinese logicians of antiquity would say). Before founding society in the same stroke as signs and communication, they are the precondition of the latter's existence, as they constitute the living entity within its species, with its needs, its elementary apperceptions and communication, distinguishing between the instinctual drives of life and death. It affects primal repression. An ultimate danger for identity, but also supreme power of symbolic instance thus returning to matters of its concern. Sublimation here is both eroticizing without residue and a disappearance of eroticism as it returns to its source.

The speaker reaches this limit, this requisite of sociality, only by virtue of a particular, discursive practice called "art." A woman also attains it (and in our society, *especially*) through the strange form of split symbolization (threshold of language and instinctual drive, of the "symbolic" and the "semiotic") of which the act of giving birth consists. As the archaic process of socialization, one might even say civilization, it causes the childbearing woman to cathect, immediately and unwittingly, the physiological operations and instinctual drives dividing and multiplying her, first, in a biological, and finally, a social teleology. The maternal body slips away from the discursive hold and immediately conceals a cipher that must be taken into account biologically and socially. This ciphering of the species, however, this pre- and transsymbolic memory, makes the mother mistress of neither begetting nor instinctual drive (such a fantasy underlies the cult of any ultimately feminine deity); it does make of the maternal body the stakes of a

natural and "objective" control, independent of any individual consciousness; it inscribes both biological operations and their instinctual echoes into this necessary and hazardous *program* constituting every species. The maternal body is the module of a biosocial program. Its jouissance, which is mute, is nothing more than a recording, on the screen of the preconscious, of both the messages that consciousness, in its analytical course, picks up from this ciphering process and their classifications as empty foundation, as a-subjective lining of our rational exchanges as social beings. If it is true that every national language has its own dream language and unconscious, then each of the sexes—a division so much more archaic and fundamental than the one into languages—would have its own unconscious wherein the biological and social program of the species would be ciphered in confrontation with language, exposed to its influence, but independent from it. The symbolic destiny of the speaking animal, which is essential although it comes second, being superimposed upon the biological—this destiny *seals off* (and in women, in order to preserve the homology of the group, it *censures*) that archaic basis and the special jouissance it procures in being transferred to the symbolic. Privileged, "psychotic" moments, or whatever induces them naturally, thus become necessary.

Adapted from J. Kristeva, *Desire in Language: A Semiotic Approach to Literature and Art.* © 1980 by Columbia University Press.

1. What is the main idea of the passage?

A) People need insight into the inscription into the memory of the biological foundation of the species, which recording precedes consciousness and the attainment of language.

B) The repression of the memory of the biological foundation of the species and the transference of that foundation to language that takes place in the maternal body during childbirth produces jouissance and is also necessary to communication and the social order.

C) Pregnant women are separate from communication and the social order until they give birth, at which point their bodies are reprogrammed to repress their memories of the biological foundation of the species.

D) By being positioned as a border or boundary, the mother is at risk of becoming psychotic because of the need to bifurcate her needs and desires.

2. By the term "enceinte" (paragraph 2) the author most likely means:

A) partition.
B) conceived or conception.
C) meaningless or meaninglessness.
D) a protective wall around a town or protected by such a wall.

3. Which of the following statements about regression is most strongly supported by the passage?

A) An "enceinte" woman may experience it.
B) A psychotic woman may experience it.
C) It constitutes an artistic act.
D) It is suggested by a loss of language.

4. The author refers to peace in the second paragraph in order to describe:

A) the libido.
B) regression.
C) the balancing tendency of jouissance.
D) the eradication of distinction.

5. The author contends that language:

A) is the basis for the instinctual drives.
B) is the primary means of awareness of the biological destiny of the species.
C) is not as intrinsic as gender.
D) manifests itself in the unconscious.

PRACTICE PASSAGE 4

The pessimism of the 14th century grew in the 15th to the belief that man was becoming worse, an indication of the approaching end. As described in one French treatise, a sign of this decline was the congealing of charity in human hearts, indicating that the human soul was aging and that the flame of love which used to warm mankind was sinking low and would soon go out. Plague, violence, and natural catastrophe were further signals.

With the English occupying the French capital, courage had sunk low. Frenchmen did not lack who were ready to accept union under one crown as the only solution to incessant war and economic ruin. In most, however, resistance to the English tyrants and "Goddams," as they were called, was axiomatic, but it was uncoordinated and leaderless. The Dauphin was weak and spiritless, captive of unscrupulous or passive ministers. Unheralded, the courage came from society's most unlikely source—a women of the commoner's class.

The phenomenon of Jeanne d'Arc—the voices from God who told her she must expel the English and have the Dauphin crowned King, the quality that dominated those who would normally have despised her, the strength that raised the siege of Orleans and carried the Dauphin to Reims—belongs to no category. Perhaps it can only be explained as the answer called forth by an exigent historic need. The moment required her and she rose. Her strength came from the fact that in her were combined for the first time the old religious faith and the new force of patriotism. God spoke to her through the voices of St. Catherine, St. Michael, and St. Margaret, but what he commanded was not chastity not humility nor the life of the spirit but political action to rescue her country from foreign tyrants.

The flight of her meteor lasted only three years. Captured in May 1430, she was sold to the English, tried as a heretic by the Church in the service of the English, and burned at the stake. Her condemnation was essential to the English because she claimed to have been moved by God, and if the claim were not disallowed, God, the arbiter in the affairs of men, would have been shown to have set His face against the English dominion of France. Neither Charles VII, who owed her his crown, nor any of the French made any effort to ransom or save her, possibly from nobility's embarrassment at having been led to victory by a peasant village girl.

Jeanne d'Arc's life and death did not instantly generate a national resistance; nevertheless, the English thereafter were fighting a losing cause, whether they knew it or not. The Burgundians knew it. The installation of Charles as anointed King of France, with a re-inspired army, changed the situation, the more so as the English were distracted by rising frictions under an infant King. Within a year, by action of an energetic new Constable, Paris was regained for the King, a signal to the realm of re-unification to come. No one could have said that the spark lit by the Maid of Orleans had become a flame, for her significance is better known to history than it was to contemporaries, but renewed hope and energy was in the air.

Adapted from B.W. Tuchman, *A Distant Mirror: The Calamitous 14th Century*. © 1987 by Ballantine Books.

1. Which of the following traits are described as contributing positively to the influence Jeanne d'Arc wielded on the political and military struggles in 15th century France?

   I.   Being a commoner
   II. Patriotism
   III. Courage

A) II only
B) I and II only
C) II and III only
D) I, II, and III

2. Given the historical climate, the author suggests that if Jeanne d'Arc had never existed:

A) it is probable that some other leader would have emerged to help unite the French people against the English.
B) it is likely that the English would eventually have succeeded in occupying all of France.
C) it is possible that France would have experienced an increase of plagues and natural disasters.
D) it is possible that the French people would soon have given up on the possibility of unity under a single sovereign.

3. Based on the account given in the passage, if instead of coming from a village Jeanne d'Arc had been a nun in a convent, born into a wealthy family, who began to hear voices and became a political and military force, then we might reasonably expect that:

A) her rallying cry would have a more devotional religious aspect and be less oriented towards French nationalism.

B) the English would find her more respectable (though still politically dangerous) and so be less inclined to attack her as a heretic.

C) Charles VII would have been more inclined to offer the English payment to win her release and prevent her execution.

D) news of her execution would have more quickly contributed to the French unification and courage needed for success against the English.

4. The author's claim that Jeanne d'Arc combined in her person religious faith and a new patriotism receives additional support from which of the following claims in the passage?

A) In the years following her death, it became clear that the English occupation could not be sustained.

B) It was critical for the English who captured her not just to execute her but also to delegitimize her claims to hear the voice of God.

C) The French nobility was uncomfortable with the political power she wielded despite her humble origins.

D) From the time she began to gain widespread attention, it was less than two years before she had led major military victories and made possible the coronation of the King.

5. The author's assertion that the English, after Jeanne d'Arc's execution, were fighting a losing battle would be most strengthened by which of the following additional historical facts?

A) Jeanne d'Arc in 1428 had led the successful attack on Orleans, which directly preceded and allowed the coronation of Charles two months later.

B) Immediately after Jeanne d'Arc's death, the war grew more brutal as the English became frustrated at the refusal of the French armies and people to succumb.

C) Many of the French common people did believe that the voices Jeanne d'Arc heard came from God and continued, after her death, to regard her as a symbol of faith and unity.

D) In 1435, the Duke of Burgundy, who previously had allied his armies with the English forces, united the French region of Burgundy with the young king Charles and sealed an alliance against the English.

6. The passage suggests that Jeanne d'Arc was abandoned to the English by the French because of discomfort concerning the fact that a commoner had contributed so much to their victories. An alternative explanation of her abandonment by the French that also is compatible with the rest of the information provided in the passage could most reasonably be that:

A) in the 15th century, the class differences between the nobility and the rural village populations were so extreme that it was unthinkable for aristocrats to be dependent on commoners.

B) the claim by a woman to hear the word of God was interpreted as a threat to the authority of the Catholic church, on which the French aristocracy founded its position and power.

C) Jeanne d'Arc's mingling of religious faith and French nationalism was widely seen as inappropriate and dangerous by both the French aristocracy and the broader population.

D) the French leadership believed that her death would not generate a significant resistance to the English occupation.

PRACTICE PASSAGE 5

By the late twentieth century, our time, a mythic time, we are all chimeras, theorized and fabricated hybrids of machine and organism; in short, we are cyborgs. The cyborg is our ontology; it gives us our politics. The cyborg is a condensed image of both imagination and material reality, the two joined centres structuring any possibility of historical transformation. In the traditions of "Western" science and politics—the tradition of racist, male-dominated capitalism; the tradition of progress; the tradition of the appropriation of nature as a resource for the productions of culture; the tradition of reproduction of the self from the reflections of the other—the relation between organism and machine has been a border war. The stakes in the border war have been the territories of production, reproduction, and imagination. This [essay] is an argument for *pleasure* in the confusion of boundaries and for *responsibility* in their construction. It is also an effort to contribute to socialist-feminist culture and theory in a postmodernist, non-naturalist mode and in the utopian tradition of imagining a world without gender, which is perhaps a world without genesis, but maybe also a world without end. The cyborg incarnation is outside salvation history. Nor does it mark time on an oedipal calendar, attempting to heal the terrible cleavages of gender in an oral symbiotic utopia or post-oedipal apocalypse. As Zoe Sofoulis argues in her unpublished manuscript on Jacques Lacan, the most terrible and perhaps the most promising monsters in cyborg worlds are embodied in non-oedipal narratives with a different logic of repression, which we need to understand for our survival.

The cyborg is a creature in a post-gender world; it has no truck with bisexuality, pre-oedipal symbiosis, unalienated labour, or other seductions to organic wholeness through a final appropriation of all the powers of the parts into a higher unity. In a sense, the cyborg has no origin story in the Western sense—a "final" irony since the cyborg is also the awful apocalyptic *telos* of the "West's" escalating dominations of abstract individuation, an ultimate self untied at last from all dependency, a man in space. An origin story in the "Western," humanist sense depends on the myth of original unity, fullness, bliss, and terror, represented by the phallic mother from whom all humans must separate, the task of individual development and of history, the twin potent myths inscribed most powerfully for us in psychoanalysis and Marxism. Hilary Klein has argued that both Marxism and psychoanalysis, in their concepts of labour and of individuation and gender formation, depend on the plot of original unity out of which difference must be produced and enlisted in a drama of escalating domination of woman/nature. The cyborg skips the step of original unity, of identification with nature in the Western sense. This is its illegitimate promise that might lead to subversion of its teleology as star wars.

The cyborg is resolutely committed to partiality, irony, intimacy, and perversity. It is oppositional, utopian, and completely without innocence. No longer structured by the polarity of public and private, the cyborg defines a technological polis based partly on a revolution of social relations in the *oikos*, the household. Nature and culture are reworked; the one can no longer be the resource for appropriation or incorporation by the other. The relationships for forming wholes from parts, including those of polarity and hierarchical domination, are at issue in the cyborg world. Unlike the hopes of Frankenstein's monster, the cyborg does not expect its father to save it through a restoration of the garden; that is, through the fabrication of a heterosexual mate, through its completion in a finished whole, a city and cosmos. The cyborg does not dream of community on the model of the organic family, this time without the oedipal project.... The main trouble with cyborgs, of course, is that they are the illegitimate offspring of militarism and patriarchal capitalism, not to mention state socialism. But illegitimate offspring are often exceedingly unfaithful to their origins. Their fathers are, after all, inessential.

Adapted from D. Haraway, *Simians, Cyborgs, and Women: The Reinvention of Nature.* © 1991 by Routledge.

1. How does the author feel about Western science and politics?

A) She is critical about their traditions.
B) She feels that while they have negative qualities, they have contributed positively to the structure of our world.
C) She feels that without them, the cyborg would have nothing to rail against.
D) The author's opinions on Western science and politics are indiscernible.

2. Why, based on the passage, does the author say "Their fathers are, after all, inessential" in the final paragraph?

A) To emphasize her critique of the concept of the cyborg
B) To further her feminist agenda by asserting that men are inessential in parenting
C) To suggest that the origins of cyborgs are inconsequential and will likely be subverted by the existence of cyborgs
D) To advocate that in a post-gender world, fathers and mothers will be irrelevant since we will be able to reproduce with the help of machines

3. Which of the following statements comes closest to expressing the author's feelings about cyborgs?

A) They have some positive attributes but also severe flaws.
B) They represent a significant disadvantage of humans' obsession with technology and machines.
C) They embody many contradictions and may ultimately be a positive thing.
D) They are monsters to be feared.

4. Which of the following qualities can be attributed to cyborgs, according to the passage?

   I.   They are part organism.
   II. They strive for organic wholeness.
   III. They are innocent.

A) I only
B) I and II only
C) II and III only
D) I, II, and III

5. What is the primary purpose of this passage?

A) To critique Western civilization for being racist and infused with male-dominated capitalism.
B) To advocate that we all become cyborgs by interfacing with machines.
C) To assert a utopian world-view whereby we transcend our history by setting up clear parameters between humans and machines, people and nature.
D) To introduce and describe the concept of the cyborg and to suggest that the confusion of boundaries this creature presents can be a source of pleasure.

PRACTICE PASSAGE 6

There is no final system for the interpretation of myths, and there never will be any such thing. Mythology has been interpreted by the modern intellect as a primitive, fumbling effort to explain the world of nature; as a production of poetical fantasy from prehistoric times; as a repository of allegorical instruction; as a group dream; and as God's Revelation to his children. Mythology is all of these. The various judgments are determined by the viewpoints of the judges. For when scrutinized in terms not of what it is but of how it functions, of how it has served mankind in the past, of how it may serve today, mythology shows itself to be as amenable as life itself to the obsessions and requirements of the individual, the race, the age.

Rites of initiation and installation teach the lesson of the essential oneness of the individual and the group; seasonal festivals open a larger horizon. As the individual is an organ of society, so is the tribe or city only a phase of the mighty organism of the cosmos. It has been customary to describe the seasonal festivals of so-called native peoples as efforts to control nature. This is a misinterpretation. The dominant motive in all truly religious (as opposed to black-magical) ceremonies is that of submission to the inevitable destiny—and in the seasonal festivals this motive is particularly apparent. No tribal rite has yet been recorded which attempts to keep winter from descending; the rites all prepare the community to endure, together with the rest of nature, the season of the terrible cold.

Symbolizations of continuity fill the world of the mythologically instructed community. From the standpoint of the way of duty, anyone in exile from the community is a nothing. From the other point of view, however, this exile is the first step of the quest. We think of ourselves as Americans, children of the twentieth century. Yet such designations do not tell what it is to be man. What is the core of us? What is the basic character of our being?

The problem of mankind today is precisely the opposite to that of men in the comparatively stable periods of those great mythologies which now are known as lies. Then the meaning was in the group, none in the self-expressive individual; today no meaning is in the group—none in the world: all is in the individual. With this we come to the final hint of what the specific orientation of the modern hero-task must be, and discover the real cause for the disintegration of all of our inherited religious formulae. The center of gravity of the realm of mystery has definitely shifted.

For primitive hunting peoples, the great human problem was to become linked psychologically to the task of sharing the wilderness with these beings. Through acts of literal imitation—such as today appear only on the children's playground—an effective annihilation of the human ego was accomplished and society achieved a cohesive organization. Today all of these

mysteries have lost their force; their symbols no longer interest our psyche. The notion of a cosmic law, which all existence serves and to which man himself must bend, has long since passed through the mystical stages and is now simply accepted in mechanical terms as a matter of course.

The descent of the sciences from the heavens to the earth (from astronomy to biology), and their concentration today on man himself (in anthropology and psychology), mark the path of a transfer of the focal point of human wonder. Not the animal world, not the miracle of the spheres, but man himself is the crucial mystery. Man is that alien presence with whom the forces of egoism must come to terms, through whom society is to be reformed. Man, understood however not as "I" but as "Thou": for the ideals of no tribe, race, continent, social class, or century can be the measure of the wonderful divine existence that is the life in all of us. The modern hero cannot, indeed must not, wait for his community to cast off pride, fear, and misunderstanding. It is not society that is to guide and save the creative hero, but precisely the reverse.

Adapted from J. Campbell, *The Hero with a Thousand Faces*. © 2008 by the Joseph Campbell Foundation.

1. The author's purpose in discussing winter rituals is primarily:

A) to argue that various tribes and communities show significant resemblances in their ritual practices.
B) to emphasize how rituals, for ancient peoples, helped them to tolerate hardship.
C) to help correct the misinterpretation that rituals actually allowed ancient peoples to control the weather and other aspects of the physical world.
D) to reinforce with an example the claim that rituals principally emphasize connectedness with nature rather than opposition.

2. Elsewhere this author writes that the great world religions no longer meet humanity's requirements because they are associated with factions, propaganda, and self-congratulation. Which statement in the passage would most strengthen this claim?

A) Symbolizations of continuity fill the world of the mythologically instructed community.
B) The ideals of no tribe, race, continent, social class, or century can be the measure of the wonderful divine existence that is the life in all of us.
C) The notion of a cosmic law has long since passed through the mystical stages and is now accepted in mechanical terms.
D) Mythology shows itself to be as amenable as life itself to the obsessions and requirements of the individual, the race, the age.

3. Which of the following most corresponds to the author's understanding of what mythology is and how we should, in the modern world, best interpret it?

A) Despite the beliefs of ancient peoples, mythology is essentially falsehood, and so contemporary people will need to look for truth in science instead.
B) Mythology will be properly understood today as one way in which we connect our communities to the broader cosmos and submit to changes in the wider world.
C) One consistent danger of mythology is that it can encourage certain obsessions, and so can contribute to damaging communal norms.
D) Mythology is highly malleable, and so will perform different functions for different communities, though consistently addressing issues of how individual, community, and cosmos interact.

4. In the final paragraph, the author says that man should be understood as "Thou" rather than as "I." By this, the author likely means that:

A) the proper understanding of mankind should be as broad and inclusive as possible, so that it may unite different communities.
B) individualism tends to lead us toward egoism and to undermine communal altruism.
C) it would be better to embrace older concepts of the self and resist the modern individualistic tendency.
D) the essential mystery of humankind is how one individual connects face-to-face with another individual.

5. Which of the following examples best parallels the shift, described in paragraph 4, from ancient people to contemporary mankind?

A) In her early works, a painter tended to use a fairly narrow range of colors, preferring very subtle contrasts. In her later works, the range of colors has broadened considerably, heightening the contrasts and adding an element of urgency to the painting.
B) In her early works, a painter employed very traditional techniques, adapting methods passed down from great masters of the past. In her more recent works, she has further adapted and in doing so has developed a much more individual and distinctive style that is instantly recognizable as her own.
C) In her early works, a painter created intense effects by uniting all of the various elements on the canvas, emphasizing their coherence through repetition. In her later works, she instead emphasized differences and incongruities, separating out certain elements, with the effect that the viewer's attention could be directed beyond the canvas altogether.
D) In her early works, a certain painter created each painting with a specific well-defined theme that stood alone. In her later works, she has created groups of paintings that work together to create a more complicated and nuanced set of meanings.

6. Which of the following ritual activities would most call into question the author's argument concerning the most central motive of traditional religious ceremony?

A) Research into the myths of a particular tribal society reveal a shift over time from myths focusing on a single divine being to myths describing a community of divinities working in concert.
B) Many ancient tribes practiced highly formalized ceremonies designed to produce rain during droughts or during the recurring dry season that would occur each year.
C) In a certain tribal dance, the principal dancer takes on the role of a wolf that first menaces the tribe but then later is reabsorbed into the tribe, becoming human but maintaining certain wolf-like traits.
D) Certain indigenous groups today continue to celebrate traditional rituals oriented around celebrating the beginning of spring and the hope for a bountiful growing season.

Chapter 9
Critical Analysis and
Reasoning Skills
Practice Section
Solutions

SOLUTIONS TO PRACTICE PASSAGE 1

1. **D**   This is an Analogy question.

    Note: The impulse to broaden the market contradicts the impulse to constantly upgrade products, with the second impulse dominating. The correct answer needs to match this relationship.

    A: No. In this case, the two impulses or goals are not contradictory.

    B: No. This answer choice matches some of the themes of the passage but does not reference two contradictory impulses. When answering Analogy questions, make sure to focus on the logic of the relevant part of the passage, not the content alone.

    C: No. There is no conflict between the two impulses described in this example. One goal is to lower tuition for all students, and the other is to attract students by offering zero-tuition scholarships to some students.

    D: Yes. In this situation, one impulse or goal is to expand enrollment (parallel to broadening the market for computers), while the other is to increase in tuition to cover costs of an improved athletic program (parallel to upgrading products to compete for high-end customers). The second impulse, which offers competitive advantage, is dominant and would undermine the first impulse.

2. **B**   This is a Weaken question.

    Note: The question asks you to weaken the claim that differences in access to computers represent an important aspect of contemporary social inequality. Look for an answer choice that gives the strongest evidence that a difference in access to computers does NOT constitute or contribute to social inequality.

    A: No. This answer choice does not address *individual* access to computers, and therefore has no effect on the author's argument.

    B: Yes. This answer choice suggests that contemporary Westerners have nearly equal (almost universal) access to computing functions and so undermines the argument that differing access to computers produces inequality.

    C: No. The lack of documentation would not be convincing evidence that such a link does not exist. Therefore, it does not have a significant negative impact on the author's argument. Furthermore, the passage argument concerns adult access to computers in the home (i.e., "access to jobs and business opportunities"), not access for children at school, which may not produce similar effects.

    D: No. This would strengthen the argument that the benefits of computer technology are tied to income level. On Weaken questions, always look out for wrong answers that do the opposite of what the question requires.

3. **C**   This is an Inference EXCEPT question.

    A: No. This fits the passage theme of minimal communication.

    B: No. This fits the passage themes of limited personal attention and problems with medical treatment.

    C: Yes. This contradicts the passage assertion that personal attention from the doctor is rare.

    D: No. This fits the passage theme that those with more money receive more attention and better medical care.

4. **A**   This is a Strengthen question.

Note: In paragraph 2 the author claims "In the United States, which has never had a national health service and does not pretend to distribute medical resources equally, the prospects for achieving social justice are far worse." The correct answer will be the choice that provides the strongest support for this claim that achieving social justice within the U.S. health care system will be very difficult.

A: **Yes. The author argues that marketplace pressure and heath care costs are the main reasons why social justice is lacking in this area. This answer choice affirms that these pressures will increase in the future, strengthening the claim that social justice will difficult to achieve.**

B: No. This answer choice confirms a link in the passage between personal attention and health care, but it does not directly support any claim related to social justice or unequal availability of services. Therefore, it doesn't address the issue raised in the question. Make sure to keep your focus on the claim cited in the question stem.

C: No. This answer choice does the opposite; it would undermine the author's reasoning concerning persisting social inequality (given that declining costs would offer greater improved access to low income people).

D: No. This answer choice suggests that health in general might improve, but it is not directly relevant to claims about ongoing social inequality. The issue is not information about health issues, but rather access to health care. To the extent that this choice tangentially affects the author's argument about social justice, it would tend to weaken, not strengthen it.

5. **B**   This is an Inference Roman numeral question.

I: **True. The passage argues in paragraph 2 that personal attention, the most significant component of health care, will inevitably be distributed unfairly.**

II: False. The passage says that companies feel pressured to create new technologies but not that consumers feel pressured to adopt them.

III: **True. In the final paragraph, education is included as one of several categories in which persistent inequality of opportunity must be addressed.**

6. **B**   This is a New Information/Strengthen/Weaken question.

Note: The point of the new information is that Internet access correlates directly with treatment of certain diseases. In the passage, Internet access is linked to improved social equality in general, including health care. Look for an answer choice that links these ideas correctly.

A: No. The author argues that low income people have less access to the Internet. If increased affordability provides greater access, it would somewhat strengthen (only somewhat, as you don't know that seeking treatment equates with actual access to effective treatment), not weaken, the author's argument.

B: **Yes. If there is in fact a causal connection between more access to the Internet and better health, this would strengthen the author's overall claim that such access encourages social equality in health care and other areas.**

C: No. If the connection described is coincidental, it would neither strengthen nor weaken any claim the author makes in the passage. This does not, for example, indicate that the health or economic opportunities of these people are not improving in other ways.

D: No. On one hand, if wealthy people who already have easy Internet access are also seeking treatment more often, it would indicate that increased financial access to the Internet had little to do with it. However, the author does not argue that affordability of the Internet is the only (or even a main) factor in whether or not people seek care. Notice as well that this choice says nothing about actual access to effective care or to improved health outcomes.

7.   **A**   This is an Analogy question.

   Note: In the last paragraph, the author of the passage states both that the problems of unequal computer access cannot be fully addressed without larger social changes and that improving computer access may help address some of those larger issues of social inequality. Look for an answer choice that parallels both of these aspects.

   A: **Yes. In this scenario, an effective minimum wage cannot be fully instituted without also addressing wider issues, but improving the minimum wage is presented as a good first step for addressing those broader issues.**

   B: No. In this scenario, exercise is described as having potential negative outcomes. This does not parallel the relationship in the passage.

   C: No. In this scenario, there is no suggestion that cameras cannot be fully implemented without addressing other social issues.

   D: No. In this scenario, there is no indication that addressing housing as a first step will help with addressing other aspects of social inequality.

SOLUTIONS TO PRACTICE PASSAGE 2

1.   **B**   This is a Weaken question

   Note: The third paragraph presents Chomsky's argument that, since essential human nature relates to mind and not to body or to material possessions, capitalism represents a perversion of that nature. Look for an answer choice that would directly *challenge* this argument.

   A: No. Chomsky does criticize corporate greed as a negative outcome of capitalism, but this is not relevant to the basic argument that capitalism, a system focused on acquiring material possessions, is a perversion of human nature, which should be separate from possessions.

   B: **Yes. If capitalism itself is fundamentally connected to freedom then, by Chomsky's own reasoning in the second paragraph, capitalism would be in keeping with human nature, not a corruption of human nature.**

   C: No. The practical difficulties of socialism are not relevant to a claim about capitalism and human nature.

   D: No. That a capitalist system encourages people to value material objects would strengthen, not weaken, Chomsky's claim that it represents a corruption of human nature, since human nature is fundamentally about mind rather than physical things. Look out for answers to a Weaken question that support rather than undermine the author's argument.

2.   **A**   This is an Analogy question.

   Note: Reason and the body are fundamentally distinct in the passage (paragraphs 1 and 2). Furthermore, the body may at times become an obstacle to reason, as in paragraph 4 where pleasure and sensuality get in the way of rational politics. Look for the answer choice that most parallels this relationship.

   A: **Yes. Here mathematics (like reason) is independent of the physical (and potentially limited or constrained) calculator or brain.**

   B: No. In this relationship, music is still fundamentally linked to physical instruments, contradicting the relationship between reason and body as it is described in the passage.

   C: No. This example emphasizes that computer "thought" is fundamentally linked to programming, merely suggesting a distinction between human-created and computer-created programming.

D: No. This example presents no fundamental separation of beauty and art. In the passage, reason is not the goal of the body. Rather, reason stands against the body.

3.   **D**   This is a Structure question.
   Note: In the first paragraph and in the reference to Chomsky as a follower of Descartes in the second paragraph, the author presents Chomsky's philosophy of language and his separation between mind and the physical as analogous and linked to Descartes' philosophy. Look for an answer choice that addresses this structural purpose.
   A: No. In this paragraph, the author presents language as analogous to reason within two distinct philosophical frameworks (Chomsky versus Descartes). The author does not argue here that language is linked to reason.
   B: No. The author does not link Descartes to Chomsky's politics.
   C: No. Although the author attributes this claim to Chomsky, it is not clear that the author agrees with it. Furthermore, Descartes is not directly connected to any claims about language.
   D: **Yes. The author states that Descartes' reason is analogous to Chomsky's language in order to clarify the centrality of language to Chomsky's understanding of human nature. Paragraph 2 affirms that Chomsky has been influenced by Descartes.**

4.   **B**   This is a Strengthen question.
   Note: The question stem asks you to strengthen the 2nd paragraph's claim that anarchy is politically ideal, an argument attributed to Chomsky on the grounds that maximum freedom is an inherent good for human nature. Look for new information that strengthens this argument.
   A: No. This information clarifies free will but is not directly relevant to the topic of political systems.
   B: **Yes. Chomsky's argument that government is inherently oppressive, and that minimizing government maximizes freedom, assumes that government does not play a significant role in preventing some people from taking away the rights and freedoms of others. This answer choice affirms that assumption.**
   C: No. This would weaken the claim, since it would suggest that anarchy does not, in fact, produce a situation of "maximum freedom" for all people. Note that this choice is essentially the opposite of choice B.
   D: No. The question of whether the government itself exercises free will is not relevant to the question of what form of political system allows human beings the maximum freedom.

5.   **A**   This is a New Information/Weaken question.
   Note: The point of the new information is that studying the brain and physical processes does in fact give insight into language, contradicting Chomsky's position in the first paragraph. The correct answer will be another claim made by Chomsky that is linked to the idea that language is separate from physical processes.
   A.   **Yes. In paragraph 4, animals are linked to the physical world, and Chomsky's denial of human beings' "animal nature" in the last paragraph is also linked to a denial of the role of the body. If all verbal communication is related to the physical functioning of the brain, this will link human and animal communication.**
   B.   No. The link between language and brain processes does suggest that the human mind has a material aspect, but this does not directly undermine the claim that human nature does not include a need for material possessions, which is the basis of Chomsky's argument against capitalism.

C. No. This is a claim made by the author of the passage rather than by Chomsky. Furthermore, Chomsky's philosophy may still be consistent even if he is wrong.

D. No. The connection of language to brain processes does not challenge the claim that all language shares a universal essence, though it may suggest that Chomsky is wrong to see the universal essence as not containing a physical component.

6. **C** This is an Inference question.
Note: The correct answer will be the title most consistent with Chomsky's views as they are described in the passage.

A: No. This article would be in favor of capitalism and acquiring material possessions (the fruits of one's labor). Chomsky is opposed to capitalism and possessions.

B: No. This title would be inconsistent with Chomsky's views as described in the passage; Chomsky understands language, reason, and free will as distinct from physical processes.

C: **Yes. In paragraph 3 Chomsky argues that human nature is fundamentally opposed to a focus on material possessions (goods) and corporate greed.**

D: No. Chomsky understands language as highly rational and structured, not free, and he does not include poetic language in his writings (last paragraph).

SOLUTIONS TO PRACTICE PASSAGE 3

Note: When a passage is this difficult to understand (and this is as hard as it gets), don't try to get a deep understanding of the text, and do use aggressive POE when answering the questions. In these solutions, we'll focus on identifying the most efficient way to eliminate each wrong answer and to recognize the "least wrong choice," even if the meaning of the text was still something of a mystery to you.

1. **B** This is a Main Point question.

A: No. This choice leaves out any reference to childbirth, which is a major theme in the passage.

B: **Yes. This is the only choice that mentions all of the major themes while remaining consistent with the passage. Of particular note is that it is the only answer choice to mention jouissance and the prerequisites of communication and the social order, which are key points in both the second and the third paragraphs.**

C: No. There is nothing in the passage about "reprogramming" after childbirth. Also, there is no suggestion that women have an actual memory of the biological foundation of the species which they then lose after childbirth. This choice takes certain references in the passage too literally.

D: No. This choice is too broad and brings in outside knowledge. It begins in a promising way, since borders and boundaries appear in the passage. However, this choice goes on to take words out of context ("need to bifurcate her needs and desires") and to misrepresent the intent of the author in discussing psychosis, which is used as an analogy rather than as a literal discussion of a mental disorder. Also note that psychosis is only mentioned twice, in passing, in the beginning and end of the passage, while this choice presents it as the major theme.

2. **A** This is an Inference question.

A: **Yes. The sentence in the passage says: "Yet, swaying between these two positions can only mean, for the woman involved, that she is within an "enceinte" *separating her from the world* of everyone else." Choice A is the only one of the first three answers to have this theme of division or separation. Try replacing "enceinte" in the passage with "partition," and the sentence appears to make sense. Choice D does have that theme of division as well, but there is no issue of a wall or town in the passage; it is talking about a pregnant woman (see also paragraph 3, which clarifies the fact that the author is talking in part about pregnancy in the second paragraph). If you keep it simple and don't over-think it, choice A can emerge fairly easily as the correct choice.**

B: No. This answer can be tempting if you speak French; "enceinte" as an adjective can mean "pregnant." However, the word in the passage is used to describe a result of pregnancy or motherhood rather than the state of being pregnant itself. Try inserting the answer into the sentence: neither "she is within a conception," nor "a conception or conceived woman" makes sense.

C: No. This choice is appealing because the passage states that "an 'enceinte' woman loses... meaning." However, this is a result of being within an "enceinte," not the meaning of "enceinte" itself.

D: No. While this choice has the theme of partition or separation, there is no mention or suggestion of a town, or of a literal wall around a town, in the passage. As with choice B, this answer can be tempting to people who speak French, but this choice doesn't correspond to the context of the word in the passage.

3. **D** This is an Inference question.

A: No. To eliminate both choices A and B, pay attention to how the author uses language to indicate what she does and does not accept as valid. In the passage she states that what a psychotic or pregnant woman experiences is seen "in the eyes of a Westerner" as regression. The next sentence begins "And yet it is jouissance," suggesting that the Westerners would be wrong, and regression is in fact not what a pregnant or psychotic woman experiences. This eliminates choices A and B.

B: No. See explanation for choice A.

C: No. The reference to art comes up in the next paragraph, in a different context. To see that it doesn't apply to the discussion of regression, it helps to note that there is a negative tone used by the author to discuss the idea of regression, while no such negative tone appears in the author's later discussion of "art" (beginning of paragraph 3).

D: **Yes. What is regressive, according to the passage is an "extinction of symbolic capabilities." Comparing the four choices, this is most similar to "loss of language" (note also the matching negative tone). You don't have to understand the meaning of "symbolic" to get the credited response for this question—the indicator words should be enough—but it would help you better understand the entire passage if you do figure out what "symbolic" means, since it recurs throughout. Its definition is hidden in the second parenthetical phrase in the second sentence of the third paragraph; there, the author suggests that "language" is associated with "the symbolic" in this passage.**

4. **C**   This is a Structure question.

    Note: The author's reference to "peace" sits within a sentence that includes several examples: "Here, alterity becomes nuance, contradiction becomes variant, tension becomes passage, and discharge becomes peace." The sentence preceding this sentence states: "And yet it is jouissance, but like a negative of the one, tied to an object, that is borne by the unfailingly masculine libido." Finally, the use of the word "this" at the beginning of the beginning of the next sentence indicates that "peace" is part of the "tendency towards equalization." All of this suggests that "peace" is related to "jouissance," and that it is not related to the "masculine libido."

    A: No. The author indicates that "peace" is related to "jouissance," and "jouissance" is the "negative" or opposite of the masculine libido.

    B: No. "Peace" is connected to "jouissance," which is contrasted with "regression" (in the same way as you saw in Question 3, choice A). What a psychotic or pregnant woman experiences is seen "in the eyes of a Westerner" as regression. The next sentence begins: "And yet it is jouissance," suggesting that the Westerners would be wrong, and regression is not jouissance. Note that when the author writes "This tendency towards equalization, *which is seen as a regressive extinction of symbolic capabilities*, does not, however, reduce differences," the phrase "which is seen as a regressive extinction of symbolic capacities" refers to the views of "Westerners" which the author rejects.

    C: **Yes. "Peace" is connected by the author to "jouissance," which is connected to "a tendency towards equalization" or balancing.**

    D: No. The author states that "this tendency towards equalization…does not, however, reduce differences" or eradicate distinctions.

5. **C**   This is an Inference question.

    Note: Language is discussed most directly in the third paragraph. To get what the author is saying is and is not true of language, pay close attention to words indicating contrasts. This will help you to eliminate choices that refer to things that are contrasted with, or distinguished from, language.

    A: No. In the second sentence of the third paragraph, the author writes: "A woman also attains [this limit] (and in our society, *especially*) through the strange form of split symbolization (threshold of language and instinctual drive, of the "symbolic" and the "semiotic") of which the act of giving birth consists." This sentence contrasts language and "instinctual drive," rather than suggesting that language is the basis for that drive.

    B: No. Toward the end of the third paragraph the author states, "If it is true that every national language has its own dream language and unconscious, then each of the sexes—a division so much more archaic and fundamental than the one into languages—would have its own unconscious wherein the biological and social program of the species would be ciphered in *confrontation with language*, exposed to its influence, but *independent from it*." This sentence suggests that the biological program or destiny of the species is independent of language.

    C: **Yes. In the third paragraph, the author claims that the division between the sexes is "so much more archaic and fundamental than" that between the national languages. Thus, gender precedes language and is more innate, or intrinsic.**

    D: No. This is given as a hypothetical in this passage—"*If* it is true that every national language has its own dream language and unconscious"—and the author does not take a side beyond that.

SOLUTIONS TO PRACTICE PASSAGE 4

1. **C**   This is a Retrieval Roman numeral question.
   I: False. Although Jeanne d'Arc was a commoner, this trait is described as unexpected (paragraph 2) and as depriving her in part of the support of the French aristocracy (paragraph 4). The passage does not state that it contributed positively to her influence.
   II: True. Paragraph 3 identifies her patriotism as a critical component of her influence.
   III: True. Paragraph 2 identifies her courage as a critical contribution.

2. **A**   This is an Inference question.
   A: **Yes. In paragraphs 2 and 3, the author describes Jeanne d'Arc as filling a role that the historical moment demanded. The French were ready for a leader and were anxious to overthrow the English. This, as well as the recognition in the last paragraph that a larger shift toward hope was not directly linked to Jeanne D'Arc, suggests that another leader (perhaps also uniting patriotism and piety) could have fulfilled a similar uniting role.**
   B: No. The passage states in the second paragraph that the French saw unity under a king as the solution to English rule, not that English rule was increasing or likely to be permanent.
   C: No. These are presented only as signs of troubling times. There is no indication that they would increase.
   D: No. The second paragraph states that the French were ready for such unity. The third paragraph suggests that the historical moment was ready for unity to come about.

3. **C**   This is a New Information/Inference question.
   A: No. The passage already indicates that Jeanne D'Arc's leadership was strongly rooted in faith. Furthermore, there is nothing in the new information that would suggest that she would be less oriented toward French nationalism.
   B: No. Her threat to the English came from her claiming divine authority. This new information would uphold that claim.
   C: **Yes. The passage speculates that one reason the French aristocracy made no move to win her release was that the nobility was embarrassed at her being a peasant (paragraph 4). The new information would remove this obstacle.**
   D: No. There is no indication in the passage that Jeanne d'Arc's status as a peasant had any relationship to the response to her death.

4. **B**   This is a Structure question.
   Note: Look for information directly linked to the claim that Jeanne d'Arc combined pro-French patriotism and faith in a distinctive way.
   A: No. That the English occupation could not endure is described as a consequence of the new French unity, but is not linked to Jeanne d'Arc's religious significance in any way.
   B: **Yes. The author explains the English motivation to have her condemned by the church as a direct outgrowth of her claims that God wanted a united France under a French king (paragraph 4).**
   C: No. The aristocrats' discomfort is not linked in any way to her patriotism or faith.
   D: No. Although her rapid success is remarkable, the passage does not directly connect this to her combination of patriotism and faith.

5. **D** This is a Strengthen question.

Note: The question asks for new historical evidence that would most strengthen the claim that England was going to lose. Look for new information directly relevant to this claim.

A: No. This fact shows her military leadership but is not relevant to what would happen after her death.

B: No. That the English were frustrated and brutal does not provide direct evidence that they were likely to lose the war. Note that this information does not say that the French people were resisting more strongly than they had before.

C: No. This information does relate to Jeanne d'Arc's continuing influence, but it is not directly relevant to the outcome of a military struggle.

D: **Yes. This is concrete evidence that the military ground was shifting for England as the newly united French forces were gaining strength.**

6. **B** This is a variation on a Weaken question.

Note: The question stem asks for an explanation of Jeanne d'Arc's abandonment by the French nobility that is different from the fact that they were discomfited by her being a commoner. Look for a logical alternative explanation that does NOT contradict any other statements made in the passage.

A: No. This is, in effect, the same explanation as that offered in the question stem, that they did not like that she was a commoner.

B: **Yes. The idea that they were threatened by her claim to religious authority is an alternative explanation that fits the rest of the facts of the passage.**

C: No. The passage states that her combination of patriotism and faith in fact made her influential and effective, so this explanation would contradict the facts of the passage.

D: No. This provides no alternative explanation for the fact that the French abandoned her to certain death at the hands of the English. Given that the French were fighting the English, they would have no reason for taking an action that would not help them in that fight, unless there was some other motivation for those actions.

SOLUTIONS TO PRACTICE PASSAGE 5

Note: This passage text represents the level of the most difficult material you will see in the CARS section. However, the questions are doable if you focus on basic aspects of the passage: tone and structure. In particular, note the author's positive tone toward cyborgs, her negative tone toward "Western science and politics," and the contrast between the concept of the cyborg and more "traditional" ways of looking at the world. Don't try to understand every reference in the passage, many of which are not fully explained (e.g., "salvation history" or "oedipal calendar" in paragraph 1). Keep your focus on the basics, and you can make your way through the questions at a reasonable pace.

1. **A** This is a Specific Attitude question.

A: **Yes. In paragraph 1, the author calls Western science and politics racist and says they have a tradition of male-dominated capitalism, among other things; immediately afterwards, she advocates a socialist-feminist, post-gender point of view. (Note the wording the author uses to express her own opinion: "This [essay] is an argument for pleasure in the confusion of boundaries...It is also an effort to contribute to....") She is therefore criticizing the traditions of Western science and politics.**

CRITICAL ANALYSIS AND REASONING SKILLS

B: No. Nowhere in the passage does the author suggest that Western science and politics' net effect has been positive. Rather, the author expresses a negative attitude toward Western science and politics; she is arguing that these views should be replaced (see paragraph 1).

C: No. While in the last paragraph, the author acknowledges that cyborgs are the "illegitimate children" of "militarism and patriarchal capitalism," and while she does suggest an opposition between cyborgs and "Western" capitalism, she does not go so far as to say that Western science and politics are the *only* things in opposition to cyborgs.

D: No. The author uses a negative tone in her discussion of Western science and politics in the first paragraph. See the explanation for choice A above.

2. **C** This is a Structure question.

A: No. Be sure to read carefully. While this quotation is close in terms of location in the passage to the author's statement about "the main trouble with cyborgs" (which sounds negative), the word "But" in the sentence preceding the quotation in question signals a shift in reasoning. The author is therefore suggesting that this origin may in fact not be a drawback; cyborgs may *not* reflect or reproduce negative aspects of their origin. The "after all" in the quotation continues and supports the shift indicated by the word "But," suggesting that cyborgs' fathers, that is, militarism and patriarchal capitalism, become unimportant.

B: No. The author is not talking about parenting in general (rather, only about the origin of cyborgs), nor is she speaking literally about parenthood. Make sure not to take words out of the context of the passage.

C: **Yes. "Inconsequential" is a good synonym of "inessential." Also, saying that cyborgs are the "illegitimate offspring" of certain elements is to say those elements are their origins. By saying "illegitimate offspring are often exceedingly unfaithful to their origins" in the sentence preceding the quotation in question, the author is suggesting that there is potential for cyborgs to subvert (go against) their origins.**

D: No. This option garbles some of the language and concepts of the passage—in particular the concept of the cyborg as a hybrid of organism and machine—with irrelevant material about human reproduction. There is no discussion in this paragraph or in the passage as a whole of actual human reproduction (i.e., making babies). As with choice B, make sure not to take vocabulary for the passage out of context.

3. **C** This is an Attitude question.

A: No. The author expresses an overall positive attitude toward cyborgs. While the author does refer to the "main trouble" with cyborgs in the last paragraph (that is, their origin), she goes on to suggest that this may in fact not be a significant problem, since "offspring are often exceedingly unfaithful to their origins."

B: No. Nowhere in the passage does the author discuss humans' obsession with technology and machines, nor does she suggest that cyborgs represent a negative consequence of such an obsession. Make sure not to bring in outside knowledge or opinion (or science fiction movies that you may have seen).

C: **Yes. At the end of the first paragraph, the author indicates that in the cyborg world, some of the most terrible monsters are also the most promising: this suggests a contradiction. Furthermore, in the final paragraph she calls cyborgs "oppositional." Finally, by suggesting that we are all cyborgs (paragraph one), that the concept of cyborg stands against "Western" traditions of racism, etc., and that her essay is a call for a different way of seeing things, based on the concept of the cyborg, the author is suggesting that cyborgs are positive things.**

D: No. This answer is too limited. While the author, at the end of the first paragraph, talks about "terrible" monsters in the cyborg world, this answer does not reflect the positive language ("promising monsters") featured in the same section of the passage. There is also no discussion of a need to fear cyborgs. Rather, you need to understand them and how the concept of the cyborg relates to the nature of our culture (paragraph 1).

4. **A** This is a Retrieval question.
   I: **True. See the first sentence of the passage: "…we are all chimeras, theorized and fabricated hybrids of machine and organism; in short, we are cyborgs."**
   II: False. The author states the opposite. In the second paragraph, she says that the cyborg "has no truck with…seductions to organic wholeness."
   III: False. In the final paragraph, the author says that cyborgs are "completely without innocence."

5. **D** This is a Primary Purpose question.
   A: No. While this is in the passage (paragraph 1), it is only part of the author's argument, not the whole of it (for example, where are the cyborgs in this choice?).
   B: No. There is no call to action for us to become cyborgs; in fact, in the opening sentences of the passage the author says that we are already all cyborgs.
   C: No. This choice garbles the language of the passage to make a statement that actually opposes the author's central point, which is that we should find "*pleasure* in the confusion of boundaries" (paragraph one). Note that the cyborg is a hybrid or combination of "machine and organism" (paragraph 1); that is, neither one nor the other. One potential point of confusion is that the author opposes the "myth of original unity" (paragraph 2) and rejects the idea of "attempting to heal the terrible cleavages of gender in an oral symbiotic utopia" (paragraph 1). This does not mean, however, that the author is arguing for maintaining or creating boundaries or parameters. Rather, she is arguing that such clear boundaries (machine/organism, male/female, etc.) don't exist in the first place.
   D: **Yes. The author explicitly tells us her purpose in the first paragraph: "This [essay] is an argument for *pleasure* in the confusion of boundaries and for *responsibility* in their construction. It is also an effort to contribute to socialist-feminist culture and theory in a postmodernist, non-naturalist mode and in the utopian tradition of imagining a world without gender, which is perhaps a world without genesis, but maybe also a world without end." Since she spends most of the passage discussing cyborgs, this is also a crucial element: The cyborg is central to this confusion of boundaries discussed by the author.**

SOLUTIONS TO PRACTICE PASSAGE 6

1. **D** This is a Structure question.
   Note: The winter rituals are presented in paragraph 2 as an example of the dominant themes of ceremony, submission to destiny, and communal unity, in contrast with the misinterpretation directly prior. Look for the answer choice that describes this structural function.
   A: No. This is not the author's argument in this paragraph, so this answer choice does not address the logical purpose of the cited reference.
   B: No. Although the author indicates that ritual probably does do that, this is not the purpose of the author in mentioning these rituals. Rather, the author's argument in this part of the passage is that ritual was not intended as a means of controlling nature.

C: No. This example does help correct a misinterpretation, but this answer choice describes the misinterpretation inaccurately. There was no suggestion that people did control the weather, only that according to some (misguided) interpretations they were attempting to.

D: **Yes. This example establishes ritual as functioning to prepare the community "with the rest of nature" to submit and also links back to the beginning of the paragraph in which the author describes rites as connecting community and cosmos.**

2. **B** This is a New Information/Strengthen question.
Note: The main point of the new information is that traditional religions are too attached to particular groups and narrow purposes to function as they should. Look for an answer choice that comes from the passage and supports this idea.

A: No. This statement somewhat weakens the new claim. If mythology focuses on continuity, it would undermine the author's new claim that great religions are linked to factions and narrow propaganda.

B: **Yes. This claim from paragraph 6 argues that no system attached to some particular social group is religiously adequate. This would strengthen the author's claim that world religions associated with particular factions cannot meet humanity's requirements.**

C: No. This statement addresses a contrast between a mystical or mechanical understanding of humanity's relationship to the cosmos. This shift is not directly relevant to the author's new claim concerning the limitations of a religion focused on factions and particular groups.

D: No. This statement somewhat weakens the new claim by indicating that mythologies adapt to fit the requirements of each age. The new claim states that religions cannot meet the requirements of the current age.

3. **D** This is an Inference question.

A: No. The author does discuss that many contemporary people choose to look at mythology as lies (paragraph 5), but the author's argument is that mythology has a function that adapts in the contemporary world.

B: No. This answer choice matches the discussion of ritual in the second paragraph, but this is a description the author offers of how ceremony functioned in the past. It is not a description of the current role of mythology.

C: No. The tone of the passage toward mythology is positive. There is no suggestion that mythology is dangerous.

D: **Yes. In the first paragraph, the author describes various functions mythology has performed and describes its adaptable nature. The rest of the passage explores relationships of individual, community, and cosmos.**

4. **A** This is an Inference question.
Note: In context, this statement is part of a description of the significance in the contemporary world of exploring the nature of the individual human being, separate from particular communities, in order to guide us toward a broader understanding of our connection to what is universal.

A: **Yes. The author seeks a mythology not limited by specific communities or factions, but one which will reach a more universal, divine truth.**

B: No. The author is not criticizing individualism here, but is instead being restricted to a particular community or outlook.

C: No. This answer choices reverses the author's point that the contemporary world requires a more individual-oriented mythology than the ancient world did.

D: No. There is no discussion here of an encounter between two individuals.

5. **C**   This is an Analogy question.

  Note: The shift in paragraph 4 is described as a reversal. Formerly, meaning was in the group not the individual. Now no meaning is in the group, all is in the individual. Find the answer choice that parallels this shift.

  A: No. There is no shift from a smaller range to a larger range described in the passage.

  B: No. The shift here is described as a continuation rather than a reversal, and it is not properly a contrast between group and individual.

  C: **Yes. This shift captures a shift from focusing on the communal, shared aspects, to a focus on individual meanings with a larger purpose.**

  D: No. This shift represents a reversal of the relationship, moving from the individual to the group, rather than vice versa.

6. **B**   This is a Weaken question.

  Note: According to the author, the dominant motive in religious rituals (paragraph 2) is submission to destiny and creating unity, not controlling nature. Therefore, the correct answer will suggest that controlling nature IS in fact the motive.

  A: No. This shift in the portrayal of divine beings is not directly relevant to the function of the myths or the motives of ceremonies linked to them.

  B: **Yes. This ritual explicitly seeks to control nature and alter the normal weather pattern (the recurring dry season). This challenges the author's claim that it is a misunderstanding to see ceremonies as attempting to control nature.**

  C: No. This ritual would fit the passage theme of rituals uniting communities with nature.

  D: No. This ritual practice would strengthen the author's description in paragraph 2 about how rituals relate to communities and to nature.

Part III

The Science Sections

Chapter 10
Science Sections Overview

10.1 SCIENCE SECTIONS OVERVIEW

There are three science sections on the MCAT:

- Chemical and Physical Foundations of Biological Systems
- Biological and Biochemical Foundations of Living Systems
- Psychological, Social, and Biological Foundations of Behavior

The Chemical and Physical Foundations of Biological Systems section (Chem/Phys) is the first section on the test. It includes questions from General Chemistry (about 30%), Physics (about 25%), Organic Chemistry (about 15%), Biochemistry (about 25%), and Biology (about 5%). Further, the questions often test chemical and physical concepts within a biological setting: for example, pressure and fluid flow in blood vessels. A solid grasp of math fundamentals is required (arithmetic, algebra, graphs, trigonometry, vectors, proportions, and logarithms); however, there are no calculus-based questions.

The Biological and Biochemical Foundations of Living Systems section (Bio/Biochem) is the third section on the test. Approximately 65% of the questions in this section come from biology, approximately 25% come from biochemistry, and approximately 10% come from Organic and General Chemistry. Math calculations are generally not required on this section of the test; however, a basic understanding of statistics as used in biological research is helpful.

The Psychological, Social, and Biological Foundations of Behavior section (Psych/Soc) is the fourth and final section on the test. About 60% of the questions will be drawn from Psychology, about 30% from Sociology, and about 10% from Biology. As with the Bio/Biochem section, calculations are generally not required; however, a basic understanding of statistics as used in research is helpful.

Most of the questions in the science sections (44 of the 59) are passage-based, and each section has ten passages. Passages consist of a few paragraphs of information and include descriptions of experiments, as well as equations, reactions, graphs, figures, tables, and experimental apparatus. Four to six questions will be associated with each passage.

The remaining 25% of the questions (15 of 59) in each science section are freestanding questions (FSQs). These questions appear in approximately four groups interspersed between the passages, generally after passages 2, 5, 8, and 10. Each group contains three to five questions.

95 minutes are allotted to each of the science sections. This breaks down to approximately one minute and 35 seconds per question.

10.2 SCIENCE PASSAGE TYPES

The passages in the science sections fall into one of three main categories: Information and/or Situation Presentation, Experiment/Research Presentation, or Persuasive (or Scientific) Reasoning.

Information and/or Situation Presentation

These passages either present straightforward scientific information or they describe a particular event or occurrence. Generally, questions associated with these passages test basic science facts or ask you to predict outcomes given new variables or new information. Here is an example of an Information/Situation Presentation passage:

> Figure 1 shows a portion of the inner mechanism of a typical home smoke detector. It consists of a pair of capacitor plates which are charged by a 9-volt battery (not shown). The capacitor plates (electrodes) are connected to a sensor device, D; the resistor R denotes the internal resistance of the sensor. Normally, air acts as an insulator and no current would flow in the circuit shown. However, inside the smoke detector is a small sample of an artificially produced radioactive element, americium-241, which decays primarily by emitting alpha particles, with a half-life of approximately 430 years. The daughter nucleus of the decay has a half-life in excess of two million years and therefore poses virtually no biohazard.

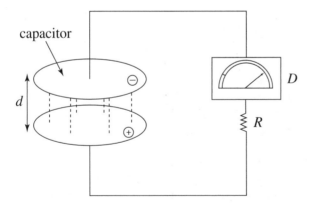

Figure 1 Smoke detector mechanism

> The decay products (alpha particles and gamma rays) from the ^{241}Am sample ionize air molecules between the plates and thus provide a conducting pathway which allows current to flow in the circuit shown in Figure 1. A steady-state current is quickly established and remains as long as the battery continues to maintain a 9-volt potential difference between its terminals. However, if smoke particles enter the space between the capacitor plates and thereby interrupt the flow, the current is reduced, and the sensor responds to this change by triggering

the alarm. (Furthermore, as the battery starts to "die out," the resulting drop in current is also detected to alert the homeowner to replace the battery.)

$$C = \varepsilon_0 \frac{A}{d}$$

Equation 1

where ε_0 is the universal permittivity constant, equal to 8.85 $\times 10^{-12}$ C^2/(N·m^2). Since the area A of each capacitor plate in the smoke detector is 20 cm^2 and the plates are separated by a distance d of 5 mm, the capacitance is 3.5×10^{-12} F = 3.5 pF.

Experiment/Research Presentation

These passages present the details of experiments and research procedures. They often include data tables and graphs. Generally, questions associated with these passages ask you to interpret data, draw conclusions, and make inferences. Here is an example of an Experiment/Research Presentation passage:

The development of sexual characteristics depends upon various factors, the most important of which are hormonal control, environmental stimuli, and the genetic makeup of the individual. The hormones that contribute to the development include the steroid hormones estrogen, progesterone, and testosterone, as well as the pituitary hormones FSH (follicle-stimulating hormone) and LH (luteinizing hormone).

To study the mechanism by which estrogen exerts its effects, a researcher performed the following experiments using cell culture assays.

Experiment 1:

Human embryonic placental mesenchyme (HEPM) cells were grown for 48 hours in Dulbecco's Modified Eagle Medium (DMEM), with media change every 12 hours. Upon confluent growth, cells were exposed to a 10 mg per mL solution of green fluorescent-labeled estrogen for 1 hour. Cells were rinsed with DMEM and observed under confocal fluorescent microscopy.

Experiment 2:

HEPM cells were grown to confluence as in Experiment 1. Cells were exposed to Pesticide A for 1 hour, followed by the 10 mg/mL solution of labeled estrogen, rinsed as in Experiment 1, and observed under confocal fluorescent microscopy.

Experiment 3:

Experiment 1 was repeated with Chinese Hamster Ovary (CHO) cells instead of HEPM cells.

Experiment 4:

CHO cells injected with cytoplasmic extracts of HEPM cells were grown to confluence, exposed to the 10 mg/mL solution of labeled estrogen for 1 hour, and observed under confocal fluorescent microscopy.

The results of these experiments are given in Table 1.

Experiment	Media	Cytoplasm	Nucleus
1	+	+	+
2	+	+	+
3	+	+	+
4	+	+	+

Table 1 Detection of Estrogen (+ indicates presence of Estrogen)

After observing the cells in each experiment, the researcher bathed the cells in a solution containing 10 mg per mL of a red fluorescent probe that binds specifically to the estrogen receptor only when its active site is occupied. After 1 hour, the cells were rinsed with DMEM and observed under confocal fluorescent microscopy. The results are presented in Table 2.

The researcher also repeated Experiment 2 using Pesticide B, an estrogen analog, instead of Pesticide A. Results from other researchers had shown that Pesticide B binds to the active site of the cytosolic estrogen receptor (with an affinity 10,000 times greater than that of estrogen) and causes increased transcription of mRNA.

Experiment	Media	Cytoplasm	Nucleus	Estrogen effects observed?
1	G only	G and R	G and R	Yes
2	G only	G only	G only	No
3	G only	G only	G only	No
4	G only	G and R	G and R	Yes

Table 2 Observed Fluorescence and Estrogen Effects (G = green, R = red)

Based on these results, the researcher determined that estrogen had no effect when not bound to a cytosolic, estrogen-specific receptor.

Persuasive (Scientific) Reasoning

These passages typically present a scientific phenomenon, along with a hypothesis that explains the phenomenon, and may include counterarguments as well. Questions associated with these passages ask you to evaluate the hypothesis or arguments. Persuasive Reasoning passages in the science sections of the MCAT tend to be less common than Information Presentation or Experiment-based passages. Here is an example of a Persuasive Reasoning passage:

Two theoretical chemists attempted to explain the observed trends of acidity by applying two interpretations of molecular orbital theory. Consider the pK_a values of some common acids listed along with the conjugate base:

acid	pK_a	conjugate base
H_2SO_4	< 0	HSO_4^-
H_2CrO_4	5.0	$HCrO_4^-$
H_2PO_4	2.1	$H_2PO_4^-$
HF	3.9	F^-
HOCl	7.8	ClO^-
HCN	9.5	CN^-
HIO_3	1.2	IO_3^-

Recall that acids with a $pK_a < 0$ are called strong acids, and those with a $pK_a > 0$ are called weak acids. The arguments of the chemists are given below.

Chemist #1:

"The acidity of a compound is proportional to the polarization of the H—X bond, where X is some nonmetal element. Complex acids, such as H_2SO_4, $HClO_4$, and HNO_3, are strong acids because the H—O bonding electrons are strongly drawn towards the oxygen. It is generally true that a covalent bond weakens as its polarization increases. Therefore, one can conclude that the strength of an acid is proportional to the number of electronegative atoms in that acid."

Chemist #2:

"The acidity of a compound is proportional to the number of stable resonance structures of that acid's conjugate base. H_2SO_4, $HClO_4$, and HNO_3 are all strong acids because their respective conjugate bases exhibit a high degree of resonance stabilization."

Mapping a Passage

"Mapping a passage" refers to the combination of on-screen highlighting and scratch paper notes that you take while working through a passage. Typically, good things to highlight include the overall topic of a paragraph, unfamiliar terms, italicized terms, unusual terms, numerical values, hypotheses, and experimental results. Scratch paper notes can be used to summarize the paragraphs and to jot down important facts and connections that are made when reading the passage or as questions are answered. More details on passage mapping will be presented in the subject-specific chapters.

10.3 SCIENCE QUESTION TYPES

Questions in the science sections are generally one of three main types: Memory, Explicit, or Implicit.

Memory Questions

These questions can be answered directly from prior knowledge, with no need to reference the passage or question text. Memory questions represent approximately 25 percent of the science questions on the MCAT. Usually, Memory questions are typically found as FSQs. They can also be tucked into a passage, but this is far less common. Here's an example of a Memory question:

Which of the following acetylating conditions will convert diethylamine into an amide at the fastest rate?

A)   Acetic acid / HCl
B)   Acetic anhydride
C)   Acetyl chloride
D)   Ethyl acetate

Explicit Questions

Explicit questions can be answered primarily with information from the passage, along with prior knowledge. They may require data retrieval, graph analysis, or making a simple connection. Explicit questions make up approximately 35–40 percent of the science questions on the MCAT; here's an example (taken from the Information/Situation Presentation passage):

The sensor device *D* shown in Figure 1 performs its function by acting as:

A) an ohmmeter.
B) a voltmeter.
C) a potentiometer.
D) an ammeter.

Implicit Questions

These questions require you to take information from the passage, combine it with your prior knowledge, apply it to a new situation, and come to some logical conclusion. They typically require more complex connections than do Explicit questions, and they may also require data retrieval, graph analysis, etc. Implicit questions usually require a solid understanding of the passage information. They make up approximately 35–40 percent of the science questions on the MCAT; here's an example (taken from the Experiment/Research Presentation passage):

If Experiment 2 were repeated, but this time exposing the cells first to Pesticide A and then to Pesticide B before exposing them to the green fluorescent-labeled estrogen and the red fluorescent probe, which of the following statements will most likely be true?

A) Pesticide A and Pesticide B bind to the same site on the estrogen receptor.
B) Estrogen effects would be observed.
C) Only green fluorescence would be observed.
D) Both green and red fluorescence would be observed.

10.4 ATTACKING THE QUESTIONS

More detail on question attack will be presented in the individual science subject chapters, but here's a brief overview of the most useful techniques:

- Using Process of Elimination (POE) is the best way to attack any MCAT question. Every answer choice that you eliminate increases your probability of choosing the correct answer. Roman numeral questions are particularly good to answer using POE.
- Do the passages within a section and the questions within a passage in the order that you want; easiest first, harder later. You don't get any more points for a hard question than you do for an easy one.
- Make sure the answer you choose actually answers the question and isn't just a true statement.
- Don't get tripped up in the LEAST/EXCEPT/NOT questions. These questions ask you to pick the incorrect or false statement.
- Remember that there cannot be two correct choices, thus if two answers say the same thing, they can both be eliminated.
- For calculations, use approximations whenever possible, and make sure you take units into consideration.
- Don't leave any question blank; there is no guessing penalty on the MCAT.

10.5 A FINAL THOUGHT

The next few chapters will address each science subject on the MCAT, presenting some of the nuances for that particular subject. However, the fact that you are using this book indicates that you are already scoring fairly well, which means that you are probably already mapping your passages and know how to tackle the questions effectively. We don't want to insult you by presenting information that is too basic, thus the chapters are intended primarily to give you an overview, not a great amount of detail.

Following each subject's overview chapter are FSQs and practice passages; most at a high level of difficulty. We know you want to hone your skills on the toughest material out there. Don't forget there is an additional full-length practice test in the Online Companion to this book found at www.PrincetonReview.com/Cracking, and don't forget to analyze your results using the skills you learned in Chapters 5 and 6.

Chapter 11
Biology and Biochemistry on the MCAT

11.1 BIOLOGY AND BIOCHEMISTRY ON THE MCAT

Biology and Biochemistry are by far the most information-dense subjects on the MCAT. MCAT Biology and Biochemistry topics span seven different semester-length courses (biochemistry, molecular biology, cell biology, microbiology, genetics, anatomy, and physiology). Further, the application of this material is potentially vast; passages can discuss anything from the details of some biochemical pathway to the complexities of genetic studies, to the subtleties of a condition caused by a missing or malfunctioning enzyme, to the nuances of an unusual disease. Fortunately, biology and biochemistry are the subjects that MCAT students typically find the most interesting, and the one they have the most background in. People who want to go to medical school have an inherent interest in biology; thus this subject, although vast, seems more manageable than all the others on the MCAT.

The science sections of the MCAT have 10 passages and 15 freestanding questions (FSQs). The Biological and Biochemical Foundations of Living Systems section (Bio/Biochem) is primarily biology (65%) and biochemistry (25%). The remaining 10% are General and Organic Chemistry questions. Further, Biology questions can show up in the Psychological, Social, and Biological Foundations of Behavior section (about 10%) and in the Chemical and Physical Foundations of Biological Systems section (about 5%). Note also that about 25% of the Chem/Phys section is Biochemistry, and frequently the passages and questions are biology-based.

11.2 TACKLING A BIOLOGY OR BIOCHEMISTRY PASSAGE

Generally speaking, time is not an issue in the Bio/Biochem section of the MCAT. Because students have a stronger background in biology than in other subjects, the passages seem more understandable; in fact, readers sometimes find themselves getting caught up and interested in the passage. Often, students report having about 5 to 10 minutes "left over" after completing the section. This means that an additional minute or so can potentially be spent on each passage, thinking and understanding.

Passage Types as They Apply to Biology and Biochemistry

Experiment/Research Presentation: Biology and Biochemistry

This is the most common type of Biology or Biochemistry passage. It typically presents the details behind an experiment along with data tables, graphs, and figures. Often these are the most difficult passages to deal with because they require an understanding of the reasoning behind the experiment, the logic to each step, and the ability to analyze the results and form conclusions. A basic understanding of biometry (basic statistics as they apply to biology and biochemistry research) is necessary.

Information/Situation Presentation: Biology and Biochemistry

This is the second most common type of Biology or Biochemistry passage on the MCAT. These passages generally appear as one of two variants: either a basic concept with additional levels of detail included (for example, all the detail you ever wanted to know about the electron transport chain), or a novel concept with ties to basic information (for example, a rare demyelinating disease). Either way, Biology and Biochemistry passages are notorious for testing concepts in unusual contexts. The key to dealing with these passages is to, first, not become anxious about all the stuff you might not know, and second, figure out how the basics you do know apply to the new situation. For example, you might be presented with a passage that introduces hormones you never heard of or novel drugs to combat diseases you didn't know existed. First, don't panic. Second, look for how these new things fit into familiar categories: for example, "peptide versus steroid" or "competitive inhibitor." Then answer the questions with these basics in mind.

That said, you have to know your basics. This will increase your confidence in answering freestanding questions, as well as increase the speed with which to find the information in the passage. The astute MCAT student will never waste time staring at a question thinking, "Should I know this?" Instead, because she has a solid understanding of the necessary core knowledge, she'll say, "No, I am NOT expected to know this, and I am going to look for it in the passage."

Persuasive Reasoning: Biology and Biochemistry

This is the least common Biology or Biochemistry passage type. It typically describes some biological or biochemical phenomenon and then offers one or more theories to explain it. Questions in Persuasive Reasoning passages ask you to determine support for one of the theories, or present new evidence and ask which theory is now contradicted.

One last thought about Biology and Biochemistry passages in general: Because the array of topics is so vast, these passages often pull questions from multiple areas of Biology and/or Biochemistry into a single, general topic. Consider, for example, a passage on renal function: Question topics could include basics about the kidney, transmembrane transport, autonomic control, blood pressure, hormones, biochemical energy needs, or a genetics question about a rare kidney disease. Or what about a passage on hemoglobin: question topics could include basics about enzymes and cooperative binding, protein structure, DNA mutations, effects of sickle cell disease, regulation of expression of the hemoglobin genes, or the data from an experiment done on sickle cell patients.

Reading a Biology or Biochemistry Passage

Although tempting, try not to get bogged down reading all the little details in a passage. Again, because most premeds have an inherent interest in biology and the mechanisms behind disease, it's very easy to get lost in the science behind the passages. In spite of having that "extra" time, you don't want to use it all up reading what isn't necessary. Each passage type requires a slightly different style of reading.

Information/Situation Presentation passages require the least reading. These should be skimmed to get an idea of the location of information within the passage. These passages include a fair amount of detail that you might not need, so save the reading of these details until a question comes up about them. Then go back and read for the finer nuances.

Experiment/Research Presentation passages require the most reading. You are practically guaranteed to get questions that ask you about the details of the experiment, why a particular step was carried out, why the results are what they are, how to interpret the data, or how the results might change if a particular variable is altered. It's worth spending a little more time reading to understand the experiment. However, because there will be a fair number of questions unrelated to the experiment, you might consider answering these first and then going back for the experiment details.

Persuasive Argument passages are somewhere in the middle. You can skim them for location of information, but you also want to spend a little time reading the details of and thinking about the arguments presented. It is extremely likely that you will be asked a question about them.

Advanced Reading Skills

To improve your ability to read and glean information from a passage, you need to practice. Be critical when you read the content; watch for vague areas or holes in the passage that aren't explained clearly. Remember that information about new topics will be woven throughout the passage; you may need to piece together information from several paragraphs and a figure to get the whole picture.

After you've read, highlighted, and mapped a passage (more on this in a bit), stop and ask yourself the following questions:

- What was this passage about? What was the conclusion or main point?
- Was there a paragraph that was mostly background?
- Were there paragraphs or figures that seemed useless?
- What information was found in each paragraph? Why was that paragraph there?
- Are there any holes in the story?
- What extra information could I have pulled out of the passage? What inferences or conclusions could I make?
- If something unique was explained or mentioned, what might be its purpose?
- What am I *not* being told?
- Can I summarize the purpose and/or results of the experiment in a few sentences?
- Were there any comparisons in the passage?

This takes a while at first, but eventually it will become second nature and you'll start doing it as you read the passage. If you have a study group you are working with, consider doing this as an exercise with your study partners. Take turns asking and answering the questions above. Having to explain something to someone else not only solidifies your own knowledge, but helps you see where you might be weak.

Mapping a Biology or Biochemistry Passage

Mapping a Biology or Biochemistry passage is a combination of highlighting and scratch paper notes that can help you organize and understand the passage information.

Resist the temptation to highlight everything! (Everyone has done this: You're reading a biology textbook with a highlighter, and then look back and realize that the whole page is yellow!) Restrict your highlighting to a few things:

- the main theme of a paragraph
- an unusual or unfamiliar term that is defined specifically for that passage (e.g., something that is italicized)
- statements that either support the main theme or contradict the main theme
- sometimes lists appear in paragraph form within a passage; highlight the general topic of the list
- relationships (how one thing changes relative to another thing)

Scratch paper should be organized. Make sure the passage number and its range of questions appears at the top of your scratch paper notes (e.g., Psg 3, Q10–14). This makes it easier to find a specific passage when looking at the review screen of the exam, which only lists question numbers. For each paragraph, note "P1," "P2," etc., on the scratch paper, and jot down a few notes about that paragraph. Try to translate biology/biochemistry jargon into your own words using everyday language (this is particularly useful for experiments). Make sure to note down simple relationships (e.g., the relationship between two variables), and if you've discovered a list in the passage (often in paragraph form), note its general topic.

Graph and Figure Analysis

Pay attention to graphs, figures, and data tables to see what type of information they present, but don't spend a lot of time analyzing at this point. For figures, note what information is being presented and look to see if anything stands out. For graphs, look at the axes, and again, look to see if anything stands out. If there is an outlier in pictures or graphs, there's a good chance you will be asked a question about it. Don't ponder *why* it's an outlier, just note that it exists. You can ponder the "why" if/when they ask the question.

Data tables, except for very simple ones, are generally large collections of numbers. Definitely do not analyze these unless you are asked a question that requires it. Below are some examples of figures and the info you could draw from them in a quick look.

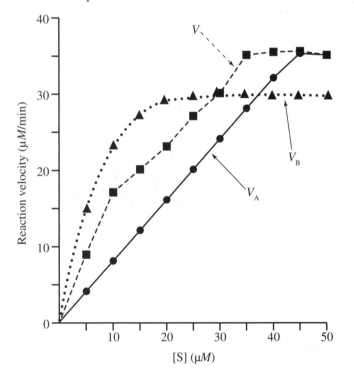

Figure 1 Graphs of data from Experiments 1, 2, and 3.

This is a straightforward V vs. [S] graph, so this is likely some kind of enzyme experiment with reaction rates of V_A and V_B lower than V. You would write " V vs. [S], V_A and V_B inhib?"

	Cardiolipin		Citrate synthase		NADH oxidase		mtDNA (copy #/ nuclear genome)	
Mean	Before	After	Before	After	Before	After	Before	After
Lean (*n* = 10)	70	109	2.4	3.2	0.45	0.63	2424	3005
Obese (*n* = 9)	72	83	3.7	5.2	0.16	0.29	2051	2210
T2DM (*n* = 11)	58	86	3.3	5.1	0.15	0.28	2150	2600
Std Error	Before	After	Before	After	Before	After	Before	After
Lean (*n* = 10)	6.1	5.2	0.2	0.4	0.1	0.12	150	300
Obese (*n* = 9)	7.9	4.8	0.3	0.5	0.05	0.1	350	375
T2DM (*n* = 11)	6.5	7.3	0.2	0.5	0.04	0.08	315	250

Table 1 Mean (upper rows) and standard error (lower rows) measurements for markers
of ETC activity, in relative units normalized to creatine kinase activity

There is a LOT of data presented here. A quick glance shows that they are comparing different markers, between three groups of individuals (lean, obese, and T2DM) before and after something. Nothing beyond that immediately jumps out, so you might note "Table 1, bef/aft data for lean, obese, diabetic."

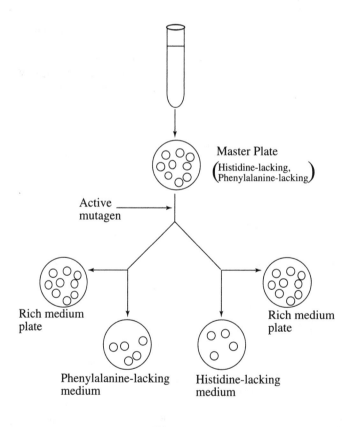

Figure 1

This looks like some kind of bacterial plating experiment, using different media. What jumps out here is that there are fewer colonies when there is no phenylalanine or histidine. You could note "Fig. 1 bact plating, no phe no his = ↓ colonies."

Disease	HLA Allele	Relative Risk
Type 1 Diabetes	HLA-DR3	5
	HLA-DR4	6
	HLA-DR3 + HLA-DR4	15
Autoimmune Hepatitis	HLA-DR3	14
Rheumatoid Arthritis	HLA-DR4	4
Sjögren Syndrome	HLA-DR3	10

Figure 1 Relative Risk and HLA-DR Haplotypes

This table shows the relative risk of different diseases based on the presence of a particular HLA allele. A quick glance shows the biggest relative risks are associated with HLA-DR3. You could write "HLA-DR3 ↑ most diseases."

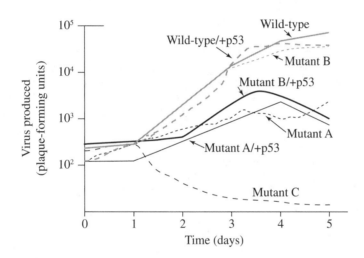

Figure 2

Mutant A adenovirus had the E1A gene deleted.
Mutant B adenovirus had the gene for E1B truncated due to the introduction of a premature stop codon.
Mutant C adenovirus had a point mutation in the gene encoding a viral capsid protein.

The axes indicate that this is a graph of viral reproduction over several days. Note that the units on the y-axis are not linear, but exponential. On a graph like this, you just want to see how different things group together. It looks like Mutant B seems to be growing just fine, as its line is very close to the wild type lines. However, when you add p53, Mutant B grows more like Mutant A, and Mutant C doesn't grow very well at all. You might note "virus vs time, exponent y-axis, wt and B high, Bp53 and A med, C poor." (Use abbreviations that make sense to you.)

Let's take a look at how we might highlight and map a passage. Below is a passage on the pentose phosphate pathway.

The pentose phosphate pathway (PPP) produces ribose-5-phosphate from glucose-6-phosphate and generates NADPH, which is used by the cell in biosynthetic pathways (such as fatty acid biosynthesis) as a reducing agent. Ribose-5-phosphate is converted to 5-phosphoribosyl-1-pyrophosphate (PRPP) by the enzyme ribose phosphate pyrophosphokinase. PRPP is an essential precursor in the biosynthesis of all nucleotides. Ribose phosphate pyrophosphokinase is inhibited by both ADP and GDP nucleotides.

The committed step in purine nucleotide synthesis is catalyzed by the enzyme amidophosphoribosyl transferase, which uses glutamine and PRPP as substrates. This enzyme is inhibited by AMP, and GMP and is activated by high concentrations of PRPP. An intermediate in purine biosynthesis is inosine monophosphate (IMP). The conversion of IMP to AMP is inhibited by AMP, and the conversion of IMP to GMP is inhibited by GMP. An essential precursor in pyrimidine biosynthesis is carbamoyl phosphate, which is generated by the enzyme carbamoyl phosphate synthase. This enzyme is inhibited by UTP and activated by ATP and PRPP. The production of CTP from UTP is inhibited by CTP. These reactions are summarized in Figure 1.

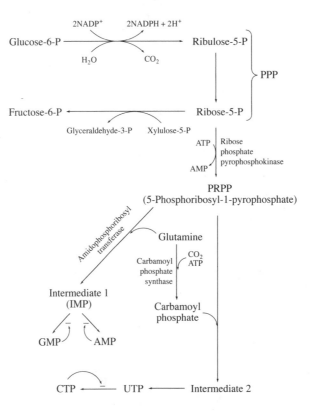

Figure 1 Biosynthetic pathway

Analysis and Passage Map

This passage is an Information Presentation passage and starts out with a paragraph about the pentose phosphate pathway. This is primarily a background paragraph and can be skimmed quickly, with a few words highlighted.

The second paragraph goes into more detail about the steps in purine and pyrimidine biosynthesis and specifically discusses some of the enzymes and their inhibitors. This paragraph presents information that is beyond what you are expected to know about the pentose phosphate pathway for the MCAT. Figure 1 shows some of the details of the pathway.

Here's what your passage map might look like:

> *P1 – pentose phosphate pathway, products and their uses*
> *P2 – committed step purines, enzyme and inhib.*
>   *precursor to pyrim., enzyme, and inhib.*
>   *Fig 1 = details of pathway*

Let's take a look at a different passage. Below and on the following page is an Experiment/Research Presentation passage.

In times of fasting, the body relies more heavily on catabolism of amino acids to produce either ketone bodies (in the case of ketogenic amino acids) or precursors of glucose (in the case of glucogenic amino acids) through a series of interactions involving an α-ketoacid intermediate. A representative reaction is shown in Figure 1.

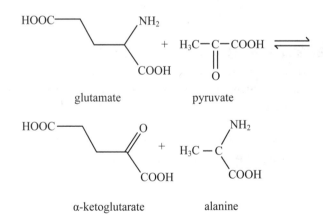

Figure 1 Interconversion of pyruvate and alanine

"Low carb" diets capitalize on this feature of metabolism to achieve a ketogenic state in which the body is chronically deprived of carbohydrate sources of energy and thus forced to produce ketone bodies from either fat or amino acids to obtain energy. Interested in changes in the makeup of energy molecules in blood during this ketogenic state, researchers measure the levels of ketone bodies, glucose, insulin, glucagon, and fatty acids at various time points after a participant begins a ketogenic diet. Their findings are shown below.

	After normal meal	Overnight fasting	2 days after starting diet	5 days after starting diet
Insulin	↑	↓	↓	↓
Glucagon	↓	↑	↑	↑
Glucose	Normal	Normal	Normal	Normal
Fatty Acids	↑	↓	↑	↑↑↑
Ketones	↓	↓	↑	↑↑↑

Figure 2   Results of experiment

Adapted from Harvey, R. A., & Ferrier, D. R. (2011). *Lippincott's illustrated reviews, biochemistry* (5th ed.). Philadelphia: Wolters Kluwer Health.

Analysis and Passage Map

This passage starts out by describing the effects of fasting on the body and how it turns to amino acid catabolism to generate ketones or glucose precursors. It mentions the involvement of an α-ketoacid intermediate; Figure 1 shows this reaction.

The second paragraph describes how "low carb" diets can lead to ketogenesis. It also describes the experiment and refers us to Figure 2 for the results of the experiment.

Here's how your map might look:

P1 – fasting, a.a. catabolism → ketones, glu. precursors
P2 – low carb diet effects, desc. of experiment
Fig 2 – keto diet causes ↑ glucagon, fats, and ketones and ↓ insulin

One last thought about passages: Remember that, as with all sections on the MCAT, you can do the passages in the order *you* want to. There are no extra points for taking the test in order. Generally, passages in the Bio/Biochem section will fall into one of four main subject groups:

- biochemistry
- other non-physiology
- physiology
- organic/general chemistry

Figure out which group you are most comfortable with and do those passages first. See Chapter 3 for general strategies for moving through each of the sections efficiently.

11.3   TACKLING THE QUESTIONS

Biology and Biochemistry questions mimic the three typical questions of the science sections in general: Memory, Explicit, and Implicit.

Question Types as They Apply to Biology

Biology and Biochemistry Memory Questions

Memory questions are exactly what they sound like: They test your knowledge of some specific fact or concept. While Memory questions are typically found as freestanding questions, they can also be tucked into a passage. These questions, aside from requiring memorization, do not generally cause problems for students because they are similar to the types of questions that appear on a typical college biology exam. Below is an example of a freestanding Memory question:

> Regarding embryogenesis, which of the following sequence of events is in correct order?
>
> A) Implantation—cleavage—gastrulation—neurulation—blastulation
> B) Blastulation—implantation—cleavage—neurulation—gastrulation
> C) Implantation—blastulation—gastrulation—cleavage—neurulation
> D) Cleavage—blastulation—implantation—gastrulation—neurulation

The correct answer to the question above is choice D. Here's another example.

ACE inhibitors are a class of drugs frequently prescribed
to treat hypertension. Captopril, a compound that is
structurally similar to angiotensin I, was developed
in 1975 as the first ACE inhibitor. When patients take
Captopril, which of the following is true about the
kinetics of their ACE?

A) V_{max} decreases, K_m remains the same.
B) V_{max} remains the same, K_m increases.
C) Both V_{max} and K_m increase.
D) Both V_{max} and K_m remain the same.

The correct answer to the question above is choice B. Here's a third example. This question is from a passage:

The genital organs of the *guevedoche* that develop at
puberty are derivatives of the mesodermal germ layer.
Which of the following is/are also derivatives of the
mesodermal germ layer?

I.   Skeletal muscle
II. Liver
III. Kidney

A) I only
B) II only
C) I and III only
D) II and III only

Note that this question includes an additional, unnecessary sentence at the beginning, but it is a Memory
question all the same. You don't need to know anything about the *guevedoche* to answer the question, and
the information in that first sentence does not help you in any way. The correct answer is choice C.

There is no specific "trick" to answering Memory questions; either you know the answer or you don't.

If you find that you are missing a fair number of Memory questions, it is a sure sign that you don't know
the content well enough. Go back and review.

Biology and Biochemistry Explicit Questions

True, pure Explicit questions are rare in the Bio/Biochem section. A purely Explicit question can be answered only with information in the passage. Below is an example of a pure Explicit question taken from
the previous pentose phosphate pathway passage:

Which of the following are products of the pentose
phosphate pathway?

I.   NADPH
II. Glycolytic intermediates
III. Ribose-5-phosphate

A) I only
B) II only
C) I and III only
D) I, II, and III

Referring back to the map for this passage, it indicates that information about the products of the pathway are in paragraph 1 and Figure 1. Paragraph 1 states that NADPH and ribose 5-phosphate are both products, and Figure 1 shows that fructose-6-P and glyceraldehyde-3-P, both of which are glycolytic intermediates, are products. The correct answer is choice D.

However, more often in this section, Explicit questions are more of a blend of Explicit and Memory; they require not only retrieval of passage information, but also recall of some relevant fact. They usually do not require a lot of analysis or connections. Here's an example of the more common type of Explicit question.

Which of the following enzymes in the liver is most active five days after starting a ketogenic diet?

A)   Hexokinase
B)   Phosphofructokinase I
C)   HMG-CoA synthase
D)   Glycogen phosphorylase

To answer this question, you first need to retrieve information from the passage about the substances that are elevated in the blood after five days on a ketogenic diet. From Figure 2 we know that fatty acids, ketones, and glucagon are elevated. You also need to remember the metabolic pathways in which the enzymes in the answer choices participate. Hexokinase and phosphofructokinase I are glycolytic enzymes, and fats and ketones are not products of glycolysis. Thus, it is unlikely that these enzymes would be very active (choices A and B can be eliminated). Glycogen phosphorylase breaks down glycogen. Fats and ketones are not the products of glycogen breakdown, so it is unlikely that glycogen phosphorylase would be very active. The correct answer is HMG-CoA synthase, choice C.

A final subgroup in the Explicit question category are graph interpretation questions. These fall into one of two types: those that ask you to take graphical information from the passage and convert it to a text answer, or those that take text from the passage and ask you to convert it to a graph. On the following page is an example of the latter type.

Which of the following represents the Lineweaver-Burk
plot of an enzyme alone (solid line) and in the presence
of an inhibitor that binds exclusively to the enzyme
active site (dashed line)?

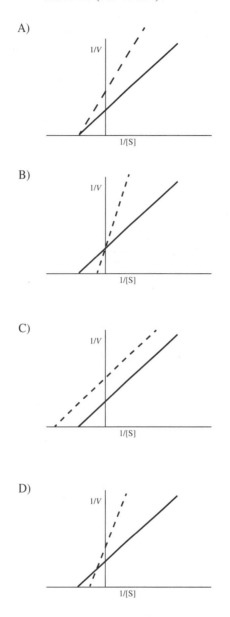

A)

B)

C)

D)

The passage for this question described how a Lineweaver-Burk plot is generated. You have to combine
that information with your knowledge about enzyme inhibitors and how they affect V_{max} and K_m. The
correct answer for this question is choice B.

If you find that you are missing Explicit questions, practice your passage mapping. Make sure you aren't
missing the critical items in the passage that lead you to the right answer. Slow down a little; take an extra
15 to 30 seconds per passage to read or think about it more carefully.

Biology and Biochemistry Implicit Questions

Implicit questions require the most thought. These require recall not only of biology and biochemistry information but also information gleaned from the passage and a more in-depth analysis of how the two relate. Implicit questions require more analysis and connections to be made than Explicit questions. Often they take the form "If...then...." Below is an example of a classic Implicit question, taken from the ketogenesis passage shown earlier.

If the researchers observed on Day 6 that the levels of fatty acids and ketones decreased while the level of insulin increased, which of the following could be assumed?

A) Protein and amino acid catabolism has increased in this participant.
B) The participant consumed a meal containing carbohydrates.
C) An increase in Krebs cycle activity would also be observed.
D) Glucagon levels would be unchanged from their levels five days after starting the ketogenic diet.

To answer this question, conclusions have to be drawn from the experiments described in the passage, and new conclusions have to be predicted based on the new circumstance. Many more connections need to be made than when answering an Explicit question. From the passage, we need to realize that the low insulin levels on Day 5, combined with high fatty acid and ketone levels in the blood, indicate that the participant is in ketosis, i.e, is burning fat as fuel. If insulin levels suddenly rise while fats and ketones fall, the participant must have eaten some carbohydrates. Protein and amino acid catabolism can result in ketone body production, according to the passage. If protein and amino acid catabolism had increased, we would expect if anything, to see an increase in ketone bodies, not a decrease (choice A is false). There is no reason to assume that Krebs cycle activity would increase; Krebs generally runs well during ketogenesis because of the acetyl CoA from fat breakdown. If the levels of fats are decreased on Day 6, then Krebs cycle activity would likely decrease as well (choice C is false). Insulin and glucagon are opposing hormones; insulin is released when blood sugar levels increase, and glucagon is released when blood sugar levels fall. If insulin is elevated, the glucagon will be decreased (choice D is false).

If you find that you are missing a lot of Implicit questions, first make sure that you are using POE aggressively. Second, go back and review the explanations for the correct answer to figure out where your logic went awry. Did you miss an important fact in the passage? Did you forget the relevant Biology or Biochemistry content? Did you follow the logical train of thought to the right answer? Once you figure out where you made your mistake, you will know how to correct it.

11.4 SUMMARY OF THE APPROACH TO BIOLOGY AND BIOCHEMISTRY

How to Map the Passage and Use Scratch Paper

1) The passage should not be read like textbook material, with the intent of learning something from every sentence (science majors especially will be tempted to read this way). Passages should be read to get a feel for the type of questions that will follow and to get a general idea of the location of information within the passage.

2) Highlighting—Use this tool sparingly, or you will end up with a passage that is completely covered in yellow highlighter! Highlighting in a Biology and/or Biochemistry passage should be used to draw attention to a few words that demonstrate one of the following:
   - the main theme of a paragraph
   - an unusual or unfamiliar term that is defined specifically for that passage (e.g., something that is italicized)
   - statements that either support the main theme or counteract the main theme
   - list topics (see below)
   - relationships

3) Pay brief attention to equations, figures, and experiments, noting only what information they deal with. Do not spend a lot of time analyzing at this point.

4) For each passage, start by noting the passage number, the general topic, and the range of questions on your scratch paper. You can then work between your scratch paper and the review screen to easily get to the questions you want to (see Chapter 3).

5) For each paragraph, note "P1," "P2," etc. on the scratch paper and jot down a few notes about that paragraph. Try to translate biology and biochemistry jargon into your own words using everyday language. Especially note down simple relationships (e.g., the relationship between two variables).

6) Lists—Whenever a list appears in paragraph form, jot down on the scratch paper the paragraph and the general topic of the list. It will make returning to the passage more efficient and help to organize your thoughts.

7) Scratch paper is only useful if it is kept organized! Make sure that your notes for each passage are clearly delineated and marked with the passage number and question range. This will allow you to easily read your notes when you come back to review a marked question. Resist the temptation to write in the first available blank space as this makes it much more difficult to refer back to your work.

Biology and Biochemistry Question Strategies

1) Remember that the content for these subjects is vast, so don't panic if something seems completely unfamiliar. Understand the basic content well, find the basics in the unfamiliar topic, and apply them to the question.

2) POE is paramount! The strikeout tool allows you to eliminate answer choices; this will improve your chances of guessing the correct answer if you are unable to narrow it down to one choice.

3) Answer the straightforward questions first (typically the memory questions). Leave questions that require analysis of experiments and graphs for later. Take the test in the order YOU want. Make sure to use your scratch paper to indicate questions you skipped.

4) Make sure that the answer you choose actually answers the question and isn't just a true statement.

5) Try to avoid answer choices with extreme words such as "always," "never," etc. In Biology, there is almost always an exception and answers are rarely black-and-white.

6) I-II-III questions: Always work between the I-II-III statements and the answer choices. Unfortunately, it is not possible to strike out the Roman numerals, but this is a great use for scratch paper notes. Once a statement is determined to be true (or false), strike out answer choices which do not contain (or do contain) that statement.

7) LEAST/EXCEPT/NOT questions: Don't get tricked by these questions that ask you to pick the answer that doesn't fit (the incorrect or false statement). Make sure to highlight the words "LEAST," "EXCEPT," or "NOT" in the question stem. It's often good to use your scratch paper and write a T or F next to answer choices A–D. The one that stands out as different is the correct answer!

8) Again, don't leave any question blank.

11.5   MCAT BIOLOGY AND BIOCHEMISTRY TOPIC LIST[1]

Biochemistry

A. Macromolecules
1. amino acid structure and classification
2. protein structure (1°–4°, peptide bond, folding, separation techniques)
3. carbohydrates (mono-, di-, and poly-saccharides)
4. lipids (fatty acids, triglycerides, phospholipids, steroids, terpenes)
5. nucleic acids (nucleotides/-sides, pyrimidines, purines)

B. Thermodynamics
1. free energy
2. spontaneous reactions and ΔG
3. endergonic and exergonic reactions
4. ATP hydrolysis and reaction coupling

C. Enzyme Structure and Function
1. substrates and specificity
2. activation energy
3. reaction coordinate graph
4. enzyme regulation (phosphorylation, feedback inhibition, allosteric regulation, zymogens)
5. Michaelis-Menten kinetics
6. inhibition (competitive, noncompetitive, uncompetitive, mixed)
7. Lineweaver-Burk plots
8. classification by reaction type

D. Cellular Metabolism
1. oxidation-reduction reactions
2. electron carriers
3. glycolysis
4. PDC/Krebs cycle
5. electron transport chain/oxidative phosphorylation
6. fermentation
7. energy counts
8. gluconeogenesis
9. glycogenesis/glycogenolysis
10. pentose phosphate pathway
11. fatty acid oxidation
12. fatty acid synthesis
13. ketogenesis
14. protein catabolism
15. regulation of biochemical pathways (enzymatic and hormonal)
16. cofactors and coenzymes

Molecular Biology

A. DNA Structure, Function, and Replication
1. double helix, deoxyribose, phosphate, bases
2. base pairing
3. role in Central Dogma
4. comparisons between eukaryotes and prokaryotes (DNA structure, packaging, and replication)
5. eukaryotic chromosomes (chromosomal proteins, centromeres, telomeres, function of telomerase)
6. mechanism of replication and enzymes involved
7. semiconservative
8. types of mutations (missense, nonsense, silent, frameshift)
9. DNA damage (oxidation, single- and double-stranded breaks, deletions, inversions, transposons)
10. DNA repair mechanisms

B. Transcription
1. Central Dogma (DNA → RNA → protein)
2. genetic code (degenerate, start and stop codons)
3. mechanism of transcription, comparison to replication
4. regulation of transcription (promoters, DNA binding proteins, transcription factors, prokaryotic operons)
5. eukaryotic mRNA (mRNA processing including capping, tailing, splicing, location, enzymes involved)
6. prokaryotic mRNA (no processing, location, enzymes involved)
7. hnRNA, siRNA, miRNA

---

[1] Adapted from *The Official Guide to the MCAT Exam (MCAT2015)*, 4th ed., © 2014 Association of American Medical Colleges.

C. Translation
1. ribosome structure (prokaryotic and eukaryotic)
2. roles of mRNA, tRNA, rRNA, and ribosome in protein synthesis
3. codon-anticodon relationship
4. wobble pairing
5. energy requirements
6. posttranslational modification of proteins

D. Lab Techniques
1. restriction enzymes, plasmids, gene cloning
2. DNA libraries, expression of cloned genes
3. analyzing gene expression and function (RT-PCR, microarrays, knockout experiments, etc.)
4. cDNA, PCR
5. gel electrophoresis
6. blotting and hybridization (Southern, northern, western)
7. DNA sequencing
8. Practical applications, safety, and ethics of DNA technology

Microbiology

A. Viruses
1. definition
2. structure, including enveloped and non-enveloped
3. relative size compared with prokaryotes and eukaryotes
4. genome (RNA and DNA genomes)
5. life cycles (lytic, lysogenic, productive, retroviral)
6. subviral particles (viroids, prions)

B. Bacteria
1. structure
2. genome and plasmids
3. classification by shape (cocci, bacilli, spirilli)
4. classification as eubacteria or archaebacteria
5. classification as aerobes or anaerobes
6. cell wall, flagella
7. binary fission for population growth
8. methods of acquiring genetic diversity (conjugation, transduction, transformation)
9. acquisition of antibiotic resistance

Cell Biology

A. Generalized Eukaryotic Cells
1. structure and function of all organelles (nucleus, nucleolus, mitochondria, rough ER, smooth ER, Golgi apparatus, lysosomes)
2. secretory pathway (transmembrane and secreted proteins)
3. plasma membrane structure and general function
4. exo- and endocytosis
5. colligative properties, osmosis/diffusion, passive and active transport, membrane potential
6. receptors and cell signaling pathways (second messengers, G-proteins)
7. cytoskeleton filaments, cilia and flagella, centrioles, MTOC
8. cell junctions (desmosomes, tight junctions, gap junctions)
9. cell cycle and mitosis, including G_0
10. regulation of cell cycle
11. apoptosis
12. cancer

Genetics and Evolution

A. Genetics
1. genes and alleles
2. genotype, phenotype, homozygous, heterozygous
3. classical dominance, incomplete dominance, codominance
4. recessiveness
5. penetrance and expressivity
6. Punnett squares, testcross
7. rules of probability (multiplication, addition)
8. Mendel's rules (segregation of alleles, independent assortment)
9. meiosis, and comparison of meiosis to mitosis
10. linkage and recombination
11. sex-linked genes
12. mutations and chromosomal rearrangements
13. Hardy-Weinberg (equations, conditions)

B. Evolution
1. natural selection and fitness
2. speciation, adaptation, competition
3. inbreeding/outbreeding
4. genetic drift

Anatomy and Physiology

A. Nervous System
1. neuron structure, including myelin and myelinating cells
2. glial cells
3. resting potential, action potential
4. propagation of action potential, saltatory conduction
5. synapses: electrical and chemical
6. summation (excitation, inhibition), frequency of firing
7. overall system function (sensory input, integration, motor output)
8. organization of nervous system
9. CNS roles (brain and spinal cord)
10. PNS (somatic and autonomic, sympathetic and parasympathetic)
11. reflexes

B. Endocrine System
1. function
2. endocrine glands and products
3. types of hormones, mechanism of action in cells, and transport in the blood
4. specificity of hormones and their actions
5. control (feedback)

C. Cardiovascular System
1. function
2. heart structure/function, pulmonary and systemic circulation
3. blood vessel structure, function, pressures, flow (arteries, veins, capillaries)
4. blood pressure (systolic, diastolic, regulation)
5. cardiac action potential, pacemaker role in heart
6. blood composition and clotting mechanisms
7. gas transport (O_2 and CO_2)
8. hemoglobin and O_2 affinity
9. nervous and endocrine control

D. Lymphatic System
1. function
2. source and composition of lymph
3. lymph nodes

E. Immune System
1. innate immunity and inflammation
2. antigen, antibody function, antibody structure
3. cells and functions (B-cells, T-cells, phagocytes)
4. mechanism of stimulation, antigen presentation (MHC I, MHC II)
5. self vs. non-self, autoimmune disease

F. Digestive System
1. alimentary canal structure and function (mouth, esophagus, stomach, small intestine, large intestine)
2. saliva, peristalsis, sphincters
3. hormones and enzymes
4. liver functions, bile
5. gallbladder function
6. pancreas, endocrine and exocrine function

G. Excretory System
1. urinary organs (ureter, bladder, urethra)
2. kidney and nephron structure
3. formation of urine, functions of parts of nephron (PCT, loop of Henle, DCT, collecting duct)
4. urine concentration, role of hormones
5. role of kidney in homeostasis (blood pressure regulation, osmoregulation, acid-base balance)

H. Muscular System
1. functions (movement, protection)
2. characteristics and structure of skeletal, cardiac, and smooth muscle
3. structure of striated muscle (T tubules, SR, actin/myosin)
4. sarcomere structure and sliding filament theory
5. role of calcium, troponin, tropomyosin
6. oxygen debt
7. nervous control of voluntary muscle
8. skeletal muscle fiber types

I. Skeletal System
1. functions (support, protection, mineral storage)
2. connective tissue, general structure/function
3. bone and joint structures, bone types (compact, spongy)
4. cartilage, ligaments, tendons
5. osteoblast/osteoclast functions
6. hormones that regulate calcium

J. Respiratory System
1. general functions (gas exchange, pH regulation)
2. structures and functions of the conduction zone and respiratory zone
3. mechanism of ventilation, structure of diaphragm, rib cage
4. lung elasticity, surface tension

K. Skin
1. functions (protection, homeostasis, osmoregulation)
2. thermoregulation
3. structure (layers, cell types, tissue types)
4. epithelial cells

L. Reproductive Systems
1. male and female structures and functions
2. spermatogenesis and oogenesis
3. menstrual cycle and hormones
4. fertilization

M. Development
1. embryonic stage (cleavage, implantation, blastulation, gastrulation, neurulation)
2. formation and fate of primary germ layers
3. fetal stage (major landmarks)
4. labor, lactation
5. determination/differentiation, cell communication
6. programmed cell death
7. stem cells

Chapter 12
Biology and
Biochemistry
Practice Section

FREESTANDING QUESTIONS

1. Myrcene is a monoterpene with a pleasant aroma found in several plants. What is the molecular formula of myrcene?

A) C_5H_8
B) $C_{10}H_{16}$
C) $C_{15}H_{24}$
D) $C_{20}H_{32}$

2. Peptoids are a class of protein mimics that differ from traditional amino acids in that the side chain is attached to the nitrogen atom rather than the α-carbon. Which of the following is possible with a peptide but would be most directly disrupted in a peptoid?

A) Hydrogen bonding
B) Salt bridges
C) Hydrophobic forces
D) Dehydration synthesis

3. A newly discovered enzyme, inhibitase, acts on its substrate using a magnesium cation cofactor. An inhibitor with several glutamic acid residues is found to bind to inhibitase at the active site. Which of the following is the double reciprocal plots that would be observed for the substrate with different concentrations of inhibitase?

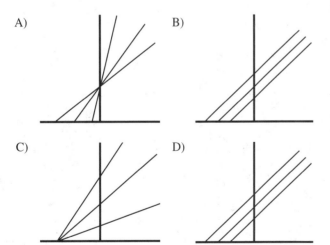

A)
B)
C)
D)

4. Oxidation of ethanol by alcohol dehydrogenase results in a change in the NAD^+/NADH ratio. This ratio consequently affects the ratio of pyruvate and lactic acid in the process of fermentation. How will the oxidation of alcohol dehydrogenase affect gluconeogenesis?

A) Increase gluconeogenesis, because of increased NAD^+ levels
B) Increase gluconeogenesis, because of decreased NAD^+ levels
C) Decrease gluconeogenesis, because of increased NAD^+ levels
D) Decrease gluconeogenesis, because of decreased NAD^+ levels

5. Small interfering RNA (siRNA) is used in a cell culture experiment to induce mRNA knockdown of a secreted protein of interest. However, the protein is still detected at high levels in the media via Western blot. What is the most likely cause of this result?

A) The siRNA sequence was designed based on an intron.
B) The sequence encoding the secreted protein was highly complex with minimally repetitive regions.
C) The siRNA was unable to leave the nucleus due to a nuclear localization signal.
D) The level of RNA polymerase in the nucleus was insufficient to induce production of the siRNA.

6. Signs of DNA damage in a cell can trigger an SOS response, leading to an escalating sequence of attempts at cellular repair. The transcription factor LexA normally inhibits this sequence of events. As the SOS response progresses, the binding affinity of LexA to its target sequences decreases. Which is the most likely relationship between how LexA binds to the SOS genes and the impact on the cell?

A) SOS genes with a high affinity for LexA are responsible for nucleotide excision repair, while those will a low affinity for LexA are responsible for arresting the cell cycle.
B) SOS genes with a low affinity for LexA are responsible for nucleotide excision repair, while those will a high affinity for LexA are responsible for arresting the cell cycle.
C) SOS genes with a high affinity for LexA are responsible for inducing somatic mutations, while those will a low affinity for LexA are responsible for double-stranded break repair.
D) SOS genes with a low affinity for LexA are responsible for inducing somatic mutations, while those will a high affinity for LexA are responsible for double-stranded break repair.

7. Two researchers each perform a separate Western blot on the same protein sample. Researcher A observes a single band but Researcher B observes two bands. Which of the following best explains the difference?

A) Researcher B added a reducing agent to the solution.
B) Researcher A added a reducing agent to the solution.
C) Researcher B added an oxidizing agent to the solution.
D) Researcher A did not add an oxidizing agent to the solution.

8. Fanconi syndrome results in impaired reabsorption at the proximal convoluted tubule. What would be an expected finding in a patient with Fanconi syndrome?

A) Hyperglycemia
B) Decreased urinary output
C) Metabolic acidosis
D) Increased amino acid reabsorption in the collecting duct

9. In a randomly mating population of 200 individuals, 102 of them carry at least one copy of the recessive allele. What is the predicted frequency of individuals in the population that are carriers for the recessive allele?

A) 0.49
B) 0.42
C) 0.51
D) 0.3

10. Multiple sclerosis (MS) is a demyelinating disease that affects the central nervous system. Which of the following cells is most likely affected in patients with MS?

A) Astrocytes
B) Schwann cells
C) Oligodendrocytes
D) Ependymal cells

11. Hyperchlorhydria is the defined as having abnormally high gastric acid levels. The cause in one particular patient is determined to be cell damage in the pancreas. Which of the following cell types is most likely affected?

A) α cells
B) β cells
C) γ cells
D) δ cells

12. Long-acting reversible contraceptives (LARCs), including the etonogestrel contraceptive subdermal implant and the levonorgestrel-releasing intrauterine device, have significantly gained in popularity. Both of these devices utilize the slow release of synthetic progesterones (known as progestins) to aid in the prevention of pregnancy. Which of the following is true of LARCs?

A) Lower serum progestin levels result in fewer systemic side effects than oral contraceptive pills.
B) Progestins increase FSH release in order to prevent ovulation.
C) Progestins increase LH release in order to prevent ovulation.
D) Progestins inhibit endogenous progesterone release, triggering sloughing of the endometrium.

13. Kartagener's Syndrome, otherwise known as primary ciliary dyskinesia, results in immotile cilia due to a defect in the dynein arm of microtubules. Which of the following outcomes would NOT be expected in patients with this disease?

A) Decreased male fertility
B) Decreased female fertility
C) Recurrent respiratory infections
D) Decreased peristalsis in the bowel

14. Proto-oncogenes like RAS, WNT, and MYC code for proteins that regulate cell division. Once activated, they become oncogenes, or tumorigenic agents. For example, RAS is a GTPase that regulates the activation of genes that control proliferation, cell adhesion, apoptosis, and cell migration. Were RAS made constitutively active via mutation as part of a malignant transformation, which of the following outcomes would NOT be expected?

A) Increased invasion of surrounding tissues
B) Increased cellular adhesion
C) Decreased apoptosis
D) Decreased differentiation

15. Which of the following best describes the mechanism by which immature B-cells are screened by the body to prevent autoimmunity?

A) Apoptosis is induced in B-cells that express MHC II.
B) B-cells produce antibodies that bind to self-antibodies, preventing them from causing any damage.
C) Immature B-cells that bind to normal cell surface proteins divide into plasma cells.
D) Apoptosis is induced in immature B-cells that bind to normal cell surface proteins.

PRACTICE PASSAGE 1

Chymotrypsin is a digestive protease which selectively hydrolyzes the peptide bond on the C-terminus of amino acids with aromatic side chains. This selectivity can be explained by a region in the protease known as the "hydrophobic pocket", which is lined with amino acid residues that participate in van der Waals interactions with the aromatic sidechains, ultimately positioning various polypeptides for cleavage by the active site.

A group of students is given Peptide A, a polypeptide of eight amino acids of unknown order. After Peptide A is digested with chymotrypsin by the students, the amino acid sequences of the resultant peptides are determined, and are named Peptide B, Peptide C, and Peptide D. The composition of the peptides after digestion are given below with standard 1-letter amino acid abbreviations:

Peptide B: A-P

Peptide C: G-C-A-F

Peptide D: E-W

In a separate experiment, the kinetics of Peptide A digestion are compared in chymotrypsin to a mutant of chymotrypsin called MutaChy. After measuring the velocity of the two enzymes at varying Peptide A concentrations at physiological pH, the students determined that the K_m value of chymotrypsin was several orders of magnitude greater than that of MutaChy.

Lastly, the students run a gel electrophoresis experiment where they load separate samples of Peptide B and Peptide D in two separate rows of a gel. Both peptides are loaded in the middle of their respective columns, directly centered between the negative and positive electrodes, as show below in Figure 1:

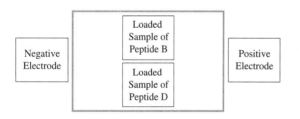

Figure 1

An electric field is then applied to the gel, buffered at a hydronium concentration of 0.1 M. This experiment is repeated multiple times but at varied concentrations of hydronium ion with each trial. During one of the trials, it was observed that Peptide B did not migrate toward either electrode; this trial was titled "Trial B". During a separate trial, students observed that Peptide D did not migrate toward either electrode; this trial was titled "Trial D".

1. Which of the following amino acids is the C-terminal amino acid of Peptide A?

A) Phenylalanine
B) Glycine
C) Proline
D) Alanine

2. The group of students hypothesize that the difference between chymotrypsin and MutaChy is that several of the hydrophobic amino acid residues located in the "hydrophobic pocket" of chymotrypsin are replaced by lysine residues in MutaChy. To test this hypothesis, they react both enzymes with the following polypeptide, called Peptide E:

A-R-R-G

If their hypothesis is true, and the K_m values for both enzymes are determined, what should be true about the K_m value of chymotrypsin relative to MutaChy?

A) K_m will be higher, because chymotrypsin has a higher affinity for Peptide E.
B) K_m will be higher, because chymotrypsin has a lower affinity for Peptide E.
C) K_m will be lower, because chymotrypsin has a higher affinity for Peptide E.
D) K_m will be lower, because chymotrypsin has a lower affinity for Peptide E.

3. In the gel electrophoresis experiments mentioned in the passage, how did the buffered concentration of hydronium ion compare between Trial B and Trial D?

A) Trial B was buffered at a higher hydronium concentration than Trial D.
B) Trial B was buffered at a lower hydronium concentration than Trial D.
C) Trial B was buffered at an equivalent concentration of hydronium to Trial D.
D) The relative hydronium concentrations of Trial B and Trial D cannot be determined.

4. Tyrosine is one of the amino acids which fit favorably into the hydrophobic pocket of chymotrypsin. The molecular formula of tyrosine is $C_9H_{11}NO_3$. What is the molecular formula of a tripeptide comprised entirely of tyrosine?

A) $C_{27}H_{33}N_3O_9$
B) $C_{18}H_{22}N_2O_4$
C) $C_{27}H_{27}N_3O_6$
D) $C_{27}H_{29}N_3O_7$

5. Which of the following hormones is most directly responsible for the release of chymotrypsin in digestion?

A) Secretin
B) Cholecystokinin
C) Insulin
D) Somatostatin

6. The amino acids that result from protein degradation by proteases can be utilized in forming which of the following:

    I.   Urea
    II. Acetyl-CoA
    III. DNA Bases

A) I only
B) I and II only
C) III only
D) I, II, and III

PRACTICE PASSAGE 2

RNA interference (RNAi) is a process by which RNA molecules inhibit gene expression. RNAi is often utilized as a cellular defense mechanism against pathogens such as viruses. First, foreign double-stranded RNA injected by a virus is cut into short fragments by the enzyme Dicer, forming small double-stranded RNA fragments called small interfering RNAs (siRNAs). One of the siRNA strands, the passenger strand, is degraded, and the complementary strand, the guide strand, is incorporated into the RNA-induced silencing complex (RISC). The guide strand is used as a template to anneal to complementary mRNA produced by the virus. Upon annealing, the endonuclease component of RISC degrades the viral mRNA.

One strategy for treating hormone refractory prostate cancer is to manipulate apoptotic resistance in cells. A group of proteins called Inhibitor of Apoptosis (IAP) proteins is hypothesized to be responsible for mediating this apoptotic resistance. A group of scientists hypothesize that knocking down three of these IAP proteins using RNAi would result in an increase in sensitivity to apoptosis.

To test the effectiveness of RNAi on protein expression, prostate cancer cells were transfected with siRNA, targeting genes associated with prostate cancer. Expression levels of targets were determined. The results of the experiments are shown below (Figure 1).

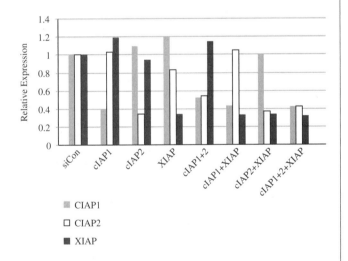

Figure 1 siRNA mediated knockdown of cIAP-1, cIAP-2, and XIAP. A non-targeting siRNA (siCon), is used as a control group.

Adapted from: Gill C, Dowling C, O'Neill AJ, et al. *Effects of cIAP-1, cIAP-2 and XIAP triple knockdown on prostate cancer cell susceptibility to apoptosis, cell survival and proliferation.* Mol Cancer. 2009; 8:39.

1. Which of the following contains the same monomeric structural elements found in RISC?

    I.   Ribosomes
    II. RNA Polymerase
    III. Nucleosomes

A) I only
B) II only
C) I and II only
D) I and III only

2. Which of the following is NOT true about apoptosis?

A) Apoptosis may result from increased expression of tumor suppressor genes such as p53.
B) Apoptosis may be triggered by either an external or internal cellular stress.
C) Apoptosis may result in gradual expansion of cellular volume leading to disassembly of the cytoskeleton.
D) The cleaving of cellular proteins by effector caspases is triggered by initiator caspases.

3. Scientists transfect cells with either Gene X or Gene X' along with siRNA targeting all three IAP proteins. Gene X encodes a nuclease that hydrolyzes siRNA targeting cIAP-2 and contains the antisense sequence 3'-TCACCCTTAATGATT-5'. Gene X' is a fusion gene containing Gene X and a downstream sequence that encodes for a nuclease that hydrolyzes siRNA targeting XIAP. According to the data in Figure 1, how will XIAP levels compare between cells infected with Gene X and Gene X'?

A) XIAP levels will be higher in cells infected with Gene X.
B) XIAP levels will be higher in cells infected with Gene X'.
C) XIAP levels will be equal in both groups of cells.
D) It cannot be determined from the information provided.

4. The first ten nucleotides that are part of the discarded RNA strand following a RISC formation has the sequence 5'-UAUUUGCGCU-3'. What are the first ten nucleotides that are part of the transcript that is ultimately degraded by RISC?

A) 5'-UAUUUGCGCU-3'
B) 5'-AUAAACGCGA-3'
C) 3'-UAUUUGCGCU-5'
D) 3'-AUAAACGCGA -5'

5. Caspase-3 is an effector caspase that helps carry out the proteolytic activity associated with apoptosis. It is a highly specific enzyme, recognizing a tetrapeptide sequence on its substrate, with a strict requirement that the first and fourth amino acids are aspartic acid residues, a hydrophobic amino acid is found at position 2, and a hydrophilic amino acid at position 3. Which of the following would NOT be found at position 2 of the caspase-3 substrate?

A) W
B) N
C) F
D) A

PRACTICE PASSAGE 3

Adrenoleukodystrophy (ALD) is a disorder which results in the accumulation of very long chain, saturated fatty acids (VLCSFAs), particularly cerotic acid, a 26-carbon long-chain saturated fatty acid, in tissues throughout the body. It is caused by mutations in ABCD1, a membrane transporter protein. Children affected by ALD can be born to parents that do not have the disease, and the most severely negatively affected tissues are the central nervous system myelin sheath, the adrenal cortex, and Leydig cells.

Lorenzo's oil is an investigational treatment for asymptomatic patients with ALD. It contains glyceryl trioleate (oleic acid, a monounsaturated fatty acid with 18 carbons) and erucic acid (a monounsaturated fatty acid with 22 carbons). These unsaturated shorter fatty acids are converted into harmless VLCSFAs by the same processing enzyme that converts saturated shorter fatty acids into harmful VLCSFAs.

ALD does not have an increased incidence in any specific country or ethnic group, but is more common in males than females. Many epidemiological studies have attempted to determine the frequency of the ALD allele the human population. A high estimate is 5%, although certain investigators have proposed a much lower value.

In order to determine which subcellular organelle is negatively affected in ALD, researchers stained a series of cells collected from an ALD donor for organelle markers. High resolution scans were taken of the cells, and stained organelles displayed dark in color. At the same time, researchers used an antibody specific for the ALD mutant protein. When co-staining occurred between the organelle marker and the ALD antibody, the cellular area turned white, thus allowing researchers to infer the organelle is likely involved in ALD.

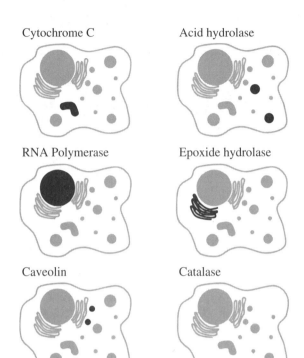

Cytochrome C   Acid hydrolase

RNA Polymerase   Epoxide hydrolase

Caveolin   Catalase

Figure 1   Cellular co-staining for subcellular markers and ABCD1^{mutant} protein

1. Compared to the β-oxidation of erucic acid, the β-oxidation of cerotic acid will yield:

A) 51 molecules of NADH and 4 additional molecules of FADH$_2$.

B) 55 molecules of NADH and 4 additional molecules of FADH$_2$.

C) Ten additional molecules of NADH and six additional molecules of FADH$_2$.

D) 27 molecules of FADH$_2$ and more than double the amount of NADH.

2. Symptoms of adrenoleukodystrophy likely include:

   I.   Progressive paralysis of the limbs
   II. High blood pressure
   III. High levels of sex steroids

A) I only
B) II only
C) I and II
D) I and III

3. A female that carries the ALD mutation is born to a couple, neither of which have ALD. What percentage of the human population will have the same genotype as the female's mother?

A) 0.25%
B) 4.75%
C) 9.5%
D) 90.25%

4. Based on Figure 1, the root cause of adrenoleukodystrophy is most similar to the root cause of:

A) cystic fibrosis, an autosomal recessive disorder caused by mutations in both copies of the cystic fibrosis transmembrane conductance regulator gene, and thus altered production of sweat, digestive fluids, and mucus.
B) Alzheimer's disease, a chronic neurodegenerative disease caused by gross atrophy of synapses in the cerebral cortex.
C) Zellweger syndrome, a rare congenital disorder characterized by the absence of functional peroxisomes in the cells of an individual.
D) acquired immunodeficiency syndrome, which is defined by having a CD_4^+ T-cell count below 200 cells per μL of blood.

5. Components of Lorenzo's oil most likely:

A) noncompetitively inhibit a transport protein located on the smooth ER membrane, thus promoting fatty acid synthesis.
B) competitively inhibit a transport protein located on the smooth ER membrane, thus promoting fatty acid synthesis.
C) noncompetitively inhibit a transport protein located on the peroxisome membrane, thus limiting fatty acid degradation.
D) competitively inhibit a transport protein located on the peroxisome membrane, thus limiting fatty acid degradation.

PRACTICE PASSAGE 4

Subarachnoid hemorrhage (SAH) is a form of stroke in which the rupture of a vessel results in the continual escape of blood from the vasculature into the subarachnoid space. Onset of the bleed will often be associated with "thunderclap headache," nausea, vomiting, altered mental status, and seizures.

Another complication commonly associated with SAH is the syndrome of inappropriate antidiuretic hormone (SIADH). Generally speaking, SIADH is believed to result from impaired regulation of ADH secretion from the pituitary gland secondary to the bleed. The net result is typically excessive secretion of ADH, resulting in excessive water retention. This leads to hyponatremia, a concentration of blood sodium below normal physiological levels (135–145 mmol/L), with increased swelling in the brain and eventual dumping of electrolytes into the blood and high urine sodium levels. Even with proper treatment, hyponatremia from SIADH can last for weeks.

One such patient was admitted to the hospital after loss of consciousness; when he regained consciousness, he experienced a severe headache. CT scan identified blood in the subarachnoid

space. β-blocker and Ca^{2+} channel blocker medications were started, isotonic saline was administered, and a ventricular drain was placed. By Day 4, the patient was trending hyponatremic and was started on NaCl tablets and eventually hypertonic saline. Clinical data throughout the hospitalization is shown below. Tolvaptan is a competitive antagonist selective for the vasopressin receptor present in the kidney.

Central pontine myelinolysis is one of the most feared complications in treating hyponatremia; it can occur when sodium is replenished too quickly. In the context of hyponatremia, neurons in the brain accommodate for the decrease in blood sodium by downregulating their own internal osmolytes to match tonicity with the extracellular fluid. When replenished too quickly, the extracellular fluid can become hypertonic with respect to the neurons, resulting in excessive water loss, cellular dysfunction, and neuronal death, particularly in the pons.

Adapted from: Laville M, Burst V, Peri A, Verbalis JG. *Hyponatremia secondary to the syndrome of inappropriate secretion of antidiuretic hormone (SIADH): clinical decision-making in real-life cases.* Clin Kidney J. 2013;(Suppl.1):i1–20.

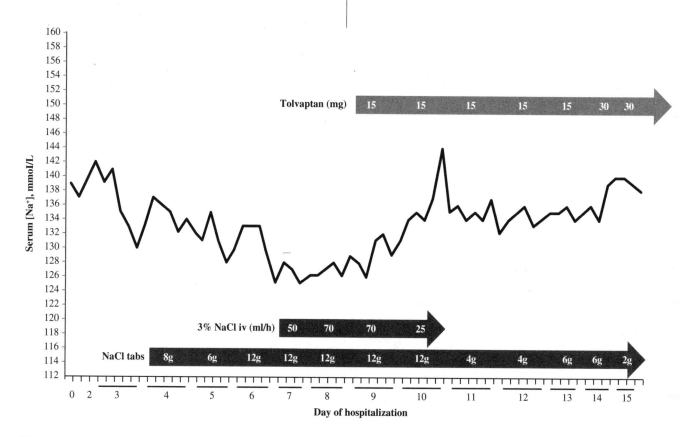

Figure 1   Serum sodium by day of hospitalization with pertinent medication dosing shown (numbers in the arrows represent the amount of medication administered, units shown above)

1. What is the most likely immediate effect of hyponatremia on the brain?

A) The increased hydrostatic pressure of hypotonic blood results in the accumulation of water in brain tissue.
B) The decreased osmotic pressure of hypotonic blood results in accumulation of water in brain tissue.
C) The increased osmotic pressure of hypertonic brain tissue results in the loss of electrolytes from the brain tissue.
D) The decreased hydrostatic pressure of hypertonic brain tissue results in the loss of electrolytes from the brain tissue.

2. Which of the following is most likely to be the primary anatomic site that provides the main driving mechanistic cause of hyponatremia in SIADH?

A) Hypothalamus
B) Anterior pituitary gland
C) Posterior pituitary gland
D) Kidneys

3. Which of the following correctly describes the mechanism of action of tolvaptan?

A) Tolvaptan competes with vasopressin for the receptor binding site and activates the vasopressin receptor when bound.
B) Tolvaptan competes with vasopressin for the receptor binding site but does not activate the vasopressin receptor when bound.
C) Tolvaptan binds to a different site as vasopressin on the vasopressin receptor but does not activate the vasopressin receptor when bound.
D) Cannot be determined with the provided information.

4. Central pontine myelinolysis can have wide-ranging effects on neurologic function; which of the following is the most likely explanation for these observations?

A) Neuronal cell death in the peripheral nervous system disrupts the ability of the brain to communicate with tissues throughout the body.
B) Widespread dehydration and lysis of neurons throughout the brain results in the disruption of neuronal functions diffusely throughout the brain and, thus, the rest of the body.
C) Most of the neurons descending from the cortex pass through the pons and their disruption results in a disconnection with the rest of the body.
D) Electrolyte abnormalities in pontine neurons inhibit the ability of action potentials to travel to and from the cortex, resulting in a transient dysregulation of neurologic function throughout the body.

5. Which of the following is the most likely explanation for the SAH patient's return to normal physiologic levels of blood sodium?

A) Repletion of blood sodium at constant levels was required to counteract excessive natriuresis and water retention.
B) Repletion of blood sodium resulted in an increase in natriuresis, requiring activation of ADH receptors by tolvaptan to increase blood sodium levels.
C) Excessive sodium repletion led to hypernatremia, requiring inhibition of ADH receptor to decrease blood sodium levels.
D) Repletion of blood sodium levels countered initially excessive natriuresis then subsequent inhibition of excessive water retention reduced dilution of blood.

PRACTICE PASSAGE 5

Excitation-contraction coupling in cardiac muscle cells translates the electrical signal of an action potential into the mechanical production of tension in the heart. After Ca^{2+} enters the intracellular fluid during an action potential, Ca^{2+} binds to a protein known as a ryanodine receptor. The ryanodine receptor is bound to a specialized membrane organelle in the cell known as the sarcoplasmic reticulum (SR), which functions solely to store Ca^{2+} for release. Binding of Ca^{2+} to ryanodine receptor triggers the release of additional Ca^{2+} from the SR into the intracellular fluid (calcium-induced calcium release). Ca^{2+} flows into the intracellular fluid through the ryanodine receptor, which functions as a channel.

Increased Ca^{2+} concentration results in binding of Ca^{2+} to troponin, leading to cardiac muscle contraction through a cross-bridge cycling mechanism similar to that of skeletal muscle. Relaxation occurs by Ca^{2+} export out of the cell by a Ca^{2+}-Na^+ antiport or back into the SR by a Ca^{2+} ATPase. To investigate the role of ryanodine receptors on heart function, scientists develop ryanodine receptor knockout. Their results are shown below in Figure 1.

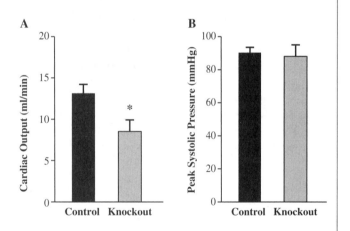

Figure 1 Ryanodine receptor knockout hearts in mice versus wild type mice. Measure of cardiac output (A) and peak systolic pressure (B). ($t = 30$ min; Control $n = 6$, RyrKO $n = 8$; $*p < 0.05$)

Substances that target the cardiac excitation-contraction coupling pathway—either directly or indirectly—can have a significant effect on heart function. Drugs derived from the foxglove plant *Digitalis purpurea* inhibit the Na^+-K^+ ATPase in cardiac muscle cells. The medication amlodipine increases arterial diameter and blocks the voltage-gated channels that allow entry of Ca^{2+} into the intracellular fluid.

Adapted from: Bround M, Asghari P, Wambolt R, et al. *Cardiac ryanodine receptors control heart rate and rhythmicity in adult mice.* Cardiovascular Research – Oxford Journals. 2012; 96. 372-380.

1. The co-permeability of the ryanodine receptor to which of the following ions would increase the rate of Ca^{2+} entry into the intracellular fluid of cardiac muscle cells?

A) K^+
B) Na^+
C) Cl^-
D) HCO_3^-

2. Positive inotropic effects increase cardiac cell contractility, while negative inotropic effects decrease it. Heart medications derived from *Digitalis purpurea* will have what inotropic effect?

A) Positive, because the ratio of extracellular to intracellular Na^+ will increase
B) Positive, because the ratio of extracellular to intracellular Na^+ will decrease
C) Negative, because the ratio of extracellular to intracellular Na^+ will increase
D) Negative, because the ratio of extracellular to intracellular Na^+ will decrease

3. Amlodipine would have which of the following effects in the body?

A) Compensating increase in calcium release from sarcoplasmic reticulum to maintain muscular contraction levels
B) Decreased magnitude of atrioventricular node depolarization
C) Increased frequency of systole
D) Increased loss of capillary fluid

4. A decrease in cardiac muscle tension relies on which of the following transport processes?

I.   Facilitated diffusion
II. Primary active transport
III. Secondary active transport

A) II only
B) III only
C) I and II only
D) II and III only

5. All of the following are true about ryanodine receptor knockout mice compared to a wild type mice EXCEPT:

A) knockout mice have similar peak systolic blood pressure.
B) knockout mice have lower heart rate.
C) knockout mice have lower stroke volume.
D) knockout mice have lower peripheral resistance.

PRACTICE PASSAGE 6

Lipodystrophy is the abnormal development or function of adipose tissue in the body. Muscular dystrophies pertain to the abnormal and often degenerative development and function of muscle tissue throughout the body. One disorder which involves both domains of pathology is Emery-Dreifuss muscular dystrophy (EDMD). EDMD primarily involves the dysfunction of lamin, a protein expressed in the nuclear envelope; pathological manifestations of this disorder accelerate later in life. The pathophysiology of this disorder depends on the disrupted function of Sterol Regulatory Element Binding Protein 1c (SREBP1c) and associated transcription factors. Though they have been more formally implicated in the regulation of lipogenic tissues in the liver and adipose tissues, they are also significantly expressed in muscle tissues as well as other tissue throughout the body. SREBP1c lipogenic activity in the liver is proposed to be induced by insulin and growth factors via the Akt pathway, as demonstrated in Figure 1.

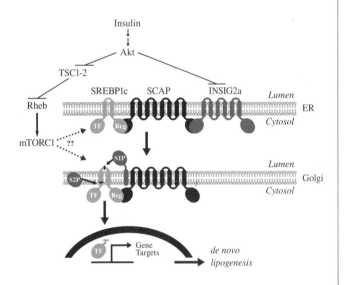

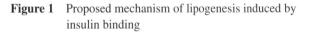

Figure 1   Proposed mechanism of lipogenesis induced by insulin binding

Insulin receptor binding is believed to activate the Akt pathway, which simultaneously suppresses the SREBP1c inhibitor INSIG2a and is theorized to activate mTORC1, which facilitates the transfer of SREBP1c from the ER to Golgi apparatus. Transcription factors (TF) for proteins required in lipogenesis then travel to the nucleus where they bind gene targets for lipogenesis.

Researchers seeking to understand the role of SREBP1c in the development of muscle tissue conducted muscle biopsies on healthy volunteers. Myoblasts were purified and differentiated myotubes (a developmental stage of muscle fiber when myoblasts fuse together) were isolated. The myotubes were then infected with recombinant adenovirus expression vectors to determine the effect of overexpression of SREBP1c. Adeno-GFP (green fluorescence protein) was used as a control. Finally, the myotubes were treated with a fluorescent-labeled anti-myosin antibody and visualized. The experiment was repeated with recombinant adenoviruses expressing either MYOG, MEF2C, or MYOD (muscle-specific transcription factors that induce expression of muscle-specific genes) in combination with Ad-GFP or Ad-SREBP1c to determine their effect on myosin expression. Imaged results are shown below in Figure 2.

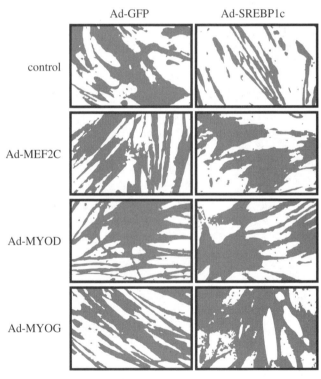

Figure 2   Immunofluorescence staining of myotube culture transfected with expression vectors (white = no staining, gray = immunostained myosin)

Figure 1 adapted from: Yecies, J.L., et al. *Akt Stimulates Hepatic SREBP1c and Lipogenesis through Parallel mTORC1-Dependent and Independent Pathways.* Cell Metabolism, 2011.

Content and data adapted from: Dessalle, K. *SREBP-1 Transcription Factors Regulate Skeletal Muscle Cell Size by Controlling Protein Synthesis Through Myogenic Regulatory Factors.* PLoS One, 2012.

1. Which of the following metabolic derangements would be expected to decrease SREBP1c activity?

A) Insulin resistance
B) Hyperglycemia
C) Hyperinsulinemia
D) Ketoacidosis

2. To which of the following standard laboratory techniques is the SREBP1c expression protocol most similar?

A) Southern blotting
B) In-situ hybridization
C) Western blotting
D) Immunohistochemistry

3. Activation of which of the following proteins will lead to increased mTORC1 activity?

   I.   Akt
  II.   TSC1-2
 III.   Rheb

A) I only
B) II only
C) I and III only
D) I, II, and III

4. Which of the following statements best characterizes the conclusion that can be drawn from the data presented in Figure 2?

A) Inhibition of SREBP1c increases myosin production, but additional induction of muscle transcription factors decreases myosin production.
B) Inhibition of SREBP1c increases myosin production, and additional induction of muscle transcription factors normalizes myosin production.
C) Inhibition of SREBP1c decreases myosin production, and additional induction of muscle transcription factors normalizes myosin production.
D) Inhibition of SREBP1c decreases myosin production, but additional induction of muscle transcription factors increases myosin production.

5. EDMD can be caused by an autosomal recessive allele, an autosomal dominant allele, and an X-linked recessive allele. Prevalence of the X-linked version is estimated to be 1 in 100,000 individuals, while prevalence of the autosomal dominant version is estimated to be three times as common as the X-linked version. A woman affected with X-linked EDMD has children with an unaffected man, and all of their children marry and have children with unaffected partners. Which of the following is NOT a true statement?

A) All of the original couple's male children will be affected by X-linked EDMD.
B) The children of the original couple have a 50% probability of being carriers of X-linked EDMD.
C) All grandchildren produced by the daughters of the original couple will be unaffected.
D) There is a 25% probability that grandchildren produced by the sons of the original couple are affected females.

Chapter 13
Biology and
Biochemistry Practice
Section Solutions

SOLUTIONS TO FREESTANDING QUESTIONS

1. **B** Terpenes are a broad class of compounds composed from isoprene units (C_5H_8). Monoterpenes, such as myrcene, consist of two isoprene units resulting in a molecular formula of $C_{10}H_{16}$ (choice B is correct). Hemiterpenes (C_5H_8), sesquiterpenes ($C1_5H_{24}$), and diterpenes ($C_{20}H_{32}$) consist of one, three, and four isoprene units, respectively (choices A, C, and D are wrong).

2. **A** In a typical protein, nitrogen atoms in peptide bonds have a hydrogen atom that is used for hydrogen bonding in secondary structure. Since the nitrogen in a peptoid has an R group attached, it would no longer have free hydrogen available for hydrogen bonding (choice A is correct). Side chains have not been eliminated, so salt bridges and hydrophobic forces are still possible (choices B and C are wrong). Dehydration synthesis can still occur, as two hydrogens remain on the amino group that can be combined with a carboxylate oxygen (choice D can be eliminated). Of note, hydrogen bonding in tertiary and quaternary structure will not be disrupted.

3. **C** The x-values of the double-reciprocal plot correspond to $1/[S]$, while the y-values correspond to $1/V$. The x-intercept of the plot will be $-1/K_m$ and the y-intercept will be $1/V_{max}$. A plot with different concentrations of inhibitase enzyme will have different values for V_{max}, because V_{max} is dependent on the concentration of enzyme. K_m will not change, because altering the concentration of enzyme does not affect that enzyme's affinity for the substrate. Thus, the correct graph is one where the x-intercept remains constant while the y-intercept changes (choice C is correct; eliminate choices A, B, and D). Note that the first two sentences of the question stem contain irrelevant information designed to confuse you.

4. **D** If ethanol is oxidized by alcohol dehydrogenase, this implies that NAD^+ is reduced to NADH, as oxidation reactions are always paired with a reduction reaction. This would decrease NAD^+ levels (choices A and C can be eliminated) and increase NADH. An increase in NADH would drive the reduction of pyruvate to lactic acid, consequently decreasing the amount of pyruvate. Since pyruvate is the starting material in gluconeogenesis, reduced pyruvate would result in a decrease in gluconeogenesis (choice B can be eliminated; choice D is correct).

5. **A** siRNAs are short (typically 20–25 base pairs) double-stranded RNAs synthesized to then silence the expression of transcribed, processed RNAs. If an siRNA were synthesized based on an intron rather than an exon, it would be targeting a sequence no longer present in the final mRNA (choice A is correct). Having a complex, minimally repetitive initial DNA sequence as a baseline would make the subsequently designed siRNA more specific and presumably more effective, not less (choice B is wrong). Nuclear localization signals are a short sequence of amino acids that aid in bringing necessary proteins to the nucleus and are not involved in siRNAs (choice C is wrong). A lack of RNA polymerase in the cell could limit the production of mRNA, but not siRNA; the lack of mRNA would then also limit secretion of the protein, not maintain it (choice D is wrong).

6. **B**   From the description, LexA is a transcription factor that represses gene activity when bound. Since the SOS response is an attempt at cellular repair, it should not induce further mutations (choices C and D can be eliminated). As the SOS response begins, the binding affinity of LexA to its target sequences decreases. Genes with a lower affinity for LexA will be released before those with a higher affinity. The goal of genomic repair is to preserve the cell where possible so the more moderate approaches will be tried first. Thus, it follows that genes with a low affinity for LexA would be those responsible for nucleotide excision repair, while those with a higher affinity for LexA would be responsible for arresting the cell cycle in the event that repair could not be achieved (choice B is correct and choice A is wrong).

7. **A.** A reducing agent can cleave disulfide bonds in a protein. If the protein were a heterodimer connected by disulfide bonds, the addition of a reducing agent by Researcher B could separate the two subunits, yielding two bands. Since Researcher A did not add a reducing agent, only one band would be observed (choice A is correct). If Researcher A had added a reducing agent, it would not explain the band patterns observed by the two researchers as (choice B is wrong). Adding an oxidizing agent leads to the formation of disulfide bonds. The formation of a disulfide bond would not explain why Researcher B obtained two bands (choice C is wrong). Similarly, if Researcher A did not add an oxidizing agent, it still does not explain why researcher B obtained two bands (choice D is wrong).

8. **C**   The proximal convoluted tubule is responsible for the reabsorption of numerous solutes and metabolites including glucose, amino acids, bicarbonate, and phosphorous. With impaired reabsorption in Fanconi syndrome, patients can develop hypoglycemia since glucose would not be reabsorbed normally (choice A is wrong) and metabolic acidosis due to poor reabsorption of bicarbonate (choice C is correct). Normally, water passively follows the reabsorption that occurs in the proximal convoluted tubule. In Fanconi syndrome, this is disrupted and a greater volume of fluid remains in the nephron resulting in greater urinary output (choice B is wrong). Amino acid reabsorption takes place largely in the proximal convoluted tubule, whereas the collecting duct is involved in selective reabsorption of electrolytes and water (choice D is wrong).

9. **B**   This problem requires use of the Hardy-Weinberg equation. Individuals that carry at least one copy of the recessive allele are either heterozygous or homozygous recessive. Therefore, $2pq + q^2 = 102/200 = 0.51$, and $p^2 = 1 - 0.51 = 0.49$, so $p = 0.7$. Since $p + q = 1$, $q = 1 - 0.7 = 0.3$. The proportion of carriers is equal to $2pq$, which is $2(0.7)(0.3) = 0.42$ (choice B is correct and choices A, C, and D are wrong).

10. **C**   The myelin in the central nervous system is formed by oligodendrocytes (choice C is correct). Schwann cells form the myelin in the peripheral nervous system (choice B is wrong). Astrocytes and ependymal cells are both found in the CNS, but neither has a role in producing or maintaining myelin (choices A and D are wrong).

11. **D** The δ cells produce somatostatin, which inhibits many digestive processes including the secretion of gastrin. If these cells are damaged, somatostatin levels will be decreased and gastrin levels will be increased, leading to excess release of stomach acid (choice D is correct). α cells and β cells release glucagon and insulin, respectively, and neither is involved with gastric acid (eliminate choices A and B). The pancreas does not contain any γ cells (eliminate choice C).

12. **A** LARCs prevent pregnancy via numerous mechanisms. By virtue of their mechanism of delivery, both the subdermal implant and hormone-releasing intrauterine devices result in lower serum progestin levels and fewer systemic side effects than generally experienced with oral contraceptive pills (choice A is correct). Administration of exogenous progestins would result in a fall in gonadotropins via negative feedback, not an increase (choices B and C are wrong), and it is this suppression of LH that prevents ovulation. Progesterone is normally responsible for the conversion of the endometrium to the secretory phase, and its withdrawal is what triggers the sloughing of the endometrium during menstruation. With an exogenous progesterone supply (in the form of progestins), the progesterone level will be maintained and the endometrium will not be lost (choice D is wrong).

13. **D** Peristalsis is driven by the rhythmic contraction of smooth muscle in the walls of the bowel; this process is regulated by the autonomic nervous system and has nothing to do with ciliary contraction (choice D would not be expected and is the correct answer choice). Generalized ciliary dysfunction in a patient diagnosed with Kartagener's syndrome would result in the broad disruption of functions that depend on proper ciliary movement. In females, oviductal cilia are primarily responsible for moving the ovum down the fallopian tubes to allow fertilization; ciliary dysfunction would reduce the chance that the egg would be fertilized (choice B would be expected and can be eliminated). Cilia are also utilized by the respiratory tract to clear mucus from the lungs and bronchi; ciliary dysfunction would lead to poor clearance of infectious agents from the respiratory tract (choice C would be expected and can be eliminated). Motility of sperm, a key determinant of male fertility, is highly dependent on the flagellum that drives sperm toward the egg. The question stem states that the condition is due to a defect in the dynein arm of microtubules, a structure that is also critical for flagellar movement. It is a reasonable to assume that if the defective dynein prevents ciliary movement, it would also prevent flagellar movement (choice A would be expected and can be eliminated).

14. **B** Consistent qualities among malignant growths are the increased invasion of surrounding tissues (choice A would be expected and can be eliminated), decreased cellular adhesion (choice B would NOT be expected and is the correct answer choice), decreased apoptosis (choice C would be expected and can be eliminated), and decreased differentiation (choice D would be expected and can be eliminated). This is accomplished by rapid mitosis, degradation of the extracellular matrix, downregulation of normal apoptosis, and, generally speaking, the predominance of the specific cell line that received the mutation.

15. **D** If immature B-cells bind to normal cell surface proteins, apoptosis is induced (choice D is correct). If apoptosis were induced in MHC II-expressing B-cells, then all B-cells would be killed, since they are professional antigen-presenting cells and express MHC II (choice A is wrong). While antibodies that bind to other antibodies are a target for many drugs that treat autoimmune diseases, the body does not produce these endogenously (these would also technically be self-antigens; choice B is wrong). If immature B-cells that bind to normal cell surface antigens divided into plasma cells, this would result in the production of antibodies to self-antigens, causing autoimmune diseases, not preventing them (choice C is wrong).

SOLUTIONS TO PRACTICE PASSAGE 1

1. **C**   Chymotrypsin cleaves at the C-terminus of aromatic amino acids, two of which—tryptophan (W) and phenylalanine (F)—are in peptide A. Thus, in order to produce the three resultant peptides mentioned in the passage, there are only two possibilities for the original sequence of peptide A: E-W-G-C-A-F-A-P, or G-C-A-F-E-W-A-P. Regardless of which of these two options was actually peptide A, the C-terminus in both cases will always be proline (choice C is correct, and choices A, B, and D can be eliminated).

2. **C**   This is a 2x2 type of question. K_m and affinity have an inverse relationship such that higher K_m values imply lower affinity for a substrate and vice versa (choices A and D can be eliminated). If several of the hydrophobic residues located in the hydrophobic pocket of chymotrypsin are replaced by lysine residues in MutaChy, the pocket will be lined with positive charges, as lysine is a basic amino acid. If the students experiment using Peptide E, which has two arginines (which will also be positively charged at physiological pH), then the lysine-lined pocket of MutaChy will repel Peptide E due to Coulomb's Law. This repulsion will cause MutaChy to have a lower affinity for Peptide E than chymotrypsin. Thus, chymotrypsin will have a higher affinity for Peptide E (choice B can be eliminated), and consequently a lower K_m value (choice C is correct).

3. **B**   The dipeptides Peptide B and Peptide D will not migrate through the gel when the peptides are at their isoelectric point. The isoelectric point is the pH such that the net overall charge for a peptide is zero. For peptides with acidic amino acid side chains, the isoelectric point will be lower than that of a peptide with only neutral or basic side chains. Comparing Peptide B and Peptide D, Peptide D has a glutamic acid residue and thus is a more acidic peptide than Peptide B. Consequently, the isoelectric point for Peptide D will be lower. If the isoelectric point for Peptide D is lower, the pH at which it shows no migration will be lower, and thus the concentration of hydronium will be higher for Peptide D. Thus, the trial at which Peptide B did not move was buffered at a lower hydronium concentration than when Peptide D did not move (answer choice B is correct; answer choices A, C, and D can be eliminated).

4. **D**   A tripeptide is a peptide that consists of three amino acids. If the tripeptide is comprised entirely of tyrosine, the peptide will comprise of three tyrosine amino acids linked together, thus there will be $9 \times 3 = 27$ carbons total in the tripeptide (choice B can be eliminated). During peptide bond formation, a molecule of water is lost in dehydration. If the amount of atoms in tyrosine is simply multiplied by three, $C_{27}H_{33}N_3O_9$ is the molecular formula. However, this does not take into account the loss of water (choice A can be eliminated). Since the peptide has three amino acids, this implies that two peptide bonds were formed, and thus two water molecules were lost (choice D is correct and choice C can be eliminated.)

5. **B**   This is a memory-based question. Since chymotrypsin is a protease, the correct hormone will be the one that stimulates the production of proteases in the digestion process. Secretin stimulates the exocrine portion of the pancreas to secrete bicarbonate (choice A can be eliminated). Insulin stimulates the removal of glucose from the blood for storage as glycogen and fat (choice C can be eliminated). Somatostatin inhibits many digestive processes, and inhibits the release of hormones such as secretin and cholecystokinin (choice D can be eliminated and choice B is correct). Cholecystokinin (also known as CCK) is a hormone that acts on the pancreas, thereby stimulating the release of many pancreatic digestive proteases such as chymotrypsin.

6. **D** First, note that in the answer choices, both Items II and III appear twice, so start by analyzing one of those. This will allow you to eliminate two choices at once. Item II is true: Amino acids resulting from peptide digestion can be used as precursors for creating many other metabolites in the body. Individual amino acids are further degraded into the amine group and the carbon skeleton. The carbon skeleton be first converted to pyruvate and then to acetyl-CoA, or directly to acetyl-CoA for some amino acids (choices A and C can be eliminated). Since both remaining answer choices include Item I, Item I must be true and we can focus on Item III. Item III is also true: The amine group of the amino acids can be used to form nitrogen containing compounds such as DNA bases (choice B can be eliminated and choice D is correct). It can also be excreted as urea (Item I is true).

SOLUTIONS TO PRACTICE PASSAGE 2

1. **A** RISC contains both single stranded RNA and an endonuclease, and hence is comprised of RNA and protein. The monomeric units of RNA and protein are ribonucleotides and amino acids, respectively. Item I is true, as ribosomal subunits consist of both rRNA and proteins (choice B is wrong). Item II is false, as RNA polymerase is a protein that uses a DNA template; RNA is not part of its structure (choice C is wrong). Item III is false because nucleosomes do not consist of RNA, but rather are made of DNA wound around proteins (choice A is correct; choice D is wrong).

2. **C** The correct answer is the statement that is false. While apoptosis leads to the disassembly of the cytoskeleton, the cell does not gradually expand, but rather shrinks in size during apoptosis (choice C is correct; choices A, B, and D are wrong). The rest of the statements are all true about apoptosis.

3. **C** If Gene X encodes a nuclease that degrades siRNA targeting cIAP-2 expression, only cIAP-1 and XIAP targeting siRNA will remain in transfected cells. Cells transfected with Gene X' have that same gene, plus they encode for nucleases that degrade cIAP-2 and XIAP targeting siRNA. However, only one of these nucleases—the same gene originally in Gene X—will be translated. This is because the inserted sequence of Gene X' is downstream of Gene X and the mRNA of Gene X (transcribed from the antisense strand) will contain the region 5'-TCAGGGAAUUACUAA-3'. Upon translation, a stop codon (UAA) will be reached before the inserted gene mRNA can be translated. Therefore, in both cells transfected with Gene X and Gene X', only nucleases degrading siRNA targeting cIAP-2 will be ultimately translated. Consequently, XIAP levels for both groups of cells be the same (choice C is correct; choices A, B, and D are wrong).

4. **A** The discarded RNA strand following RISC formation is complementary to the strand that remains on the RISC. Therefore, the strand that remains on the RISC will have the sequence 3'-AUAAACGCGA -5'. Because this strand has to anneal to the mRNA transcript to degrade it, the mRNA strand will have the complementary sequence 5'-UAUUUGCGCU-3' (choice A is correct; choices B, C, and D are wrong). Of note, the mRNA transcript that is degraded by RISC is actually the exact same sequence as the strand that is initially discarded by RISC.

5. **B** The question states that a hydrophobic amino acid is found at position 2. Tryptophan (W), phenylalanine (F), and alanine (A) are all hydrophobic, but asparagine (N) is hydrophilic, and would not be found at position 2.

SOLUTIONS TO PRACTICE PASSAGE 3

1. **A**   The passage says that cerotic acid is a 26-carbon long-chain saturated fatty acid. It will undergo 12 cycles of β-oxidation to generate 13 molecules of acetyl-CoA, 12 NADH and 12 $FADH_2$. After the acetyl-coa molecules go through the Krebs cycle, 39 molecules of NADH and 13 molecules of $FADH_2$ will be formed. This leads to a total of 51 NADH and 25 $FADH_2$ (eliminate choices B and D). The passage also says that erucic acid is a monounsaturated fatty acid with 22 carbons. It will undergo 10 cycles of β-oxidation to generate 11 molecules of acetyl-CoA, 10 NADH and 10 $FADH_2$. After the acetyl-coa molecules go through the Krebs cycle, 33 molecules of NADH and 11 molecules of $FADH_2$ will be formed. This leads to a total of 43 NADH and 21 $FADH_2$. Thus, cerotic acid will give 51 – 43 = 8 additional molecules of NADH and 25 – 21 = 4 additional molecules of $FADH_2$ (eliminate choice C; choice A is correct).

2. **A**   The passage says that ALD affects the central nervous system myelin sheath, the adrenal cortex, and Leydig cells. Item I is true: A damaged myelin sheath could lead to progressive paralysis of the lower limbs (eliminate choice B). Item II is false: The adrenal cortex secretes aldosterone, which increases blood pressure. If this tissue is negatively affected by ALD, it likely will not secrete normal levels of aldosterone, thus causing decreased blood pressure in ALD patients (eliminate choice C). Item III is false: Sex steroids are produced by the adrenal cortex and also (in males) by the Leydig cells. If ALD affects these negatively, levels of sex steroids should be low (eliminate choice D; choice A is correct).

3. **B**   The passage says that children affected by ALD can be born to parents that do not have the disease; this means the condition is caused by a recessive allele. The passage also says that ALD is more common in males than females, suggesting it is an X-linked trait. If you let X^A = the normal allele, and X^a = the ALD allele, the female in the question stem must have a $X^A X^a$ genotype, and her parents must be $X^A Y$ (father) and $X^A X^a$ (mother). This is the only option for normal parents generating a carrier female. The passage says that the frequency of X^a in the human population is estimated to be approximately 5%; this means that $q = 0.05$, and $p = 1 – 0.05 = 0.95$. Approximately 50% of humans are female, and of those, you need to calculate the frequency of the $X^A X^a$ genotype. In other words, the probability of being female $\times 2pq = (0.5) \times (2)(0.95)(0.05) = (0.5) \times (0.1)(0.95) = (0.5) \times (0.095) = 0.0475$, or 4.75% (choice B is correct).

4. **C**   The cells in Figure 1 are being stained for mitochondria (via cytochrome C), lysosomes (via acid hydrolase), the nucleus (via RNA polymerase), the smooth endoplasmic reticulum (via epoxide hydrolase, although this is not a protein you are responsible for knowing for the MCAT), vesicles (via caveolin, also a protein you are not responsible for recognizing), and peroxisomes (via catalase). The passage says that when an organelle marker and the antibody against the ABCD1^{mutant} protein co-stain, the organelle will turn white and will thus disappear. This only occurs with catalase staining. This means that the protein responsible for ALD localizes to the peroxisome. The passage says the organelle of interest is negatively affected by ALD (choice C is correct). There is no mention of exocrine secretions in the passage (eliminate choice A). The neurodegenerative disease focuses on synapses, which are not mentioned in the passage (eliminate choice B). AIDS is caused by a virus, which does not match the root cause of ALD (eliminate choice D).

5. **D** Recognize the opportunity to do a 2x2 elimination. The passage states that the fatty acids in Lorenzo's oil are converted into harmless VLCSFAs by the same enzyme that converts saturated shorter fatty acids into harmful VLCSFAs. This means they must bind the active site, similar to a competitive inhibitor (eliminate choices A and C). To determine the organelle of interest, focus on the experimental data in Figure 1; the cells in Figure 1 are being stained for mitochondria (via cytochrome C), lysosomes (via acid hydrolase), the nucleus (via RNA polymerase), the smooth endoplasmic reticulum (via epoxide hydrolase, although this is not a protein you are responsible for knowing for the MCAT), vesicles (via caveolin, also a protein you are not responsible for recognizing), and peroxisomes (via catalase). The passage says that when an organelle marker and the antibody against the ABCD1^{mutant} protein co-stain, the organelle will turn white and will thus disappear. This only occurs with catalase staining. This means that the protein responsible for ALD localizes to the peroxisome (eliminate choice B; choice D is correct).

SOLUTIONS TO PRACTICE PASSAGE 4

1. **B** Key physiologic derangements occurring with a sudden loss of sodium in the blood is an osmotic process—not hydrostatic (choices A and D can be eliminated). A quick decrease in blood levels of sodium (the major electrolyte in the blood) will result in a decrease in the osmotic pressure of the blood, resulting in the passage of water from the blood stream into the tissues via osmosis (choice B is correct). While brain tissue is effectively hypertonic with respect to the blood in this context, the question asks specifically about immediate effects of hyponatremic blood; changes in brain tissue electrolytes would occur after equilibrium is sought by osmosis (choice C is wrong).

2. **A** The passage states that hyponatremia in SIADH lasts for weeks and that dysregulation of ADH secretion is the most likely culprit; thus, it is most likely that hypothalamic dysfunction leads to persistent, excessive release of ADH (choice A is correct). The anterior pituitary gland is not involved in the release or regulation of antidiuretic hormone release (choice B is wrong). While posterior pituitary dysfunction could result in excessive, dysregulated release of antidiuretic hormone, this gland stores ADH synthesized by the hypothalamus and could not produce the persistent, weeks-long SIADH (choice C is wrong). In the context of the passage, while the kidneys are acted upon by excessive ADH synthesized by the hypothalamus and released by the posterior pituitary, they do not give rise to the phenomenon (choice D is wrong).

3. **B** According to the passage, tolvaptan is a competitive antagonist of the vasopressin receptor. As a competitive antagonist, tolvaptan competes with vasopressin for the same binding site (choice C is wrong) but does not activate the receptor (choice A is wrong; choice B is correct). Choice D is wrong, as the mechanism of action of tolvaptan can be determined from the information provided in the passage.

4. **C** The pons' position at the top of the brainstem means that much of the neurologic fibers passing in and out of the brain must pass through this structure; disruption of the neurons at this point will have wide-ranging effects on the function of the peripheral nervous system (choice C is correct). While more disseminated neurologic damage is possible with rapid

corrections of hyponatremia, the passage describes central pontine myelinolysis as primarily caused by damage in the brain (CNS, not PNS, so choice A is wrong). While it is possible for rapid correction of hyponatremia to result in more broadly disseminated damage throughout the brain, the disorder presented in the question stem refers specifically to damage in the pons (choice B is wrong). Though electrolyte derangements are no doubt implicated in neurologic dysfunction in this context, the problem identified in the stem (neuronal death) is more permanent than transient disruption of neuronal conductivity (choice D is wrong).

5.   D   In the context of confirmed SAH, this patient required a large amount of sodium repletion via both hypertonic (triple concentrated) saline and oral salt tabs to counter natriuresis and with eventual administration of tolvaptan to counter water retention (blood dilution) (choice D is correct). Repletion of sodium was not constant. The sodium was administered in increasing amounts during the early part of the hospitalization then subsequently tapered toward the end (choice A is wrong). The patient was administered with tolvaptan, which is described in the passage to be a competitive antagonist of the vasopressin receptor. This lead to inhibition (not activation) of ADH receptors (choice B is wrong). According to the passage, normal physiological blood sodium levels are between 135–145 mmol/L. According to Figure 1, the patient's blood sodium levels never exceeded this range (the patient was never hypernatremic; choice C is wrong).

SOLUTIONS TO PRACTICE PASSAGE 5

1.   A   According to the passage, the sole function of the SR is to store and release Ca^{2+}, which implies that the concentration of all other ions in the SR is low. If the SR were permeable to any other ion, the concentration gradient would favor the movement of the ion form the intracellular fluid into the SR. As calcium ions diffuse down their concentration gradient from the lumen of the SR into the intracellular fluid, a negative electrical gradient forms within the lumen of the SR. To alleviate this negative gradient, the ryanodine receptor should be permeable to a cation, which will act as a counter-ion and flow into the SR lumen (choices C and D are wrong). Sodium and potassium could both act as counterions, but since the concentration of potassium is higher than sodium inside the cell, there is a greater gradient for potassium and faster relief any negative charge created in the SR lumen (choice A is correct; choice B is wrong).

2.   B   As stated in the passage, heart medications derived from *Digitalis purpurea* inhibit the Na^+-K^+ ATPase. This ATPase pumps three sodium ions out of the cell, so inhibition will increase concentration of sodium inside the cell, decreasing the ratio of intracellular to extracellular concentrations (choices A and C are wrong). To relax heart muscle, a Ca^{2+} is exported out of the cell and Na^+ into the cell (because the porter is an antiport, as mentioned in the passage). However, since the extracellular sodium outside the cell is decreased due to the medication, there will not be as strong of a gradient to allow sodium influx to relax the muscle, leading to more contractility (choice B is correct; choice D is wrong).

3. **D** As stated in the passage, amlodipine increases arterial diameter, thereby increasing blood flow through the arteries. A larger volume of blood will increase the hydrostatic pressure, forcing more fluid out of the capillaries (choice D is correct). Without calcium to bind to the ryanodine receptor, calcium cannot be released from the SR (choice A is wrong). Amlodipine interferes with voltage gated calcium channels, which will decrease the rate of AV node depolarization, not the magnitude of the depolarization (choice B is wrong). If AV node action potential rates decrease, there will be decreased frequency of systole (choice C is wrong).

4. **D** Item I is false. Facilitated diffusion is a type of passive diffusion which does not rely on ATP, however, both the Ca^{2+}-Na^+ antiport and the Ca^{2+} ATPase use ATP, either directly or indirectly (choice C is wrong). Item II is true. A decrease in muscle tension requires a decrease of intracellular calcium, which relies on the Ca^{2+}-Na^+ antiport in addition to the Ca^{2+} ATPase. The direct use of ATP in transporting ions against their concentration gradient, as in the Ca^{2+} ATPase pumping calcium outside of the cell against its gradient is an example of primary active transport (choice B is wrong). Item III is true. The Ca^{2+}-Na^+ antiport uses the sodium gradient created by the Na^+-K^+ ATPase to move calcium out of the cell against its gradient, and thus uses ATP indirectly—an example of secondary active transport (choice A is wrong; choice D is correct).

5. **D** Based on Figure 1, the knockout mouse has a significantly lower cardiac output. To compensate for this, the mouse would most likely have increased total peripheral resistance, so that blood pressure can remain closer to normal (choice D is correct). The increase of total peripheral resistance is a common homeostatic compensation mechanism during hemorrhages, where cardiac output is dropped rapidly. According to Figure 1, the knockout mouse has the same peak systolic blood pressure to the wild type (choice A is wrong). Since cardiac output is directly proportional to heart rate and stroke volume, and the knockout mouse has a lower cardiac output, it is likely to have a lower heart rate and stroke volume (choices B and C are wrong).

SOLUTIONS TO PRACTICE PASSAGE 6

1. **A** The proposed mechanism depicted in Figure 1 demonstrates that SREBP1c activity is triggered by the Akt pathway, which is initiated by insulin binding to its receptor. Since insulin increases SREBP1c activity, the opposite, insulin resistance, must decrease its activity (choice A is correct; choice C is wrong). Excess glucose in the blood (hyperglycemia) would trigger the release of insulin and, subsequently, activation of SREBP1c (choice B is wrong). Ketoacidosis is often observed in the context of insulin deficiency or insulin resistance and is therefore likely to be associated with decreased levels of SREBP1c activity, however, this is not implicated as a cause with the information provided (choice D is wrong).

2. **D** The researchers used a radiolabeled anti-myosin antibody to image myotubes present in their samples; this means of identifying a specific protein is essentially an immunohistochemistry technique (choice D is correct). The substrate of interest was not a nucleic acid (choice B is wrong), and the imaging data shown in Figure 2 was not obtained by a blotting technique (choices A and C are wrong).

3. **C** Since both Items II and III are found in two of the answer choices, it's wise to start with one of those. Item II is false: Activation of TSC1-2 will lead to increased inhibition of Rheb, which is then unable to increase mTORC1 activity (choices B and D can be eliminated). Since choices A and C both include Item I, it must be true, so you can focus on Item III. Item III is true: Activation of Rheb will directly increase mTORC1 activity (choice A can be eliminated; choice C is correct). Note that Item I is true: According to Figure 1, activation of Akt will lead to increased inhibition of TSC1-2. Inhibition of TSC1-2 will stop the inhibition of Rheb, which will then stimulate mTORC1 activity.

4. **B** The immunofluorescence data in Figure 2 demonstrates that, when SREBP1c is over-expressed in the absence of additional muscle transcription factors, myosin production is decreased. Compare Ad-GFP and Ad-SREBP1c in the top line of Figure 2 (control). Cells expressing SREBP1c show less staining, indicating less myosin (choices C and D are wrong). However, once the muscle transcription factors are introduced (Ad-MEF2C, Ad-MYOD, and Ad-MYOG), myosin production returns closer to normal but doesn't obviously increase (the 2nd, 3rd, and 4th lines, comparing Ad-GFP and Ad-SREBP1c, look about the same; choice B is correct, and choice A is wrong).

5. **C** For X-linked EDMD, let X^E represent the normal dominant allele and X^e represent the recessive allele. The original affected woman must have the genotype X^eX^e, and her unaffected partner's genotype is X^EY. All of their daughters will be carriers (X^EX^e), and all of their sons will be affected (X^eY, choices A and B are true statements and can be eliminated). If the daughters of the original couple (X^EX^e) have children with unaffected males (X^EY), there is a 25% probability of producing unaffected granddaughters (X^EX^E), a 25% probability of producing carrier granddaughters (still unaffected, X^EX^e), a 25% probability of producing unaffected grandsons (X^EY), and a 25% probability of producing affected sons (X^eY, choice C is NOT true and the correct answer choice). If the sons of the original couple (X^eY) have children with unaffected females there are two possible crosses (because unaffected females can be homozygous dominant or heterozygous): $X^eY \times X^EX^E$ (cross A) or $X^eY \times X^EX^e$ (cross B). None of the children from cross A would be affected (0% probability); all males would be X^EY and all females would be X^EX^e. For cross B, there is a 25% probability of producing an affected male (1/2 probability dad donates a Y and 1/2 probability mom donates X^e) and a 25% probability of producing an affected female (1/2 probability dad donates X^e and 1/2 probability mom donates X^e). You have to consider both possible crosses, so we must use the Rule of Addition: the probability of cross A OR cross B = (probability of cross A) + (probability of cross B) − (probability of cross A AND cross B) = (0) + (1/4) − (0 × 1/4) = 1/4 − 0 = 1/4 probability (choice D is a true statement and can be eliminated).

Chapter 14
General Chemistry on
the MCAT

14.1   GENERAL CHEMISTRY ON THE MCAT

Although General Chemistry is sometimes remembered as a daunting topic from college, the MCAT does not test the fine details of General Chemistry. Rather, the focus of this section is on having a strong knowledge of chemistry fundamentals, and manipulating that knowledge to adapt to different scenarios presented in passages and questions. The passages often contain information that recapitulates basic chemistry knowledge, and they may present additional information that builds on fundamental concepts.

The majority of the G-Chem questions will not be based on rote memory, but will require you to retrieve information from the passage and use some deductive reasoning skills. Thus, in order to succeed in this section, you not only need solid knowledge of fundamental principles of chemistry, but also strong critical reasoning and reading comprehension skills. These three components may be stressed differently depending on the passage type.

The science sections of the MCAT have 10 passages and 15 freestanding questions (FSQs). General Chemistry will make up about a third of the questions in the Chemical and Physical Foundations of Biological Systems section. The remaining questions will be on Physics (25%), Organic Chemistry (15%), and Biochemistry (25%). In addition, about 5% of the questions on the Biological and Biochemical Foundations of Living Systems section will be General Chemistry.

14.2   PASSAGE TYPES AS THEY APPLY TO G-CHEM

Information/Situation Presentation

These passages assume knowledge of basic scientific concepts, and also present new information that builds on these basic concepts. The new information may be presented in a way that is very similar to how it would appear in a textbook or other scientific reference. The questions may be about basic scientific facts that you already know, but often the passage will present topics or subtopics with which you are unfamiliar. Information/Situation Presentation passages can be intimidating, as they often explore topics in a greater level of detail than the scope of your MCAT preparation, and they may be wrapped in a Biology or Biochemistry package, adding complexity to the passage text and figures, even though the questions are likely to test fundamental general chemistry concepts. However, keep in mind that the whole point of these types of passages is to force you to use critical reasoning and apply your basic scientific knowledge to new topics. It is not to see how much advanced scientific coursework you have memorized. Therefore, it is important when you see a passage on, say, molecular orbital theory, that you don't think to yourself, "Oh no!! I forgot to study molecular orbital theory!!!" Rather, look at the information in the passage, and consider how your knowledge about more basic chemical concepts, such as electron configurations and bonding, can be applied in order to answer the questions. The new information in the passage can supplement your basic knowledge.

This type of passage may also present information in the context of a specific situation, such as the results of a research study or an experiment. In this case, the questions may ask you to distinguish between data that supports or refutes the result being presented. In some passages, an apparently contradictory or erroneous result is presented and questions may ask what mistakes could have been made over the course of the experiment to cause such a result. Thus, these passages require to you think critically about the importance of each chemical and physical element of an experiment. Note however, that they do not present the steps of an experiment in great detail; that style is reserved for Experiment/Research Presentation passages.

Experiment/Research Presentation

These passages present an experimental set up in great detail; they describe the rationale behind an experiment, how it is set up and executed, and its results. In these passages you are often asked to analyze data given in the form of charts and graphs. In addition, questions may ask you how the results of the experiment would differ if a certain variable were changed; this requires you to think critically about the role of each element of the experiment. In this passage type, be careful not to gloss over important experimental details as you retrieve information from the passage. Be aware that details such as units can make the difference between answering a question correctly or incorrectly, and be vigilant about these experimental details as you work through the questions and look back to the passage.

Persuasive Argument

In a Persuasive Argument passage, two perspectives on a problem are presented. It may be different researchers putting forth two different methodologies for conducting an experiment, or two different explanations for an experimental result or phenomenon.

The questions may ask how the authors came to develop different perspectives, or ask you to evaluate the credibility of each of their arguments. Persuasive Argument passages are the least common passage type in G-Chem.

14.3 READING A G-CHEM PASSAGE

Reading a G-Chem passage is not like reading a scientific paper or a textbook. That is, you are not reading thoroughly and trying to understand the relevance of each sentence, as the passage will likely contain details beyond the scope of the questions.

Instead, your goal is to take no more than 60 seconds and skim the passage in order to determine the general topic area being tested and create a brief passage map before moving on to the questions. To do this as efficiently as possible, focus on the first sentence of each paragraph and any bolded or italicized words. In addition, chemical equations and figures may provide insight as to the general topic of the passage. For example, if you see a titration curve, it is likely that the passage will test acid-base chemistry.

G-Chem passages often include complex graphs and data tables. Avoid the temptation to analyze this data on your first pass through the passage. Rather, wait until you find a question that requires the use of the data in the graph or table, then analyze the data in the context of that question. This approach is more efficient and productive than trying to preemptively interpret data.

The bottom line: You can always go back and reread more details from the passage. Furthermore, not all of the details from the passage are necessary to answer the questions. Therefore, it is a waste of your time to read and attempt to thoroughly understand the passage the first time you read it.

14.4   MAPPING A G-CHEM PASSAGE

Highlighting Text

As you skim through a G-Chem passage to get a feel for the type of questions that might follow, take note of the general location of information within the passage. The highlighting tool is a useful way to visually note a few key words that relate to the general topic of the passage or some unusual or new term that is introduced. Highlight sparingly, and use the scratch paper to make more detailed notes. An example of a highlighted passage is shown below. This is an Information Presentation passage:

The batteries that start an automobile or power flashlights are devices that convert chemical energy into electrical energy. These devices use spontaneous oxidation-reduction reactions (called half-reactions) that take place at the electrodes to create an electric current. The strength of the battery, or electromotive force, is determined by the difference in electric potential between the half cells, expressed in volts. This voltage depends on which reactions occur at the anode and the cathode, the concentrations of the solutions in the cells, and the temperature. The cell voltage, E, at a temperature of 25°C and nonstandard conditions, can be calculated from the Nernst equation, where $E°$ is the standard potential, n denotes the number of electrons transferred in the balanced half reaction, and Q is the reaction quotient.

$$E = E° - \frac{0.0592}{n} \log_{10} Q$$

Equation 1

The lead storage battery used in automobiles is composed of six identical cells joined in series. The anode is solid lead, the cathode is lead dioxide, and the electrodes are immersed in a solution of sulfuric acid. As each cell discharges during normal operation, the sulfate ion is consumed as it is deposited in the form of lead sulfate on both electrodes, as shown in Reaction 1:

Reaction 1:

$$Pb(s) + PbO_2(s) + 4\,H^+(aq) + 2\,SO_4^{2-}(aq)$$
$$\downarrow$$
$$2\,PbSO_4(s) + 2\,H_2O(l)$$

Each cell produces 2 V, for a total of 12 V for the typical car battery. Unlike many batteries, however, the lead storage battery can be recharged by applying an external voltage. Because the redox reaction in the battery consumes sulfate ions, the degree of discharge of the battery can be checked by measuring the density of the battery fluid with a hydrometer. The fluid density in a fully charged battery is 1.2 g/cm³.

Half-reaction	E° (V)
$F_2(g) + 2e^- \rightarrow 2F^-(aq)$	+2.87
$Cl_2(g) + 2e^- \rightarrow 2Cl^-(aq)$	+1.36
$Cu^+(aq) + e^- \rightarrow Cu(s)$	+0.52
$Cu^{2+}(aq) + 2e^- \rightarrow Cu(s)$	+0.34
$Zn^{2+}(aq) + 2e^- \rightarrow Zn(s)$	–0.76
$Al^{3+}(aq) + 3e^- \rightarrow Al(s)$	–1.66
$Li^+(aq) + e^- \rightarrow Li(s)$	–3.05

Table 1 Standard Reduction Potentials at T = 25°C

Note that only a few words are highlighted. In the first paragraph, "batteries," and "spontaneous oxidation-reduction," relate to the general topic of the passage, and they serve as a reminder that batteries contain a spontaneous redox reaction. The second paragraph identifies the two electrode in the battery and, in the last paragraph, the voltage and density of a car battery are highlighted. Since these are specific and unusual pieces of information, they might come up in a question.

Rather than highlighting large portions of the passage as you skim it, use your scratch paper to create a simple passage map to help organize where different types of information are in the passage. Scratch paper is only useful if it is kept organized! Make sure that your notes for each passage are clearly delineated and marked with the passage number and range of questions on your scratch paper. This will allow you to easily read your notes when you come back to review a marked question. Resist the temptation to write in the first available blank space, as this makes it much more difficult to refer back to your work.

As you skim the passage, note the subject of each paragraph and any key words or values. A well-constructed passage map makes it easier and more efficient to go back and retrieve specific information as you work through the questions. Here is an example of a passage map for the passage shown above:

P1 – Batteries, general information, background
P2 – Specifics car batteries
P3 – Recharge car battery, Red. Pot Table 1

As you can see, your passage map does not need to be particularly detailed, nor should it be, as reading and mapping the passage should only take a minute of your time. However, this does provide a valuable framework for efficiently locating information within the passage. You may find that highlighting the text in a General Chemistry passage is enough of a framework and reference for you, however, and many test-takers are just as successful without writing any information down on their scratch paper until they actually get into the specifics of the questions.

Let's look at another passage and how to map it. This is an Experiment/Research Presentation passage:

Two cube-shaped compartments, X and Y, each with a volume of one cubic meter, were used in several experiments to study the properties of gases. Compartment X was fitted with a piston of negligible mass which fit snugly against the walls of the container. The compartments were connected by a pinhole which could be opened or closed at will (see Figure 1). The pressure and temperature could be measured in either compartment. At the start of each experiment, Compartment X contained equal molar quantities of four gases (helium, oxygen, nitrogen, and carbon dioxide), the temperature in Compartment X was 25°C and the pressure was 1 atm. Initially, Compartment Y was evacuated. The behavior of all the gases can be assumed to be ideal. (Note: 1 atm ≈ 105 Pa.)

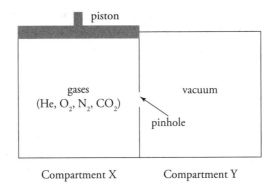

piston

gases
(He, O_2, N_2, CO_2)

vacuum

pinhole

Compartment X   Compartment Y

Figure 1   Experimental apparatus

Experiment 1:

With the pinhole closed, the temperature of the gases in Compartment X was gradually increased to 50°C, and the pressure of the gas inside the compartment was measured.

Experiment 2:

With the pinhole closed, the piston was gradually lowered into Compartment X until it had dropped a distance of 0.5 m. The pressure of the gas in the container was then measured.

Experiment 3:

The pinhole was opened, and the pressure change in each compartment was measured until equilibrium was reached.

Here, the highlighter tool can be used to emphasize that this passage is about the behavior of gases. Any time a passage is about gases, it's useful to know if the gas behaves in a real or ideal manner; therefore, the phrase "assumed to be ideal" is also highlighted. In experimental passages, if important details jump out at you on your initial skim of the passage, it's useful to highlight them. For example, Figure 1 makes it fairly obvious that compartment X contains four gases, while compartment Y is a vacuum with no gas, however, the "equal molar quantities" of the four gases in compartment X is a useful detail to highlight. Here's how you might map this passage on your scratch paper:

P1 – Experimental setup
E1 – Temp change, constant V
E2 – Pressure change
E3 – Pressure change, equilibrium

As was true of our last passage map, the main purpose is to create an outline so that it will be easier to retrieve necessary information as you work through the questions. Since this is an Experiment Presentation passage, the map points out the location of the main experimental details. Note that on the first pass, it is not important to note the specific details of each individual experiment on your scratch paper, though quickly highlighting new experimental conditions, such as temperature, etc. can be helpful. If possible, however, it may be helpful to note the general variable being changed.

Let's look at one more example of passage mapping. This passage is a Persuasive Argument Passage:

Two theoretical chemists attempted to explain the observed trends of acidity by applying two interpretations of molecular orbital theory. Consider the pK_a values of some common acids listed along with the conjugate base of each acid:

acid	pK_a	conjugate base
H_2SO_4	< 0	HSO_4^-
H_2CrO_4	5.0	$HCrO_4^-$
H_3PO_4	2.1	$H_2PO_4^-$
HF	3.9	F^-
HOCl	7.8	ClO^-
HCN	9.5	CN^-
HIO_3	1.2	IO_3^-

Recall that acids with a $pK_a < 0$ are called strong acids, and those with a $pK_a > 0$ are called weak acids. The arguments of the chemists are given below.

Chemist #1:

"The acidity of a compound is proportional to the polarization of the H—X bond, where X is some nonmetal element. Complex acids, such as H_2SO_4, $HClO_4$, and HNO_3 are strong acids because the H—O bonding electrons are strongly drawn towards the oxygen. It is generally true that a covalent bond weakens as its polarization increases. Therefore, one can conclude that the strength of an acid is proportional to the number of electronegative atoms in that acid."

Chemist #2:

"The acidity of a compound is proportional to the number of stable resonance structures of that acid's conjugate base. H_2SO_4, $HClO_4$, and HNO_3 are all strong acids because their respective conjugate bases exhibit a high degree of resonance stabilization."

For a Persuasive Argument passage, the goal of passage mapping and highlighting is to identify the issue being addressed, and the main points of each of the opposing lines of reasoning. This can be accomplished using the highlighter tool to emphasize that the passage is about "trends of acidity," and that Chemist #1 attributes the behavior of acids to "polarization of the H—X bond," while Chemist #2 focuses on "number of stable resonance structures."

In this case, a passage map would be very similar to the results achieved by highlighting. However, keep in mind that the very act of writing things down helps clarify it in your head:

P1/Main issue: Trends of acidity, using MO theory
Chemist #1: acidity ∝ # of EN atoms; polarization of H—X bond
Chemist #2: acidity ∝ # of res. struct. for conj. base.

14.5 FIGURE AND TABLE ANALYSIS

Figures, graphs, data tables, and both algebraic and chemical equations are generally the sources of information you'll need to answer the majority of the General Chemistry questions on the MCAT. Your goal as you skim through each passage, is to get a general sense of the type of information that is presented in these figures to give you some insight into what types of questions you might be asked. Don't spend too much time analyzing information that you might not need to use in the passage. Instead, jot down any information on your scratch paper that will help you return to the important details quickly when a question seems to require passage information. What follows are some examples of figures/tables/equations you might see in a G-Chem passage and the type of information you might note about them after a brief glance.

Experimental Equipment

For figures that represent an experimental set up, read any titles that might be given, the labels on equipment, and take note of any information that stands out. Don't spend too much time trying to figure out what's going on in a picture that seems very new to you, as you'll likely waste a lot of time without a question to direct you to the relevant information. Just get a general sense of what variables are being tested or what the goal of the experiment is before jumping into the questions. On the other hand, in cases where the equipment is very familiar to you and the intent of the experiment is obvious, pause long enough to see if there are any tweaks or exceptions that the MCAT is throwing into the mix that might trip you up.

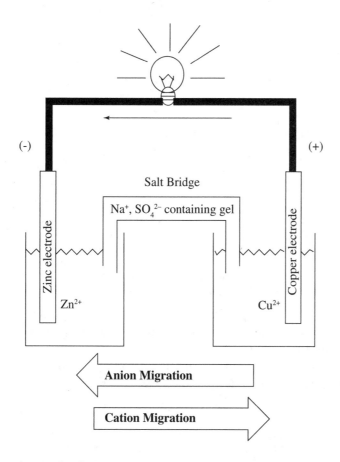

For example, the electrochemical cell above should look very familiar to you, but take just a second to pay attention to the labels in the figure to confirm any assumptions you might make. The glowing light bulb suggests a spontaneous reaction, but the electrode signs in conjunction with the arrows that show the direction of ion migration are what allow you to jot down "galvanic cell" on your scratch paper. Importantly, note that the unlabeled arrow by the light bulb represents current direction, not e^- flow. It's best to note some more detail about the electrodes to keep your sign conventions straight. Something like "Zn = anode/ox, Cu = cathode/red)" would be a good reference.

Graphs

For graphs (which are generally also labeled as Figures), read the titles, axes labels, units, and any legends provided. Note if any obvious trends exist or what type of relationship the variables plotted might have. Don't spend any time trying to analyze or quantify relationships at this point. You'll be more efficient doing so if/when a specific question asks you about this level of detail, and you'll know exactly where to start looking.

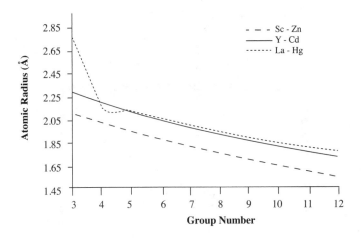

Figure 1 Atomic radii of *d*-block elements by period

For this graph, you should note from the title and legend that the three lines represent different rows of transition metals on the periodic table, so you might need to call it up on screen for this passage. You should also note that while the slopes of all three lines are similar, lines 2 and 3 from the legend are nearly identical, except for the big dip from group 3 to 4. This is likely an important feature of the graph, so be on the lookout for a question asking about something anomalous.

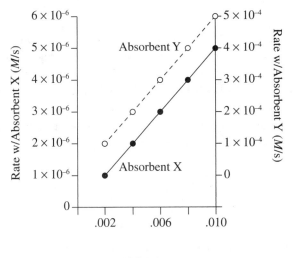

Figure 2 CO_2 scrubbing at 25°C

For this graph, you should take note that each straight line is associated with a different vertical axis, and that each axis has a different order of magnitude for its rate values. If you choose to attack this passage immediately, you might not jot anything down, but if you skip it for later, you might note on your scratch paper "left = X (10^{-6}), right = Y (10^{-4})".

Tables

Data tables are generally straightforward and tend to either summarize experimental results or list properties of different chemical species, like pK_a values, standard reduction potentials, thermodynamic values, etc. In either case, read the table titles as well as column or row headings, and take note of any units presented with the values. If experimental data is given, jot down any obvious trends that jump out at you quickly. For the latter type of table, don't spend any time analyzing or internalize the values until you read a question that requires another look at them.

Metal	Bath A	Bath B	Bath C
Magnesium	V	V	X
Lead	OO	OO	V
Iron	M	S	X
Aluminum	V	M	X
Copper	OO	OO	V
Silver	OO	OO	M
Zinc	V	V	X
Cobalt	M	M	X
Tin	M	M	V
Mercury	OO	OO	M

Table 1 Rates of gas evolution

This table shows relative degrees of gas evolution based on an experiment described in the text of the passage. Note that the key for the table itself is not near the data, but was buried in the text of the passage preceding the table. This would be appropriate information to highlight as you skim the passage. Even without the key shown here, you might note (since the OO jumps out a bit) on your scratch paper "baths A&B usu. same; bath C usu. diff."

Mole percent of Ammonia at Equilibrium					
Temp (°C)	Pressure (atm)				
	10	50	100	500	1000
200	51	74	82	94	98
300	15	39	52	80	93
400	4	15	25	56	80
500	1.2	6	11	26	57

For this set of experimental data, first note the variables that affect mole percent of NH_3 at equilibrium are pressure and temperature. Since this table has a lot of numbers you shouldn't focus on them too much, but a fairly quick glance should make the relationships between the variables clear. On your scratch paper jot down "as P↑, mole %↑; as T↑, mole %↓."

Compound	ΔH_t° (kJ/mol)	ΔG_t° (kJ/mol)	S° (J/K mol)
C(s)	0.0	0.0	5.7
$H_2O(g)$	−241.8	−228.6	188.7
CO(g)	−110.5	−137.1	197.6
$H_2(g)$	0.0	0.0	130.6

Table 1 Thermodynamic Data for Reactants and Products in Water Gas Reaction

This data table shows reference values for thermodynamic properties of the elements and compounds found in the water gas reaction given in the passage, not experimentally derived data. A calculation question of some sort based on these numbers is likely. The column headings show the properties and units presented, and you should either highlight, if the screen lets you, or jot down "S = J and H/G = kJ." You might also note that while pure elements have 0 values for H and G, they are non-zero values for S.

Equations

Equations can be of two different types in a G-Chem passage. You could be given some sort of quantitative (algebraic) relationship, which you may or may not be familiar with, or you might be given one or more chemical reactions. In both cases, they will be offset from the text and will clearly be labeled with an equation or reaction number, making them easy to find when you need to refer to them. Because of this, it's often unnecessary to highlight the equations themselves. However, the text around these equations will generally give you more detail about the equations, and flagging this information is a much better use of your highlighter.

$$D_{(A-B)} = \frac{1}{2}[D_{(A-A)} + D_{(B-B)}] + \alpha(\chi_A - \chi_B)^2$$

Equation 1

A complex algebraic expression such as this is likely new information the MCAT does not expect you to already know, so be sure to pay attention to surrounding text and highlight what each variable represents. Chances are a question will ask you to apply your outside knowledge and use this equation in some way.

Step 1 (slow)	$CO_2(g) + H_2O(l) \rightleftharpoons H_2CO_3(aq)$
Step 2 (moderate)	$H_2CO_3(aq) + NaOH(aq) \rightarrow NaHCO_3(aq) + H_2O(l)$
Step 3 (fast)	$NaHCO_3(aq) + Ca(OH)_2(s) \rightarrow CaCO_3(s) + NaOH(aq) + H_2O(l)$

In this case, the series of equations represents the chemical reactions of a mechanism, for which the overall reaction was given in the passage. Don't spend any time focused on any reactant or product, but do note that Step 1 is an equilibrium, while Steps 2 and 3 are not, and that Step 1 is also the slow (rate-determining) step.

As you can see from the examples above, effective passage-mapping requires a combination of highlighting and jotting down notes in an organized fashion on your scratch paper. The best way to improve your passage mapping, and to determine which combination of these skills works best for you, is to practice, practice, practice.

14.6 TACKLING THE QUESTIONS

In general, G-Chem questions require a combination of basic knowledge, passage retrieval, and critical reasoning. The more difficult G-Chem questions tend to weigh the last two skills more heavily. Therefore, if you have a sound basis in the fundamental principles of General Chemistry, it is safe to assume that a tough question will be best addressed by looking back to the passage for information that is either explicitly stated or implied.

In the section on passage mapping, we reviewed an Information/Situation Presentation passage on batteries and redox reactions. We will draw on questions from this passage in order to illustrate the different question types.

Memory Questions

These questions test background knowledge and require you to recall a specific definition or relationship. Memory questions are most often freestanding questions, and only rarely will they be within a set of questions that accompany a passage. When they are, they will help you complete a passage more quickly since there is no information retrieval required that will slow you down. For example, a question from the car battery passage shown above asked:

> If the reaction in a concentration cell is spontaneous in the reverse direction, then:
>
> A) $Q < K$, ΔG for the forward reaction is negative, and the cell voltage is positive.
> B) $Q < K$, ΔG for the forward reaction is positive, and the cell voltage is negative.
> C) $Q > K$, ΔG for the forward reaction is negative, and the cell voltage is positive.
> D) $Q > K$, ΔG for the forward reaction is positive, and the cell voltage is negative.

In order to answer this question correctly, you need to know the connection between ΔG and spontaneity. A spontaneous reaction has a negative ΔG, and a nonspontaneous reaction has a positive ΔG. Since the reaction is spontaneous in the reverse direction, it must be nonspontaneous in the forward direction. Therefore, the ΔG of the forward reaction is positive, eliminating choices A and C. Alternatively, you could know that cell voltage applies to the forward direction, and that a nonspontaneous cell has a negative voltage, also eliminating choices A and C.

To distinguish between choices B and D, you must have a fundamental understanding of equilibrium and Le Chatelier's Principle. The reaction quotient, Q, always approaches the equilibrium constant, K, and if $Q > K$, the reaction will be pushed in the reverse direction, toward the reactants side of the equilibrium, in order to decrease the value of Q. Thus, since the question says the reaction is spontaneous in the reverse direction, Q must be greater than K. This makes choice D the best answer.

Also, note that this question asks about concentration cells, which are not mentioned in the passage, and therefore this problem is essentially a free-standing question.

Explicit Questions

Explicit questions require direct retrieval of information from the passage. Sometimes, the answers to Explicit questions are definitions or relationships that are clearly stated in the passage. However, these types of questions may also require some background knowledge or a simple step of logical reasoning. Here is another example from the car battery redox passage shown above:

Of the following, which is the best reducing agent?

A) Li^+
B) Li
C) Cl^-
D) F^-

To answer this question, you must have fundamental knowledge of redox definitions and relationships, but you also need to retrieve information from the passage. The best reducing agent is the species that has the highest oxidizing potential, and Table 1 gives the reduction potentials for these reagents. However, you also need the knowledge that the oxidation potential is the same as the reduction potential, but with the opposite sign. Since the oxidation of Li has the highest positive potential (3.05 V), Li is the strongest reducing agent.

The best way to approach Explicit questions is to refer to your passage map or highlighting to find the location of the information you need. Then, go back to the passage and read that section in greater detail. There are two instances when retrieval of information for Explicit questions can be especially tricky. First, in research study passages, be cautious when retrieving information from tables and graphs. Rather than simply pulling data directly from the figures, be sure to read the text just before and after the figures as well, as it may contain important information that changes the way the data should be interpreted. Second, when a passage goes into greater detail about a subject that you already have fundamental knowledge of, avoid the temptation to answer questions directly from memory. Often, these types of passages will provide some obscure detail or anomalous situation that will be tested in the questions and require you to retrieve information from the passage in order to select the correct answer.

Implicit Questions

Implicit questions require you to work through two or more steps of critical reasoning based on your background knowledge and information given in the passage. In other words, the answer is not directly stated in the passage, but is implied by the information provided. The distinction between an Implicit and an Explicit question can be subtle, as both require you to retrieve information from the passage, and Explicit questions may also require you to make a simple critical reasoning decision. The difference is that in Implicit questions, the reasoning step required is not as direct or obvious, and more than one step is usually required. Here's an example.

> When a lead storage battery recharges, what happens to the density of the battery fluid?
>
> A) It decreases to 1.0 g/cm^3.
> B) It increases to 1.0 g/cm^3.
> C) It decreases to 1.2 g/cm^3.
> D) It increases to 1.2 g/cm^3.

First, information on the density of the battery fluid must be retrieved from the passage. Our passage map tells us that specific information on car batteries can be found in paragraph two and reviewing the highlighted text reveals that in the third paragraph of the passage, it states that the density of fluid in a fully charged battery is 1.2 g/cm^3. Therefore, as the battery is recharging, its density is approaching this value, eliminating choices A and B.

The difference between choices C and D is whether the density of the solution is increasing or decreasing to 1.2 g/cm^3 during recharge. To determine this, we can look for additional information in the passage that may relate to changing density of the battery fluid. The second paragraph of the passage states that as the battery discharges, sulfate ions are consumed and deposited in the form of lead sulfate. The removal of ions from solution implies that the amount of mass in the solution is going down, and therefore its density is also decreasing. Therefore, density is decreasing during discharge and increasing during recharge. This makes choice D the best answer.

The key step here is focusing on the differences among answer choices. What can be difficult about approaching Implicit questions is that it is often hard to determine which information is supposed to "imply" something about the answer. Zeroing in on differences among the answer choices can help you determine which information from the passage is most relevant, and it may help you rephrase what the question is really asking. Also, note that the first step of our analysis, eliminating the choices with 1.0 g/cm^3 density, was basically just answering an Explicit question via direct passage retrieval. Many Implicit questions begin this way, and it is much easier to eliminate answer choices first based on explicit information than it is to try to make a decision based on implicit information.

14.7   SUMMARY OF THE APPROACH TO GENERAL CHEMISTRY

How to Map the Passage and Use Scratch Paper

1) The passage should not be read like textbook material, with the intent of learning something from every sentence (science majors especially will be tempted to read this way). Skim through the paragraphs to get a feel for the type of questions that will follow, and to get a general idea of the location of information within the passage.

2) Highlighting—Use this tool sparingly, or you will end up with a passage that is completely covered in yellow highlighter! Highlighting in a General Chemistry passage should be used to draw attention to a few words that demonstrate one of the following:

   - the main theme of a paragraph
   - important predictions or conclusions about an experiment
   - any unusual or unfamiliar terms that are defined specifically for that passage (like something that is italicized)

3) Pay brief attention to equations, figures, and experiments, noting only what information they deal with (i.e., read titles, axes, and column/row headings). Do not spend a lot of time analyzing at this point, as you can come back and look more closely at this information if a question requires it.

4) Scratch paper is only useful if it is kept organized! Make sure that your notes for each passage are clearly delineated and marked with the passage number and range of questions on your scratch paper. This will allow you to easily read your notes when you come back to review a marked question. Resist the temptation to write in the first available blank space, as this makes it much more difficult to refer back to your work.

General Chemistry Question Strategies

1) Remember that POE is paramount! The strikeout tool allows you to eliminate answer choices; this will improve your chances of guessing the correct answer if you are unable to narrow it down to one choice.

2) Answer the straightforward questions first. Leave questions that require analysis of experiments and graphs for later. Take the test in the order YOU want. Make sure to use your scratch paper to indicate questions you skipped.

3) Make sure that the answer you choose actually answers the question, and isn't just a true statement.

4) I-II-III questions: Always work between the I-II-III statements and the answer choices. Unfortunately, it is not possible to strike out the Roman numerals, but this is a great use for scratch paper notes. Once a statement is determined to be true (or false), strike out answer choices that do not contain (or do contain) that statement.

5) LEAST/EXCEPT/NOT questions: Don't get tricked by these questions that ask you to pick the answer that doesn't fit (the incorrect or false statement). It's often good to use your scratch paper and write a T or F next to answer choices A–D. The one that stands out as different is the correct answer. Don't forget that you can also highlight information in the question stem, so draw attention to the LEAST/EXCEPT/NOT in the question so you don't forget!

6) 2x2 style questions: These questions require you to know two pieces of information to get the correct answer, and are easily identified by their answer choices, which commonly take the form A because X, B because X, A because Y, B because Y. Tackle one piece of information at a time, which should allow you to quickly eliminate two answer choices.

7) Ranking questions: When asked to rank items, look for an extreme—either the greatest or the smallest item—and eliminate answer choices that do not have that item shown at the correct end of the ranking. This is often enough to eliminate one to three answer choices. Based on the remaining choices, look for the other extreme at the other end of the ranking and use POE again.

8) If you read a question and do not know how to answer it, look to the passage for help. It is likely that the passage contains information pertinent to answering the question, either within the text or in the form of experimental data.

9) If a question requires a lengthy calculation, mark it and return to it later, particularly if you are slow with arithmetic or dimensional analysis.

10) Again, don't leave any question blank, and when randomly guessing, choose the same letter for every question unless you have already eliminated it.

14.8   MCAT GENERAL CHEMISTRY TOPIC LIST[1]

Stoichiometry
A.   Metric units
B.   Density
C.   Molecular weight
D.   Mole concept, Avogadro's number
E.   Empirical formulas vs. molecular formulas
F.   Percent composition by mass
G.   Reactions and chemical equations
    1.   writing and balancing chemical equations
    2.   limiting reactants and theoretical yields
H.   Oxidation states

Atomic Nucleus
A.   Atomic number, atomic weight
B.   Neutrons, protons, isotopes
C.   Nuclear forces, binding energy
D.   Radioactive decay
    1. α, β, γ decay
    2.   half-life, exponential decay, semi-log plots

Electronic Structure[2]
A.   Orbital structure of H, principle quantum number n
B.   Number of electrons per orbital, use of Pauli Exclusion Principle
C.   Ground and excited states
D.   Paramagnetism and diamagnetism
E.   Conventional notation for electronic structure (electron configuration)
F.   Emission and absorption line spectra
G.   The Bohr model of an atom
H.   Effective nuclear charge
I.   Heisenberg Uncertainty Principle
J.   Photoelectric effect

The Periodic Table
A.   Alkali metals
B.   Alkaline earth metals
C.   Halogens
D.   Noble gases
E.   Transition metals
F.   Representative elements
G.   Metals and nonmetals
H.   Oxygen group

Periodic Trends
A.   Valence electrons
B.   First and second ionization energies
C.   Electron affinity
D.   Electronegativity
E.   Electron shells and sizes of atoms and ions

Bonding
A. σ and π bonds
B.   Hybrid orbitals and respective geometries
C.   VSEPR theory, prediction of molecular shape
D.   Lewis dot symbols
E.   Resonance and formal charge
F.   Polarity and relationship to electronegativity
G.   Multiple bonding, relationship to length/strength

Phases
A.   Intermolecular forces
    1.   Hydrogen bonding
    2.   Dipole interactions
    3.   London dispersion forces (van der Waal's forces)
B.   Phase transitions
C.   Phase diagrams, pressure vs. temperature
D.   Heats of phase change

---

[1]   Adapted from *The Official Guide to the MCAT Exam (MCAT2015)*, 4th ed., © 2014 Association of American Medical Colleges.

[2]   The AAMC categorizes many of the items in this list as Physics topics, but these concepts are also relevant to General Chemistry.

Gases

A. Units of volume, temperature, and pressure
B. Molar volume at 0°C and 1 atm = 22.4 L/mol
C. Ideal gases and the Ideal Gas Law
D. Kinetic molecular theory of gases
E. Other gas laws (Henry's, Boyle's, Charles', Avogadro's)
F. Deviation of real-gas behavior from Ideal Gas Law
G. Partial pressure, mole fraction
H. Dalton's Law of Partial Pressures

Solutions

A. Units of concentration
B. Common ions in solution: names, formulas, charges (e.g., PO_4^{3-})
C. Hydration
D. Electrolytes
E. Colligative property—osmotic pressure

Kinetics

A. Reaction rates, dependence on temperature and concentration
B. Rate-determining step
C. Activation energy and transition state
D. Catalysts
E. Rate laws, rate constants, reaction order
F. Reaction coordinate graphs
G. Kinetics vs thermodynamics in a reaction

Equilibrium

A. Equilibrium constant and reaction quotient
B. Law of Mass Action
C. Le Châtelier's principle
D. Solubility product constant , K_{sp}
E. The ion product
F. Common ion effect, its use in laboratory separations
G. Complex ion formation, solubility, and pH effects

Acids and Bases

A. Lewis, Brønsted-Lowry, definition of acid, base
B. Conjugate acids and bases
C. Strong acids and bases, common examples
D. Weak acids and bases, common examples
E. Equilibrium constants K_a and K_b (pK_a and pK_b)
F. Ionization of water and $K_w = [H^+][OH^-] = 10^{-14}$ at 25°C
G. pH definition and calculations
H. Hydrolysis of salts of weak acids or bases
I. Buffers, definitions and concepts, influence on titration curves
J. Neutralizations
K. Titrations
   1. Indicators
   2. Interpretation of titration curves

Thermodynamics

A. Thermodynamic system, state function
B. "Zeroth" Law (concept of temperature)
C. First law, conservation of energy
D. Second law, entropy as disorder, variation across phases
E. Enthalpy of reaction
   1. Hess's Law
   2. Standard enthalpies of formation
   3. Bond dissociation energy
F. Reaction energy diagrams, endothermic and exothermic reactions
G. Free energy and spontaneity, connection to equilibrium
H. Calorimetry, heat capacity, specific heat

Redox and Electrochemistry

A. Oxidation/reduction reactions
   1. Common oxidizing and reducing agents
   2. Disproportionation reactions
B. Galvanic cells
   1. Half-reactions, cathode vs. anode
   2. Reduction potentials, cell potential
   3. Direction of electron flow
   4. Nernst equation
   5. Concentration cells
C. Electrolytic cells
   1. Electrolyte
   2. Electron flow
   3. Electrolysis, Faraday's Law
D. Redox titrations
E. Batteries (lead storage and Ni/Cd)

Chapter 15
General Chemistry
Practice Section

FREESTANDING QUESTIONS

1. Recently, the noble gas reagent KrF_2 has been used to induce the formation of other compounds in extreme oxidation states. What is the most likely role for KrF_2 in these reactions?

   A) Photosensitizer
   B) Reducing agent
   C) Oxidizing agent
   D) Source of $F_2(g)$

2. The anti-cancer drug cisplatin is a neutral compound with the formula $Pt(NH_3)_2Cl_2$. What is the valence electron configuration of the platinum atom in this drug?

   A) $6s^2\ 5d^8$
   B) $6s^2\ 5d^6$
   C) $6s^0\ 5d^{10}$
   D) $6s^0\ 5d^8$

3. The free energy of hydrogen bond formation between two water molecules at 298 K is near –8.4 kJ/mol. Of the following choices, which of the following represents the most likely result of the same measurement at 333 K?

   A) –1.7 kJ/mol
   B) –0.88 kJ/mol
   C) –0.84 kJ/mol
   D) –0.53 kJ/mol

4. In experiments monitoring the rate of ethanol elimination from the blood, it was found that the rate of elimination was invariant with time. Which of the following statements explains this observation?

   A) Ethanol elimination follows first-order kinetics.
   B) Ethanol elimination follows zero-order kinetics.
   C) Ethanol elimination follows second-order kinetics.
   D) Ethanol elimination follows inverse first-order kinetics.

5. Recently, a new compound ($Cs[H_2NB_2(C_6F_5)_6]$) was synthesized wherein the Cs ion was 16-coordinate. What characteristic of the Cs ion enables the formation of such a large number of interactions?

   A) Its exceptionally high positive charge
   B) Its exceptionally large electronegativity
   C) Its exceptionally negative electron affinity
   D) Its exceptionally large ionic radius

6. Magnetite (Fe_3O_4) is the biosynthetic mineral thought to allow certain organisms the ability to sense the magnetic field lines of the Earth. If the biosynthetic pathway involves a coprecipitation of ferrihydrite ($Fe(OH)_3$) and ferrous oxide (FeO), assuming no redox activity during precipitation, what must be the overall ratio of ferrihydrite to ferrous oxide in the reaction?

   A) 1 ferrihydrite : 2 ferrous oxide
   B) 2 ferrihydrite : 1 ferrous oxide
   C) 2 ferrihydrite : 3 ferrous oxide
   D) 3 ferrihydrite : 2 ferrous oxide

7. Diborynes, a recently discovered class of compounds, are characterized as having a triple bond between two boron atoms with similar orbital make up to the triple bonds in alkynes and N_2. Which types of bonds constitute the three bonds between the boron atoms?

   A) 2 π bonds and 1 σ bond
   B) 1 π bond and 2 σ bonds
   C) 1 π bond, 1 σ bond, 1 δ bond
   D) 3 π bonds

8. If the following conversion of dental hydroxyapatite ($Ca_5(PO_4)_3(OH)$, $\Delta H_f = -3229$ kcal/mol) to fluoroapatite ($Ca_5(PO_4)_3(F)$), $\Delta H_f = -3296$ kcal/mol) by NaF is exothermic as written, what must always be true regarding the relative ΔH_f values of NaF and NaOH?

   $$Ca_5(PO_4)_3(OH) + NaF \rightarrow Ca_5(PO_4)_3(F) + NaOH$$

   A) $\Delta H_f\ (NaOH) - \Delta H_f\ (NaF) < 67$ kcal/mol
   B) $\Delta H_f\ (NaOH) - \Delta H_f\ (NaF) > 67$ kcal/mol
   C) $\Delta H_f\ (NaF) + \Delta H_f\ (NaOH) < 67$ kcal/mol
   D) $\Delta H_f\ (NaF) + \Delta H_f\ (NaOH) > 67$ kcal/mol

9. n-Butyllithium, butane deprotonated at the 1-position to form an organic anion with a lithium cation, was found to be insufficiently strong to deprotonate 2,5-dimethyltetrahydrofuran. Which of the following bases might instead be used to effect this transformation?

   A) Sodium *n*-butoxide
   B) Sodium *tert*-butoxide
   C) Triethylamine
   D) *Tert*-butyllithium

10. Fluorodeoxyglucose ($C_6H_{11}O_5{}^{18}F$, shown below) is an attractive tracer agent for positron emission tomography based on monitoring positron flux from the decay of ^{18}F ($t_{1/2}$ = 109 min) for which one of the following reasons?

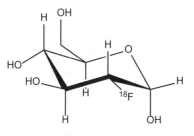

A) The exceptionally long half-life of ^{18}F allows for synthesis and storage of the tracer compound for several days prior to use.
B) The nuclear decay product of fluorodeoxyglucose in living cells is easily metabolized and removed.
C) The compound is readily sequestered in the hydrophobic portions of quickly growing cancer cells.
D) The emitted nuclear particles are sequestered within the cell, not allowing it to damage the surrounding tissues.

11. The free $[Ca^{2+}]$ in the gall bladder of a patient was determined to be 0.53 mmol/L. If the K_{sp} of $CaCO_3$ in gall bladder bile is 1.3×10^{-8}, what must be the minimum concentration of carbonate prior to the nucleation of calcite responsible for the initial formation of gall stones?

A) 22.1 mmol/L
B) 3.65 mmol/L
C) 0.024 mmol/L
D) 0.0043 mmol/L

12. Inhalation of ethyl chloride leads to symptoms resembling alcohol intoxication at a concentration of 3% (by mole) of the inhaled air. At STP, what is the minimum molar concentration of ethyl chloride at which these effects are felt?

A) 0.12 M
B) 0.03 M
C) $1.3 \times 10^{-3} M$
D) $9.7 \times 10^{-3} M$

13. The next generation of lithium ion batteries, so-called lithium air batteries, utilize lithium metal for the anode and an inert cathode exposed to air. Which of these common gases present in air is likely to act as the electrochemically active portion of the cathode?

A) O_2
B) N_2
C) Ar
D) H_2

14. In a recent study, sodium ions were found to closely associate with various isomeric 1,2,3,4,5,6-hexafluorocyclohexanes. Which of the following molecules below likely showed the strongest interaction with the sodium cation?

A)
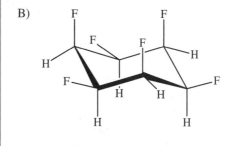

B)
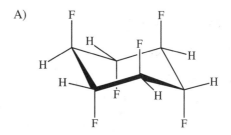

C)
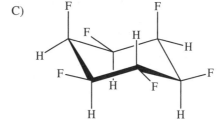

D)
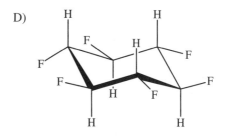

PRACTICE PASSAGE 1

CO_2 is a ubiquitous biological molecule, which is used as a carbon source for photosynthesis and produced as a waste product in cellular respiration. In the past century, the rise in man-made CO_2 has led to negative changes in Earth's climate. Scientists have been working hard to devise an effective strategy to reduce CO_2 levels. One such method involves the use of CO_2 capture with molten salts, such as $CaCO_3$. The solubility of CO_2 in molten $CaCO_3$ has been observed to exceed what would be expected from Henry's Law, $c_{CO_2} = k_H \cdot p_{CO_2}$, where c_{CO_2} is the concentration of CO_2 in the liquid, k_H is Henry's constant, and p_{CO_2} is the partial pressure of CO_2. The increased solubility is explained by a reaction of CO_2 with the carbonate ion to form pyrocarbonate:

$$CO_2 + CO_3^{2-} \rightleftharpoons C_2O_5^{2-}$$

Reaction 1

Using K_{pyro} as the equilibrium constant for Reaction 1, the apparent Henry's constant can be evaluated as:

$$k_H^{app} = \frac{1 + K_{pyro}}{k_H}$$

Equation 1

Researchers investigated the diffusion mechanism of CO_2 in $CaCO_3$ to gauge the potential for use in CO_2 capture. Typical diffusion mechanisms are based on simple mass migration phenomena. However, faster processes have been discovered, such as the Grotthuss diffusion of a proton in water (Reaction 2).

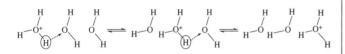

Reaction 2

Experimentally, the movement of CO_2 through $CaCO_3$ was found to be faster than that predicted by molecular diffusion. The researchers suggested the transport of CO_2 in molten carbonates occurs in a manner similar to the Grotthuss mechanism in water. The proposed mechanism (Reaction 3) involves the formation of the pyrocarbonate ion.

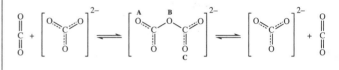

Reaction 3

Adapted from: Corradini et al., *Nature Chemistry*, 2016, *8*, 454-460.

1. One primary difference between the Grotthuss mechanism of carbon dioxide transport in carbonates and that of the diffusion of a proton in water is that:

A) in the carbonate mechanism electrophiles are moved from compound to compound, while in the water mechanism nucleophiles are moved.

B) in the carbonate mechanism nucleophiles are moved from compound to compound, while in the water mechanism electrophiles are moved.

C) the oxygen in water acts as a Brønsted acid, while the carbon in the carbonate acts as a Brønsted base.

D) the oxygen in water acts as a Brønsted base, while the carbon in the carbonate acts as a Brønsted acid.

2. If Reaction 1 was determined to be endothermic, how would an increase in temperature affect the equilibrium concentration of dissolved CO_2 in molten $CaCO_3$, assuming the change to p_{CO_2} is negligible?

A) The concentration of CO_2 would not change.
B) The concentration of CO_2 would increase.
C) The concentration of CO_2 would decrease.
D) The effect on CO_2 concentration cannot be determined from the information given.

3. Which of the following additional findings, if true, would contradict the proposed Grotthuss mechanism for CO_2 transport described in the passage?

I.   The presence of pyrocarbonate was detected in molten $CaCO_3$ during CO_2 transport.
II. After addition of ^{13}C-labeled CO_2 to molten carbonate, the only CO_2 IR stretch ever found in the sample corresponded to $^{13}C=O$.
III. The solubility of CO_2 was found to be similarly greater than expected in other molten carbonates, such as $MgCO_3$.

A) II only
B) III only
C) I and III only
D) II and III only

4. For the pyrocarbonate ion in Reaction 3, what is the best ranking of the C–O bonds from longest to shortest?

A) $C–O_A > C–O_C > C–O_B$
B) $C–O_A = C–O_C > C–O_B$
C) $C–O_B = C–O_A = C–O_C$
D) $C–O_B > C–O_A = C–O_C$

PRACTICE PASSAGE 2

Halogen bonding is a type of intermolecular force between a halogen on an organic molecule and a lone pair of electrons on a second molecule (R–X···D; R = alkyl, aryl; X = halogen; D = electron pair donor). Though crystallographically well documented, and more recently observed as important in materials and biological systems, the underlying physical forces involved in halogen bonding are not well described. Though the notion of a halogen atom bearing a partial negative charge yet acting as an electrophile is counterintuitive, examples of halogen bonds with similar strengths as hydrogen bonds, a much more easily explained electrostatic interaction, have been recently documented.

Computational quantum chemistry has emerged as an important tool in examining the foundations of halogen bonding. In a recent set of computational experiments, the bond lengths and bond strengths of various halogen bonds were calculated. Figure 1 gives the results of four such investigations. Figure 1a shows Lennard-Jones potential plots (lengths vs. energy of interaction) for a series of pentafluorobenzyl halide compounds with the nitrogen on pyridine (C_6F_5–X···NC_5H_5). Figure 1b repeats this experiment using non-fluorinated benzene (C_6H_5–X···NC_5H_5). Figure 1c gives a similar plot comparing the pyridine interactions with perfluoroiodoalkanes (R_F-I···NC_5H_5), and Figure 1d compares these bonds in perfluoro- and non-fluorinated-systems of both alkyl and aromatic character.

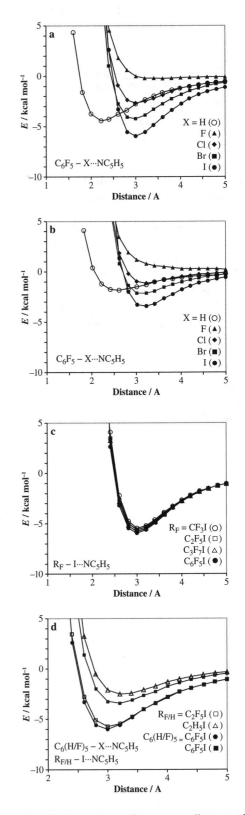

Figure 1(a–d) Comparison of energy vs. distance of the halogen bond (···)

Adapted from: S. Tsuzuki et al., *Chem. Eur. J.* **2012**, 18, 951–960.

1. When considering the halogenated series of C_6F_5X compounds, which of the following is an accurate statement?

A) The strongest halogen bonds are formed by more electropositive halogens.
B) The strongest halogen bonds are formed by more electronegative halogens.
C) The weakest halogen bonds are formed by the largest halogens.
D) The strongest halogen bonds are formed by the halogens with the most negative charge per unit area.

2. According to the calculated data, which of the following interactions are always repulsive?

A) $C_6H_5-H\cdots NC_5H_5$
B) $C_6H_5-F\cdots NC_5H_5$
C) $C_3F_7-I\cdots NC_5H_5$
D) All of the halogen/hydrogen interactions with pyridine are attractive to some degree.

3. Which of the following factors was observed to play the smallest role in determining the strength of a halogen bonding interaction?

A) The electronegativity of the halogen in the bond
B) The atomic radius of the halogen in the bond
C) The electron withdrawing/donating capacity of the organic group bearing the halogen of interest
D) The aromatic/non-aromatic nature of the organic group bearing the halogen of interest

4. In the $C_6F_5-X\cdots NC_5H_5$ system, how does the trend in C–X bond lengths (ΔL_{CX}) compare to the X···N values (ΔL_{XN}) as the halogen is changed from F to I down the halogen family?

A) The trend for ΔL_{CX} is positive; variation in bond length is smaller than the $|\Delta L_{XN}|$ values.
B) The trend for ΔL_{CX} is positive; variation in bond length is greater than the $|\Delta L_{XN}|$ values.
C) The trend for ΔL_{CX} is negative; variation in bond length is greater than the $|\Delta L_{XN}|$ values.
D) The trend for ΔL_{CX} is negative; variation in bond length is smaller than the $|\Delta L_{XN}|$ values.

5. In a subsequent computational experiment, pyridine was replaced by a proton, giving a $C_6H_5-X\cdots H^+$ complex. Which of the following most likely represents the trend in the strengths of the X···H^+ interaction for X = F, Cl, Br, and I?

A) X = I > X = Br > X = Cl > X = F
B) X = Cl > X = I > X = Cl > X = F
C) X = F > X = Br > X = Cl > X = I
D) X = F > X = Cl > X = Br > X = I

PRACTICE PASSAGE 3

The epithelium of lung alveoli consists of two main cell types: alveolar type I cells and alveolar type II cells. Type I cells cover 95% of the alveolar surface and are squamous in morphology, facilitating gas exchange between the blood and alveolar air. While comprising a much smaller percentage of the alveolar surface, the spherically-shaped type II cells constitute 60% of all alveolar epithelial cells. Type II cells serve the important function of producing surfactant to reduce the surface tension of the alveolar fluid (pH 7.4). Premature infants with insufficient pulmonary surfactant exhibit neonatal respiratory distress syndrome and are treated with oxygen under continuous positive airway pressure.

The strong surface tension in the lung alveoli is due to the hydrogen bonds between water molecules. At room temperature, water has a particularly high surface tension of 72.7 mN/m, compared with 22.1 mN/m and 19.8 mN/m for ethanol and heptane, respectively. As shown in Figure 1, the attractive forces cancel out for inner liquid molecules. However, outer molecules feel a net inward force, minimizing the surface area of the liquid. The amount of energy required to increase the surface area of a liquid is defined as the surface tension. Surface tension can be reduced with the addition of surfactant molecules by decreasing the net inward force.

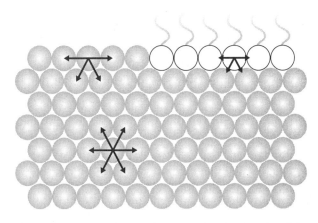

Figure 1 Attractive forces of water molecules (gray) and the effect of surfactant molecules (white)

Research was carried out to determine the efficacy of different surfactants in reducing the surface tension of water. The researchers measured the surface tension of water in the presence of tetraethylene glycol monododecyl ether ($C_{12}E_4$), *N*-dodecyl-*N*, *N*-dimethyl-3-ammonio-1-propanesulfonate (DDAPS), sodium dodecyl sulfate (SDS), and dodecyltrimethylammonium chloride (DTAC). Increased surfactant concentration was found to decrease surface tension, but only to a certain concentration (Figure 2). Charge state

at the interface was found to be a determining factor in the efficacy of the surfactant molecules. In addition, the researchers used phase-sensitive sum-frequency spectroscopy to measure the surface entropy of the liquids at the limiting concentration of each surfactant (Table 1).

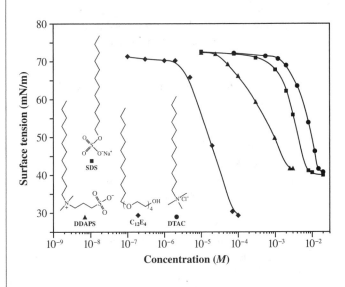

Figure 2 Surface tension of water with various concentrations of $C_{12}E_4$, DDAPS, SDS, and DTAC

Surfactant	Surface Tension (mN/m)	Entropy (mN/mK)
Pure water	72.7	0.15
$C_{12}E_4$	30.2	0.10
DDAPS	41.6	0.07
SDS	40.6	0.04
DTAC	41.6	0.02

Table 1 Surface tension and entropy at the limiting surfactant concentration

Adapted from: Hu et al., *J. Phys. Chem. B*, **2016**, *120*, 2257-2261.

1. Which of the following has the greatest surface tension?

A) $C_6H_{13}OH(l)$
B) $C_5H_{12}(l)$
C) $C_5H_{11}OH(l)$
D) $C_6H_{14}(l)$

2. Based on the passage, which of the following must be true in order for a surfactant to reduce the surface tension of water?

 I. The surfactant-surfactant interactions are weaker than the water-water interactions.
 II. The surfactant-water interactions are stronger than the water-water interactions.
 III. The surfactant-water interactions are weaker than the water-water interactions.

A) I only
B) III only
C) I and II only
D) I and III only

3. Which of the following molecules would be the most effective in treating the lung alveoli of a patient lacking endogenous pulmonary surfactant?

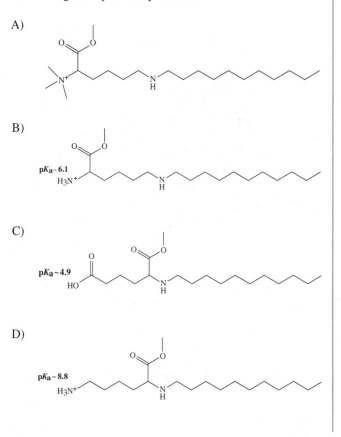

A)

B) pKa ~ 6.1

C) pKa ~ 4.9

D) pKa ~ 8.8

4. In the experiment described in the passage, which of the following is true regarding the surface enthalpy and entropy of the water upon addition of surfactant?

A) Surface enthalpy becomes less negative and surface entropy decreases
B) Surface enthalpy becomes more negative and surface entropy increases
C) Surface enthalpy becomes more negative and surface entropy decreases
D) Surface enthalpy becomes less negative and surface entropy increases

5. The primary respiratory process affected by neonatal respiratory distress syndrome is:

A) respiration, due to the inability to decrease alveolar pressure.
B) respiration, due to the inability to increase alveolar pressure.
C) ventilation, due to the inability to decrease alveolar pressure.
D) ventilation, due to the inability to increase alveolar pressure.

PRACTICE PASSAGE 4

The behavior of the noble gases is most often described in terms of their inertness toward reaction chemistries. Helium, neon, and argon, the three lightest of the family, nearly always abide by this description. However, xenon is known to deviate from the general rule, a fact illustrated by its action on biological tissues in its use as a general anesthetic. The root mechanisms at the basis of the physiological effects of Xe are not well defined. However, research has been carried out in hopes of explaining the interactions of Xe with living tissues.

In order to measure the uptake of Xe by hemeproteins, pressure cells of a known volume were charged with aqueous protein-containing solutions, and subsequently pressurized with various quantities of gaseous Xe. The amounts of gas absorbed by the solutions were determined by the decrease of pressure in the cell over an eight-hour equilibration period, as measured by an affixed manometer. The observed change in pressure ($\Delta P = P_{t=8hr} - P_{t=0}$) was then converted to moles of Xe absorbed by the solution (Δn) by the Ideal Gas Law, and corrected by a Henry's Law calculation using the number of moles of Xe absorbed by pure water (Henry's Law constant = 3×10^{-3} M/atm). This yielded the amount of Xe absorbed into the proteins. Plots of the moles of Xe absorbed per mole of protein for three different proteins at a range of equilibrium pressures and temperatures are given in Figure 1. Monitoring by UV/Vis spectroscopy indicated no differences in the spectra of proteins in the presence and absence of Xe.

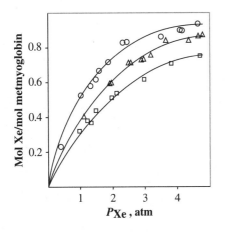

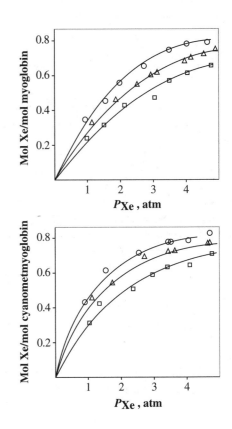

Figure 1 Xe uptake at different pressures and temperatures.
○ = 20°C; △ = 25°C; □ = 30°C

Once the amount of gas absorbed into the protein has been thus determined, a gas-solution equilibrium constant can be calculated as follows: $K_p = m_{HpXe}(m_{Hp} \cdot P_{Xe})^{-1}$. In this relation, m_{HpXe} and m_{Hp} are the molarities of xenon-bound hemeprotein and free hemeprotein, respectively, and P_{Xe} is the partial pressure of Xe in the surrounding atmosphere. Standard K_{eq} values can then be derived using the Henry's Law constants ($\sim 3 \times 10^{-3}$ M/atm) for the absorption of Xe in aqueous solutions to convert P_{Xe} into m_{Xe}. From these K_{eq} values, thermodynamic parameters for Xe absorption could be determined (Table 1).

Protein	ΔG°_{25} (kcal/mol)	ΔH°_{25} (kcal/mol)	ΔS°_{25} (eu)
Metmyoglobin	−2.9	−7.2	−14.0
Myoglobin	−2.7	−5.1	−8.0
Cyanometmyoglobin	−2.9	−9.0	−20.0

Table 1 Thermodynamic parameters for the absorption of Xe at 25°C (eu = entropy unit)

Passage adapted from: Ewing, G. J. and Maestas, S., *J. Phys. Chem.* 1970, *74*, 2341-2344.

1. If P_{Xe} of a system were to be plotted (on the x-axis) against the derived ratio of m_{HpXe} to m_{Hp} (on the y-axis), what would be the expected result?

A) A line with a y-intercept at 0, and a slope of K_{eq}
B) A line with a y-intercept at 1, and a slope of K_p
C) A line with a y-intercept at 0, and a slope of K_p
D) A line with a y-intercept at 0, and a slope of $1/K_p$

2. If the pressure cell used to determine the data in Figure 1 had a volume of 80 mL, and 10 mL of protein solution were used, what was the molarity of the Xe above a solution of myoglobin at 40% saturation at 30°C? ($R = 0.08$ L atm K^{-1} mol^{-1})?

A) 0.08 M
B) 0.007 M
C) 0.66 M
D) 1.6 M

3. What prediction can be made about the absolute value of the free energy of Xe absorption to cyanometmyoglobin at 30°C?

A) $|\Delta G^{\circ}_{30}| > 2.9$
B) $|\Delta G^{\circ}_{30}| = 2.9$
C) $|\Delta G^{\circ}_{30}| < 2.9$
D) No predictions can be made about the relationship between free energy and temperature can be made.

4. From information in the passage, which of the following is most likely a true statement?

A) Xe should be expected to actively displace bound O_2 from oxygenated hemes.
B) Interactions between Xe with the iron atom of the heme is very limited.
C) The Xe absorption process is very rapid.
D) The protein interaction energies for Xe are smaller than those expected for Ne and He.

5. A plot of the total amount of Xe in a myoglobin solution (y-axis) against P_{eq} (x-axis) is non-linear below about P_{eq} = 5 atm, but becomes linear after that point. What is the approximate slope of the linear portion of the graph?

A) 1 M/atm
B) 0.33 M/atm
C) 0.8 M/atm
D) 3×10^{-3} M/atm

PRACTICE PASSAGE 5

The phenomenon of osmosis is well understood on the large scale; however, the common equations related to predicting osmotic pressure, or similar phenomena, are derived assuming that the solutions in the system act ideally. Unfortunately, water is an exceptionally difficult medium to accurately predict in this way due to its known propensity to act non-ideally, especially at large solute concentrations. A reasonably large body of experimental work has been carried out in attempts at giving models more precise predictive power, by incorporating non-ideality into their theoretical frameworks.

The two main factors identified as areas for improving the known equations regarding osmotic phenomena are as follows: 1) explaining the differences in water clustering that occur when solutes are added, and 2) quantifying the actual dissociation (rather than the ideal dissociation) of electrolyte solutes in the solution. Pure water is a highly ordered system, with a large proportion of its molecules harnessed into tetrahedral environments by four hydrogen bonds. Since unconstrained water molecules, those not tethered with four hydrogen bonds, are more osmotically active, the molarity of these "free" molecules (n^{free}) is an important parameter, which is affected by the concentration of solutes. The ratio of free water in a pure sample to free water in a solution ($n^{free,0}/n^{free,s}$) is given the symbol ϕ^w. The effect of non-completely dissociated electrolytes is measured by the quantity ϕ^d, which is the ratio of the measured degree of salt dissociation in an electrolytic solution to the number of particles present in a hypothetical solution where the electrolyte dissociates completely ($\phi^d = i^{measured}/i^{ideal}$). In this relation, i^{ideal} is the van't Hoff factor for the salt in question (e.g., $i^{ideal}_{NaCl} = 2$).

The differences in the symmetry of free and constrained water in solution allows for the determination of their respective concentrations in solution by Raman spectroscopy, thereby allowing the experimental determination of ϕ^w. In an examination of the non-ideal osmotic effects of 2 molal solutions (2 moles solute/kg water) of four salts (NaCl, NH_4Cl, $(NH_4)_2SO_4$ and Na_2SO_4), the relative ranking of ϕ^w was determined to be $\phi^w_{NH_4Cl} > \phi^w_{(NH_4)_2SO_4} > \phi^w_{NaCl} > \phi^w_{Na_2SO_4}$. Thermodynamic measurements allowed the determination of ϕ^d, which was found to adhere to the following trend: $\phi^d_{NaCl} = \phi^d_{NH_4Cl} > \phi^d_{Na_2SO_4} = \phi^d_{(NH_4)_2SO_4}$. From these two factors, the overall osmotic potential coefficient measured (ϕ) could be accurately fit to the equation $\phi = \phi^w \cdot \phi^d$, indicating the importance of these two factors.

Adapted from Frosch et al., *J. Phys. Chem. A* **2010**, *114*, 11933–11942.

1. Which of the following is a possible ordering of the studied salt compounds in terms of their respective values of ϕ?

   A) $NH_4Cl > Na_2SO_4 > (NH_4)_2SO_4 > NaCl$
   B) $NH_4Cl > (NH_4)_2SO_4 > NaCl > Na_2SO_4$
   C) $(NH_4)_2SO_4 > NaCl > NH_4Cl > Na_2SO_4$
   D) $Na_2SO_4 > NH_4Cl > (NH_4)_2SO_4 > NaCl$

2. Attempts to make a more direct comparison between chloride salts and sulfate salts by taking measurements of the effects of an alkaline earth sulfate ($MgSO_4$) were hindered most by which one of the following factors?

   A) The larger cation (Mg vs. Na) of the alkaline earth metal caused effects with ϕ^w not seen with the alkali metals.
   B) The strong acidity of the Mg^{2+} ion in solution caused unexpected effects in the measurements.
   C) The low solubility of $MgSO_4$ prevented the formation of a 2 molal solution.
   D) The stable compound MgH_2 was rapidly produced upon dissociation of the sulfate salt in water.

3. If a value of $n^{free,0}$ was determined to be 31.6 M by Raman measurements, what is the percentage of tetrahedrally bound water molecules in pure water at any one time?

A) 31%
B) 43%
C) 57%
D) 72%

4. Hypothetically, if the values of $\phi^d_{NH_4Cl}$ and $\phi^d_{Na_2SO_4}$ were determined to be 0.9 and 0.7, respectively, and the effects of water clustering were ignored, a 2 molal solution of which of the following salt solutions would produce the greatest osmotic pressure if placed across a semi-permeable membrane from pure water?

A) Cannot be determined with the data given
B) NaCl
C) NH_4Cl
D) Na_2SO_4

5. Which of the following equilibria has the smallest value of K_{eq}?

A) $NH_4Cl(aq) \rightleftharpoons NH_4^+(aq) + Cl^-(aq)$
B) $Na_2SO_4(aq) \rightleftharpoons Na^+(aq) + NaSO_4^-(aq)$
C) $NaCl(aq) \rightleftharpoons Na^+(aq) + Cl^-(aq)$
D) $NH_4SO_4^-(aq) \rightleftharpoons NH_4^+(aq) + SO_4^{2-}(aq)$

PRACTICE PASSAGE 6

Highly lipophilic drugs often have low oral bioavailability
due to limited aqueous solubilities. To overcome this obstacle,
strategies such as ionizing these compounds with changes
in pH or the use of solubilizing additives are common. Co-
crystallization of drug compounds with other molecules,
yielding complexes with enhanced solubilities, is an attractive
technique, though effectiveness may be limited by the stability
of the interactions between the two crystal components.

Nevirapine (Table 1) is a non-nucleoside reverse transcriptase
inhibitor used in the treatment of HIV-1 infections. Co-
crystallization has been studied as a way to overcome its poor
aqueous solubility. As a weakly basic compound, the solubility
of Nevirapine is relatively high in low pH regimes. However,
this solubility falls off rapidly at higher pH. A number of
potential co-crystallization partners have been identified and
studied (Table 1).

The aqueous solubilities of the co-crystals were measured
at a range of pH values and plotted against the theoretical
solubilities determined by mathematical modeling (Figure 1).
The fit of the data to the theoretical lines provided support for
the validity of the model. In each case, the co-crystal showed
improved solubility in comparison to the drug by itself in less
acidic environments.

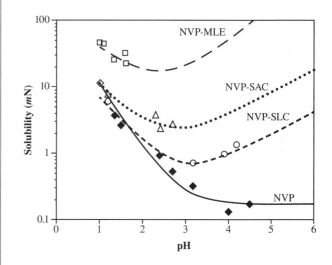

Figure 1 Experimental solubility of co-crystals vs. theoretical
solubilities at varying pH

Adapted from Kuminek et al., *Chem. Commun.* **2016**, doi: 10.1039/
c6cc00898d

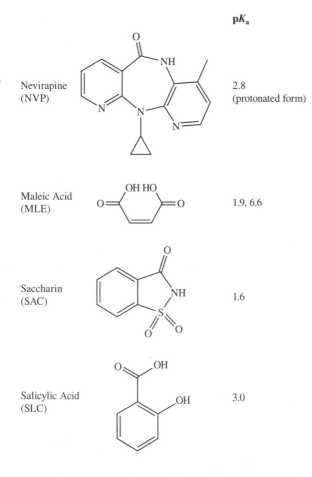

		pK_a
Nevirapine (NVP)		2.8 (protonated form)
Maleic Acid (MLE)		1.9, 6.6
Saccharin (SAC)		1.6
Salicylic Acid (SLC)		3.0

Table 1 Potential co-crystallization partners

1. Which of the following intermolecular forces is most prevalent in the association of Nevirapine with salicylic acid?

A) London dispersion forces
B) Aromatic π-π stacking
C) Hydrogen bonding
D) Dipole-dipole interactions

2. Which of the following is supported by information in the passage?

A) The complexation of additional benzene ring units to NVP results in increased solubility.
B) NVP is primarily deprotonated (anionic) at pH values greater than 3.
C) Carboxylate-bound protons are always more acidic than nitrogen-bound protons.
D) The sulfone moiety ($-SO_2-$) is exceptionally electron withdrawing.

3. How does the predominant charge state of maleic acid dissociated from NVP change upon traversing from the stomach (pH = 1.5) to the blood (pH = 7.3)?

A) It changes from –1 to –2.
B) It changes from 0 to –2.
C) It changes from 0 to –1.
D) It changes from +1 to –2.

4. The difference in the solubility behavior of NVP as compared to the NVP complexes at pH > 3 may be best explained by which of the following?

A) The existence of acidic protons on the co-crystallization partners
B) The capacity for the complexes to associate with OH^- in basic pH regimes
C) The ability of the co-crystallization partners to shield the highly hydrophobic cyclopropyl group on NVP from aqueous environments
D) The capacity of the co-crystallization partner to prevent the deprotonation of NVP at pH > 3

5. If a 1 M solution of neutral NVP was prepared in neutral water, what is the best estimate for the pH of the solution?

A) 1.2
B) 5.6
C) 8.4
D) 11.2

6. Compared to NVP, administration of NVP-SAC would most likely result in which of the following long-term effects?

A) Decreased CD_8^+ T-cell counts
B) Increased HIV viral load
C) Decreased risk of hepatotoxicity
D) Decreased risk of opportunistic infections

Chapter 16
General Chemistry
Practice Section
Solutions

FREESTANDING QUESTION SOLUTIONS

1. **C** Whereas smaller noble gases are only found in oxidation state zero, Kr can take on positive charges as in KrF_2. In this compound Kr is in the +2 oxidation state, and it will be exceptionally eager to fulfill its octet by oxidizing anything around it. This makes it a good oxidizing agent (eliminate choice B). Photosensitizers harvest energy from incoming light, and transfer this energy to other molecules. These compounds tend to be large, highly conjugated materials, often containing transition metals. Importantly, this is energy transfer, not redox, as would be required for the formation of extreme oxidation states (eliminate choice A). While it is certainly imaginable that KrF_2 might split into Kr^0 and $F_2(g)$, $F_2(g)$ is neither rare, inaccessible, or unexplored, so it stands to reason that this function would not be the root cause of "extreme oxidation states."

2. **D** The platinum in $Pt(NH_3)_2Cl_2$ is bound to four ligands, two of which (NH_3) are neutral, and two of which are anionic (Cl^-). This means that the Pt atom is in the +2 oxidation state, containing eight valence electrons (eliminate choices A and C). As electrons are ionized out of the s orbitals prior to removal from d orbitals in transition metals, choice D is the only correct choice.

3. **D** Free energy responds to changes in temperature by the equation $\Delta G = \Delta H - T\Delta S$. An increase in temperature will yield a more negative free energy if ΔS is positive. However, the process of hydrogen bond formation in the gas phase will involve a negative change in entropy, as two previously unassociated molecules will be ordered alongside one another. This means that the change in free energy with increasing temperature will be to make it more positive, leaving only choice D.

4. **B** If the rate of elimination is invariant with time, after the initial onset of ethanol elimination, then the kinetics cannot depend on the concentration of ethanol present at any given time. If the ethanol concentration did factor into the rate equation, then as the concentration of ethanol decreased (or increased, as choice D suggests) the rate would clearly change. This means that as monitored the rate must be zero-order in ethanol.

5. **D** Cesium is an alkali metal (Group 1), meaning that it only takes on a +1 ionic charge (eliminate choice A). At the far left and near the bottom of the periodic table, Cs has a rather low electronegativity (eliminate choice B). A large, negative electron affinity indicates an ion or atom that would decrease its energy through accepting an electron, which is not the case for the alkali metals (eliminate choice C). At the left and bottom of the table, Cs is an exceptionally large ion, and it is this size that allows it to make close contacts with more coordinating atoms than other species.

6. **B** With the overall formula of Fe_3O_4, the charges on the iron atoms need to sum to +8. As the iron in ferrihydrite is Fe^{3+}, and in iron oxide is Fe^{2+}, the only way to get to +8 of those listed is a 2:1 ratio of ferrihydrite to iron oxide.

7. **A** In alkynes and N_2, the central atoms (C or N) are held together by one σ bond directly on the bond axis between the atoms and two π bonds at right angles from one another. If the boron atoms in diboryne are similar to this, then choice A must be correct. In general, because σ bonds extend along the bond axis, it is very rare to have compounds where two atoms are bound to one another by more than one σ bond (eliminate choice B). Choice D is unrealistic in this case, as it is impossible to align the three orthogonal p-orbitals of the

atoms in such a way as to make 3 π bonds. One p orbital will necessarily be along the bond axis, making π bonding impossible. These first row main group elements do not have accessible d orbitals, so no δ bonds are possible (eliminate choice C).

8. **A** To determine the exothermicity of the reaction above, the following equation is written:

$$\Delta H_{rxn} = [\Delta H_f (NaOH) + \Delta H_f (Ca_5(PO_4)_3(F)] - [(\Delta H_f (NaF) + \Delta H_f Ca_5(PO_4)_3(OH)] < 0$$

$$[\Delta H_f (NaOH) - 3296 \text{ kcal/mol}] - [\Delta H_f (NaF) - 3229 \text{ kcal/mol}] < 0$$

$$[\Delta H_f (NaOH) - \Delta H_f (NaF)] - 67 \text{ kcal/mol} < 0$$

$$\Delta H_f (NaOH) - \Delta H_f (NaF) < 67 \text{ kcal/mol}$$

9. **D** A carbanion like n-butyllithium is a very strong base, and in order to deprotonate 2,5-dimethyltetrahydrofuran, an even stronger base must be found. Both of the butoxide compounds (choices A and B) rely on anionic compounds with the negative charge on oxygen. Oxygen, being more electronegative than carbon, forms more stable anions, resulting in the fact that they are weaker bases than comparable carbon anions. Triethylamine is basic, but as a neutral compound it is far less basic than the butoxides or the carbanions (eliminate choice C). *tert*-Butyllithium is a carbanion salt in which the anionic character is on the central tertiary carbon. The trend in anionic stability is known to go 1° > 2° > 3°, meaning that the tertiary anion is the most reactive. This base will, as such, act to deprotonate 2,5-dimethyltetrahydrofuran.

10. **B** The name of the technique, positron emission tomography, indicates that the decay mode of ^{18}F is positron emission, and the fact that these positrons can be monitored from outside the body indicates that choice D is incorrect. The half-life of only 109 min would require a degree of expedient usage after synthesis of the compound. After several days, the ^{18}F in the sample would be nearly entirely gone (eliminate choice A). A sugar molecule is very hydrophilic due to the many OH groups and would not be sequestered in hydrophobic environments (eliminate choice C). Choice B is correct, as the result of positron emission from ^{18}F is ^{18}O, a stable isotope of oxygen. Transmutation of F to O, and protonation in the aqueous environment, would lead to the formation of glucose, which the body is quite adept at handling.

11. **C** To answer this question, the following math may be performed:

$$K_{sp} = [Ca^{2+}][CO_3^{2-}]$$

$$1.3 \times 10^{-8} = [5.3 \times 10^{-4}] [CO_3^{2-}]$$

$$\sim(1/5) \times 10^{-4} = [CO_3^{2-}]$$

$$= 2 \times 10^{-5}$$

$$= 0.02 \text{ mmol/L}$$

12. **C** One mole of ideal gas at room temperature is occupies 22.4 L. If 3% of this were ethyl chloride, then the overall concentration would be 0.03 mol/22.4 L. With scientific notation you can write this as $(3 \times 10^{-2})/(2.24 \times 10^1)$, which will give $(3/2.24) \times 10^{-3}$. This makes choice C the best answer choice.

13. **A** The cathode is the site of reduction in the electrochemical cell. Reduction of H_2 would result in two hydrides (H^-), which is an energetically unfavorable process. In electrochemical cells, H_2 is far more often used for oxidation at the anode (eliminate choice D). Choice C may be eliminated, as reduction of this noble gas is not feasible under normal conditions. When considering both N_2 and O_2, either may be reduced, but the higher electron affinity of oxygen results in this process being far more favorable for O_2. This is readily borne out in atmospheric chemistry, where O_2 readily undergoes reduction in reactions such as combustion, while N_2 is considered largely inert.

14. **B** The interactions between sodium atoms and hexafluorocyclohexane may be classified as ion-dipole interactions. The orientation of fluorine atoms that will lead to the greatest dipole will have the strongest interactions with the ion. This will be the case when all of the fluorine atoms are on the same side of the ring, meaning they are in an all *cis* conformation (choice B is correct). Choices A and D may be eliminated, as these molecules are identical. Through a ring flip, substituents that begin axial become equatorial, and vice versa. This molecule also has all substituents in *trans* relationships to each other around the ring. Choice C will have a smaller dipole than choice B due to the one *trans* relationship indicated.

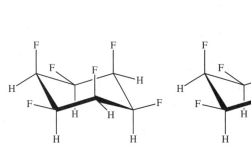

Largest Dipole Up
Choice B

Smaller Dipole Up
Choice C

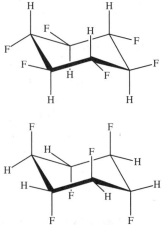

Cancelling Dipoles
Choices A and D

SOLUTIONS TO PRACTICE PASSAGE 1

1. **B** Choices C and D may be quickly eliminated, as no protons are donated nor received by the carbon in carbonate. Had the answer choice referenced a different sort of acidity, there might be a reason to think further about these choices, but the lack of mobile protons means that there is no Brønsted acid-base activity in the carbonate mechanism. In the water mechanism, protons (electrophiles) are transferred from molecule to molecule, while in the carbonate mechanism oxide (O^{2-}), a nucleophile, is passed along from molecule to molecule (eliminate choice A).

2. **B** For an endothermic reaction, heat can be considered as a reactant on the left side of the equation. An increase in temperature will shift the reaction to the right, increasing the value of the equilibrium constant. According to Equation 1, an increase in K_{pyro} will lead to an increase in k_H^{app}. By Henry's Law, an increase in k_H^{app} with a constant p_{CO_2} will lead to an increase in the concentration of dissolved CO_2.

3. **A** Item I is false. The proposed Grotthuss mechanism for CO_2 in the passage involves the formation of pyrocarbonate. The detection of the compound would not contradict the proposed mechanism (eliminate choice C). Were Item II to be observed, the mechanism would be disproved. The Grotthuss mechanism, applied to the carbonate system, involves the passage of an oxide from carbonate to CO_2, which effectively makes a new carbon atom the central atom of a newly formed CO_2 molecule. If only $^{13}C=O$ were observed, the mechanism would be incorrect. Item III is false (eliminate choice B). The passage states that the solubility of CO_2 in molten $CaCO_3$ is higher than expected, and since the solubility mechanism appears to be dependent primarily on the mechanisms enabled by the carbonate portion of the salt, there would be no reason to assume it should not be at work in other carbonate salts as well (eliminate choice D).

4. **D** In the pyrocarbonate ion, O_A and O_C are chemically equivalent. This means that their respective bonds to carbon must be of identical length (eliminate choice A). It is also true that they are not chemically equivalent to O_B, allowing for the elimination of choice C. In trying to decide which C–O bond is the longest, it is helpful to consider the double bond character of each bond in question. Both C–O_A and C–O_C have a good deal of double bond character, as the oxygen is only bound to one bonding partner, sharing a mobile electron pair with the other oxygen bound to the same carbon. The bond between carbon and O_B, on the other hand, has much less double bond character. It is possible to draw resonance structures that make one of these C–O_B bonds a double bond (placing a positive formal charge on O_B), but this resonance structure is a minor one, as opposed to the favorable resonance structures that can be drawn for double bonds to O_A and O_C. C–O_B is therefore the longest bond, and the two others are shorter and equal to one another, as stated in choice D.

SOLUTIONS TO PRACTICE PASSAGE 2

1. **A**   Figure 1 indicates that the strongest halogen bond (the deepest well in the Lennard-Jones potential) is found for the iodinated aromatic and pyridine. The brominated compound shows the second strongest, and the chlorinated the third. Since the trend in electronegativity decreases from top to bottom in the halogen family (F > Cl > Br > I), the most electropositive halogen (I) forms the strongest bond (choice A is correct; choice B can be eliminated). Since all of the halogens will have a partial charge of somewhere between 0 and −1, the largest halogens will have the lowest charge per unit area. As such, choices C and D may be mutually eliminated, as they say very similar things.

2. **B**   For an interaction to be attractive, there must be a local minimum on the energy vs. distance plot. This indicates the point where the attractive interaction overcomes the electron-electron repulsion that pushes atoms apart when they are squeezed together. If there is no minimum, and the energy of the system simply decreases as the two bonding partners move farther apart, this means that the interaction is strictly repulsive, and the two partners never form a bond. Of the listed choices, this is true for $C_6H_5–F\cdots NC_5H_5$ as can be seen in Figure 1b. The interactions in choices A and C both have minimum values, indicating a range where the interaction is attractive.

3. **D**   Figure 1a shows that the choice of halogen in the halogen bond is very important in terms of determining the strength of the halogen bond, with iodine forming the strongest bonds, and fluorine the weakest. Since both the atomic radius and electronegativity change along this series, it is impossible to say that either of these factors doesn't play a role in determining the strength of the halogen bond (eliminate choices A and B). Figure 1d indicates that halogenated organics, both alkyl and aryl, make stronger halogen bonds than non-fluorinated compounds (eliminate choice C). Figures 1c and 1d indicate that halogen bonds between electron donors and halogens on aromatic rings and alkyl chains are essentially identical, provided both are either halogenated or non-halogenated. This makes choice D correct.

4. **B**   This 2x2 question can be solved by eliminating answers wherein half of the statement is incorrect. In any system of covalent bonds (like the C–X bond in $C_6F_5–X\cdots NC_5H_5$), bond lengths will increase with increasing atomic radius of the halogen. This means that C–F < C–Cl < C–Br < C–I, and therefore the trend in ΔL_{CX} is positive going from F to I down the halogen family (eliminate choices C and D). When looking at Figure 1a, it can be seen that the lengths of the non-covalent X$\cdots$N (the bond length is given at the minimum of the curve) changes very little along the halogen family (eliminate choice A).

5. **D**   As this question is asking for ranking amongst the family of halogens, it's very unlikely a correct answer will not have the halogens in the correct order, either backward or forward (eliminate choices B and C). Choosing between choices A and D requires an investigation into the interaction at play. While in the halogen bonds discussed in the passage the halogen acts as a Lewis acid, accepting electron density from pyridine, in the $C_6H_5–X\cdots H^+$ complex, it acts as a base. The strongest electrostatic interaction from the halogen with the most electron density will prevail, and since the F on $C_6H_5–F$ is much more electronegative, and thus more highly charged than the I on $C_6H_5–I$, the fluorinated compound will show a stronger interaction with H^+. This makes choice D the correct answer.

SOLUTIONS TO PRACTICE PASSAGE 3

1. **A** The passage suggests that surface tension scales with the strength of the interactions holding the liquid molecules together at the surface. The passage also states that a small alcohol, like ethanol, has a larger surface tension than a large alkane like heptane (eliminate choices B and D). Between the two alkyl alcohols, the larger of the two (choice A) will have the greater intermolecular forces, and hence the largest surface tension.

2. **D** In order for the surfactant to form a layer at the surface of the water, but not disperse throughout the bulk of the water, a few things must be true. The first is that the surfactant-surfactant interactions must be less favorable than the surfactant-water interactions, or else the surfactant would coalesce into globules on the water surface and not spread (Item I is true; eliminate choice B). Secondly, the water-surfactant interactions must be weaker than the water-water interactions, or the surfactant would penetrate into the bulk of the water, mixing evenly (Item II is false, and Item III is true; eliminate choices A and C). This decreased attractive force between the surface layer and the layers below is the driving force behind the decrease in surface tension. These two necessities are expressed in the sizes of the arrows (force vectors) in Figure 1.

3. **B** According to Figure 2 and the text that describes charge state as a particularly important factor in the effectiveness of the surfactant, the most effective compound for reducing surface tension is the one with no charge. Zwitterions with no net charge are the second most efficient, and cationic or anionic compounds are the least efficient. The molecule in choice B has a pK_a of 6.1. At the alveolar pH of 7.4, the molecule would be predominantly deprotonated and would have no charge (choice B is correct). Choices A, C, and D can be eliminated by considering their charge states at the alveolar pH as well. The molecule in choice C would have a negative charge, while the molecule in choice D would have a positive charge. The molecule in choice A will always has a positive charge, regardless of pH.

4. **A** According to Table 1, the addition of surfactant led to a decrease in the surface entropy (eliminate choices B and D). When surfactant is added, the forces between the surface molecules are the surfactant-water interactions, which are necessarily weaker than the water-water interactions. The action of the surfactant is dependent on decreasing these forces at the surface. The decrease in the strength of the interactions results in the overall enthalpy of the surface becoming less negative (eliminate choice C).

5. **C** According to the passage, neonatal respiratory distress syndrome is the result of insufficient pulmonary surfactant. Without surfactant, the surface tension in the alveoli will remain high, leading to collapse of the alveoli. The decrease in alveolar volume results in an increase in alveolar pressure. During regular breathing, inspiration increases the alveolar volume, lowering the alveolar pressure and causing air to flow into the lungs. Without pulmonary surfactant, the alveolar volume cannot be increased as effectively (i.e., it's harder to open the alveoli) so the baby suffers from the inability to decrease alveolar pressure (eliminate choices B and D). This prevents the movement of air into and out of the lungs, a problem of ventilation (choice C is correct). Respiration is the exchange of gases, which is not impacted by neonatal respiratory distress syndrome (eliminate choice A).

SOLUTIONS TO PRACTICE PASSAGE 4

1. **C**   The passage states that the following relationship is adhered to: $K_p = m_{HpXe}(m_{Hp} \cdot P_{Xe})^{-1}$. This

    can be rearranged to give $m_{HpXe}/m_{Hp} = K_p \cdot P_{Xe}$. If thought of as the standard $y = mx + b$ form

    of a straight line, the y-intercept (b) is 0 and the slope is K_p.

2. **A**   At 40% saturation (mol Xe/mol myoglobin = 0.4) and 30°C, the middle plot in Figure 1
    says that the equilibrium pressure of Xe was 2 atm. Applying this to the Ideal Gas Law:

    $$PV = nRT$$

    $$(2 \text{ atm})(0.08 \text{ L}) = n \ (0.08 \text{ L atm K}^{-1} \text{ mol}^{-1})(303 \text{ K})$$

    $$\sim 2/300 = n$$

    $$\sim 200(10^{-2})/300 = 0.66(10^{-2}) = \sim 0.0066 \text{ mol}$$

    This can be converted to molarity by dividing by volume:

    $$0.0066 \text{ mol} / 0.08 \text{ L}$$

    $$66(10^{-4}) / 8(10^{-2})$$

    Which can be conveniently rounded to:

    $$\sim 64(10^{-4}) / 8(10^{-2})$$

    $$= 0.08 \ M$$

3. **C**   The change in free energy associated with the absorption of Xe onto cyanometmyoglobin at
    25°C is –2.9 kcal/mol, as per Table 1. Table 1 also indicates that the entropy associated with
    this phenomenon is –20.0 entropy units. Since $\Delta G = \Delta H - T\Delta S$, increasing the temperature
    should cause the $T\Delta S$ term to increase in magnitude, so the value of ΔG will be less negative,
    and thus have a smaller absolute value.

4. **B**   The passage states that the UV/Vis spectra of the proteins did not change with absorption
    of Xe. This is indicative of no interaction with the iron atom of the heme, and instead ab-
    sorption into other parts of the protein. Choice A can be eliminated, since O_2 is known to
    bind strongly to the metal, and is therefore not going to be displaced by Xe. Choice C may
    be eliminated, since equilibration over eight hours is required for the experiment. Choice D
    may be eliminated, as the passage states that the lighter noble gases tend to show far weaker
    interactions than Xe.

5. **D** As shown in Figure 1, below 5 atm the proteins absorb Xe, but above this point they are predominantly saturated. This means that Xe in solution below 5 atm is a product of both the constant absorption of Xe into the water by Henry's law, and the uptake by the protein. However, once the protein is saturated, the only new uptake will be due to Henry's Law absorption. For this system, Henry's Law would say $[Xe_{soln}] = H_{Xe}(P_{eq})$, where H_{Xe} is the Henry's Law constant for Xe in water. This is a linear plot with H_{Xe} as the slope, which is given as $3 \times 10^{-3} M$/atm in the text.

SOLUTIONS TO PRACTICE PASSAGE 5

1. **B** The final sentence of the passage states that $\phi = \phi^w \cdot \phi^d$, however, exact data is not given regarding the magnitude of the values in ϕ^w and ϕ^d. What is known is that $\phi^d_{NaCl} = \phi^d_{NH_4Cl}$ and $\phi^d_{Na_2SO_4} = \phi^d_{(NH_4)_2SO_4}$. If this information is coupled with the ϕ^w ranking ($\phi^w_{NH_4Cl} > \phi^w_{(NH_4)_2SO_4} > \phi^w_{NaCl} > \phi^w_{Na_2SO_4}$), then it may be said with certainty that $\phi_{NH_4Cl} > \phi_{NaCl}$ (eliminate choice C) and $\phi_{(NH_4)_2SO_4} > \phi_{Na_2SO_4}$ (eliminate choices A and D).

2. **C** Choice A may be eliminated, as Mg^{2+} has a smaller ionic radius than Na^+. While Mg^{2+} is a mild acid in water, it certainly cannot be considered strongly acidic, as choice B implies. Complications resulting from low levels of acidity are also ruled out by the fact that ammonium salts are used successfully. The reaction of Mg^{2+} with water will focus on the association of the electron rich oxygen atom with the Mg cation. The protons on water will never be transformed to the hydrides necessary for MgH_2 if the Mg starting material is already cationic (eliminate choice D). The ammonium and sodium salts of the respective anions were used, no doubt, because of their high solubility. Alkaline earth sulfates have notoriously limited solubilities, and a 2 molal solution would likely be impossible at the same temperatures used in the study.

3. **B** The value $n^{free,0}$ is the molarity of free (non-tetrahedrally-sequestered) water in a pure water sample. The most direct way to answer this question is to know, or to calculate, that the molarity of pure water is 55 M. By knowing that the density of water is 1000 g/L, molarity (moles/L) can be calculated thus: 1000 g H_2O/18 g/mol = ~55 mol. As 31/50 is around 0.6, the free water should be a bit less than 60%, meaning that the tetrahedrally bound water is a bit more than 40% of the sample, making choice B the best answer.

4. **D** In an ideal solution, osmotic pressure (Π) is calculated as $\Pi = MiRT$, where M is the molarity of the salt in solution, i is the ideal van't Hoff factor, R is the ideal gas constant, and T is temperature. For a real system, where water clustering is ignored, the i^{ideal} is swapped for i^{real}. Since M is 2 molal (molality and molarity are nearly identical in water) in each case, and R and T do not change, the only difference in determining Π is the value of i^{real}. The passage states that $\phi^d_{NaCl} = \phi^d_{NH_4Cl}$, so since they should have the same i^{real} value, they can both be assumed incorrect (eliminate choices B and C). Another way to consider the question is to complete the quantitative analysis as follows: since $\phi^d = i^{measured}/i^{ideal}$, $\phi^d_{NH_4Cl} = 0.9 = i^{measured}/2$, so $i^{real}_{NH_4Cl} = 1.8$. This then means that $\phi^d_{Na_2SO_4} = 0.7 = i^{measured}/3$, $i^{real}_{Na_2SO_4} = 2.1$, making choice D correct. The larger the concentration of ions in solution, the greater the osmotic pressure of a solution.

5. **D** From a chemical standpoint, it is logical to think that dissociation of NH_4^+ from $NH_4SO_4^-$ should be the least favorable of all of these dissociation reactions based on Coloumb's Law because the charge on the sulfate ion is -2 where all other anions are -1, making choice D is correct. The passage affirms this choice, as the deviations from full dissociation are observed to be the largest for the sulfate salts. Since the dissociation from the neutral salt will always be more favorable than the dissociation of the mono-anion, choice D can safely be considered the least favorable equilibrium in the forward direction.

SOLUTIONS TO PRACTICE PASSAGE 6

1. **C** Large organic systems are often subject to London dispersion forces, and aromatic systems such as those present in Nevirapine and salicylic acid are known to stack in order to maximize the overlap of their π-systems. However, neither of these forces are particularly strong in comparison to hydrogen bonding when it is available. Both molecules are capable of donating and accepting hydrogen bonds at multiple sites, making choice C best.

2. **D** It is counterintuitive to assume that additional benzene ring units (generally non-polar) would increase the aqueous solubility of NVP. While all of the complexes with NVP have regions of greater solubility than NVP alone, only the NVP-MLE complex has better solubility at all measured levels of pH, and shows the greatest solubility enhancement of the three molecules tested. MLE is also the only co-crystallization agent without a benzene unit (eliminate choice A). The lack of aqueous solubility of NVP above pH 3 means that it is likely neutral. The pK_a given in the table is valid for the protonated, conjugate acid form of NVP. Therefore, at pH

values greater than this, you would expect the deprotonated or neutral (not anionic) state to predominate (eliminate choice B). While it is generally true that carboxylate-bound protons are more acidic than those bound to neutral nitrogen atoms, the most acidic compound in Table 1 is saccharine, which contains a nitrogen-bound proton (eliminate choice C). The reason for the exceptional acidity of this proton is the inductive stabilization of the conjugate base by the highly electron withdrawing sulfone group (choice D is correct).

3. **B** The two pK_a values for the two acidic protons on MLE are given as 1.9 and 6.6. The pK_a may be considered to be the pH at which half of the acid-base sites in question are protonated and half are deprotonated. Therefore, at pH = 1.5, the predominant charge state would be 0, since this falls below either pK_a value and both COOH groups should be protonated (eliminate choices A and D). In the blood, the pH (7.3) is greater than either of the pK_a values, meaning both would be primarily deprotonated, and the charge would be –2 (choice B is correct).

4. **A** The solubility of NVP at pH levels above 3 is limited by the fact that it is a neutral compound at this pH, since it has no readily ionizable protons (the pK_a of the amide proton is far above 3). Crystallizing with compounds that bear acidic protons will allow the complex to take on a charge at pH levels above 3, and hence be more soluble in water. At pH = 3 there is very little OH^- in solution, which means that such an association cannot be a driving force for increases in solubility (eliminate choice B). A capacity to shield the cyclopropyl group from aqueous environments would not be pH dependent (eliminate choice C), and deprotonation of NVP, were it possible at pH = 3 (which it is not), would only increase its solubility (eliminate choice D).

5. **C** NVP is a weak base, with a pK_b of 11.2 ($14 - pK_a$ of the conjugate acid). With this information, a base equilibrium equation can be constructed as follows:

$$10^{-11.2} = ([NVP\text{-}H^+][OH^-]) / [NVP]$$

$$= x^2 / (1 - x)$$

Making the assumption that the value of x will be small enough to ignore in the denominator, the following approximation can be made:

$$10^{-11.2} = x^2$$

This means that $[OH^-] = 10^{-5.6}$ at equilibrium. Therefore, pOH = 5.6, and pH = 8.4 (choice C is correct). Note that $10^{-5.6} \ll 1$ and the above assumption is valid.

6. **D** Figure 1 indicates that NVP-SAC displays greater solubility than NVP across the tested pH values, which presumably would lead to greater bioavailability. Given that Nevirapine is a non-nucleoside reverse transcriptase inhibitor used in the treatment of HIV-1, increased bioavailability would result in improved anti-retroviral efficacy. This would result in improved CD_4^+ T-cell counts, a decreased viral load, and a decreased risk of opportunistic infection (choice B is wrong; choice D is correct). CD_8^+ T-cells are critical in defense against infected and cancer cells, but we are given no indication that treatment with Nevirapine would result in a decrease of CD_8^+ T-cell count (eliminate choice A). Hepatotoxicity is a significant concern in those patients being treated with Nevirapine, and increased bioavailability will result in an increase in hepatotoxic risk, rather than a decrease (eliminate choice C).

Chapter 17
Organic Chemistry
on the MCAT

Organic chemistry is the least prevalent subject tested on the MCAT, and it will make up roughly 15% of the Chemical and Physical Foundations of Biological Systems section and only about 5% of the Biological and Biochemical Foundations of Living Systems section. In the Chemical and Physical Foundations of Biological Systems section of the test, the questions will be distributed between two to four freestanding questions and either one longer passage (with five or six questions) or two shorter passages (usually with four questions each). In the Biological and Biochemical Foundations of Living Systems section, the two or three O-Chem questions are likely to be either FSQs, or mixed in with either a Biology or Biochemistry passage. Though it represents comparatively few questions, you cannot ignore Organic Chemistry if you're looking to score in a competitive range for the MCAT. The O-Chem topics covered span two college semesters' worth of material but focus most on carbonyl chemistry and laboratory techniques. For now, let's talk about what you can expect from O-Chem passages.

17.1   TACKLING A PASSAGE

In general, some sort of biologically important compound or reaction provides the context for O-Chem passages. The text of the passage might contain biologically related concepts or facts, but a sure sign that you're reading an O-Chem passage and not a Biology passage will be chemical structures, usually lots of them.

If you see chemical structures, brace yourself for O-Chem!

Your approach to reading and mapping an O-Chem passage should be a bit different than your approach for all other subjects. The reason? There is hardly ever information within the text of an O-Chem passage that will be useful or needed to answer passage-based questions. The most important information in these passages will be in the form of chemical structures from synthetic or mechanistic schemes, or experimental data from a table, graph, or figure. Often, complicated syntheses and mechanisms can be intimidating because of all the detail presented, and they can slow you down considerably if you pay too much attention to this information during your first run through the passage. Be sure to read the titles of figures or schemes to get a sense of the big picture being presented, then jump into answering the questions quickly.

17.2   O-CHEM PASSAGE TYPES

The main science passage types mentioned previously, when considered in the context of O-Chem, look something like this:

Information and/or Situation Presentation

These are the most common types of O-Chem passages, and generally present:

- A multistep synthetic scheme, a novel reaction, or atypical outcomes of reactions you might already be familiar with. Questions associated with these passages might ask you to analyze or classify the steps of the process described, or use common laboratory techniques to analyze intermediate compounds in the synthesis. You might need to justify the exceptions to the rules as described.

- A class of biologically important molecules. Questions associated with these passages could ask you to analyze the molecules with a common laboratory technique, or simply ask about their structure or their relationship to each other. You might also need to predict the reactivity of the molecules if treated with a given reagent.

- A biochemical process or mechanism. Questions here often test your understanding of the stability of intermediates and ask you to explain why the reaction occurs in the manner described. Given a new reactant, you might need to use the mechanistic steps to predict the product of a reaction.

Experiment/Research Presentation

This type of passage presents the details of an experiment or a mechanistic study, and it often includes spectroscopy data (IR or NMR) in the form of lists or tables. Questions ask you to interpret data and identify the likely pathway of reaction. You might also need to identify compounds, or simply choose the appropriate technique to achieve the desired purification or product identification.

Persuasive Reasoning

This is the least common type of O-Chem passage, but can appear as a comparison of two mechanisms that attempt to explain the outcome of a reaction. Questions ask you to evaluate the arguments presented and will likely relate to the stability of intermediates.

17.3   READING AN O-CHEM PASSAGE

You should never really *read* much of the text of an O-Chem passage, but rather, just skim through the text. Remember that most of the important information you'll use from an O-Chem passage will be in the form of the structures and data presented. O-Chem passage-based questions are often essentially free-standing questions. They require only reference to a structure given in the passage in order to answer. However, as you're skimming the passage, you won't know which structures, reaction steps, or data will be the useful bits, AND you won't be able to mark or highlight structures in any way using your on-screen tools. That means that when skimming, you should get a general sense of the importance of each figure or table by reading titles and headings, but not get bogged down in the details of the figures in any way. You want to know where to go to examine the details when a question refers you to a particular synthetic step or structure along the pathway, something the MCAT is amazingly kind enough to do in most cases.

> For the most part, info is in the figures and graphs.

While you're reading, be on the lookout for new *italicized* terms in the text to highlight, or unexpected outcomes of experiments and exceptions to rules. The MCAT will ask you to apply the science fundamentals you've studied to novel situations, so look for and highlight anything that might be out of the ordinary.

17.4　MAPPING AN O-CHEM PASSAGE

It will often be the case that the text of a passage will reproduce information presented in a more visually useful manner, such as a flowchart, reaction scheme, or mechanism. Try to focus on the structure, and resist the urge to make a lot of yellow marks in the text.

Since you cannot highlight any structures in the passage (this is unfortunate, since structures are the place you'll get most of your necessary information), remember to use your scratch paper to make note of anything related to a reaction scheme or mechanism, especially if it's taken you some time to come to your conclusion. Keep your scratch paper organized so that it will be a useful tool if you need to refer to it while checking back over your answers toward the end of the section. Label each new passage with a number on your paper, and give it an identifying title that summarizes the main point of the passage.

If you reach an important conclusion while answering questions, be sure to make note of it on your scratch paper too. For example, if a passage asks you to analyze a mechanistic study, and you determine that the first reaction described proceeds through the S_N2 mechanism, jot down "Rxn 1 = S_N2" under the passage number and title. Other questions may require this information in order to proceed, and a brief note beats wasted time reconfirming your conclusion while trying to answer a subsequent question. Your O-Chem passage map will begin to develop as you answer your questions, but before jumping into answering them, you will likely have very little to jot down.

The passage below is an example of an Information Presentation passage (of the second type described above). Note the minimal highlighting. The shaded words were seemingly important upon a first pass to identify what the passage was about and to predict the types of questions with which it might be associated. You'll find upon review of the questions, however, that nothing but structures was necessary to answer any of the passage-based questions.

The small milkweed bug, *Lygaeus kalmii*, produces and emits a number of C_5-C_8 alkenals. Some of these small, fragrant, organic molecules are used to attract conspecific males or females for mating; thus, they act as sex pheromones. Others of the molecules are strongly malodorous and are used for defense.

Collaborating scientists in Brazil, the Netherlands, and Maryland have recently developed a method of noninvasive sampling and identification of these small organic molecules from live insects. This method involves the use of gas chromatography and mass spectrometry for the separation and identification of the components of the mixture of molecules involved in the sex- and defense-pheromone response in *L. kalmii*. Several of the molecules identified in this manner are shown in Figure 1.

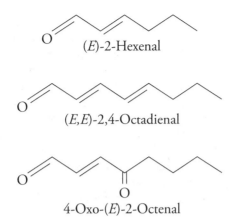

(E)-2-Hexenal

(E,E)-2,4-Octadienal

4-Oxo-(E)-2-Octenal

Figure 1 Molecules Identified Using Gas Chromatography and Mass Spectrometry

In addition to its mass spectrum, Molecule A, shown below, was also identified by its ^{1}H NMR spectrum:

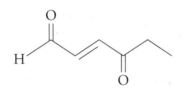

Molecule A

Remember not to get bogged down in spectroscopic data before a question specifically asks you to analyze it. Here is an example of a passage map for the passage above. This is what you might jot down on your scratch paper:

P1 – alkenals
P2 – separation and identification of alkenals
P3 – NMR data

The passage below is another example of an Information Presentation passage (of the third type described above). While the passage has much more text to wade through, only one small piece of it proves to be important in an Explicit question (addressed in detail later). Highlighted items are related to the main point of each paragraph, include new definitions, or provide examples of phenomena. The figures presented are more complex than those in the first passage, and the questions related to them are likely to be more involved as well.

Dyes are ionizable, aromatic compounds that absorb visible light due to the presence of a highly conjugated system of p orbitals. The observed color is one that is complementary to the wavelength of light absorbed by the molecule (complementary color pairs are red/green, orange/blue, and yellow/violet). Dyes bind to the materials to be colored, such as fabrics or paper, through inter- and intramolecular interactions, including hydrogen bonds, ionic interactions, covalent bonds, and coordinate covalent bonds. The stronger the interaction between dye molecule and fiber, the more permanent the color will be. When a dye covalently bonds to a fiber, it becomes a part of the fabric itself and cannot be washed away.

Two of the most common dye types are mordant dyes and direct dyes. A mordant is a polyvalent metal ion (usually Al^{3+} or Fe^{3+}) that forms a coordination complex with certain dyes. Mordants chelate to the fabric as well as the dye molecule, thereby improving their colorfastness. Mordant dyes are primarily used on protein-based fibers such as wool, silk, angora, and cashmere since the mordant can bind to the constituent amino acids of these fibers. Direct dyes are typically charged molecules, and interact with the material to be dyed through ionic forces or hydrogen bonding. As such they tend to bleed more than mordant dyes. Direct dyes are more commonly used on cellulose fibers such as cotton, linen, or hemp.

Azo dyes, a subclass of direct dyes, may be used in a dyeing technique in which an insoluble azo compound is produced directly onto or within a fiber. This is achieved by treating the fiber first with a diazonium component, followed by a coupling component. With suitable adjustment of dye bath conditions the two components react to produce the required insoluble azo dye. The coupling reagent used in the final step is typically a molecule containing either a phenolic hydroxyl group or an arylamine. The synthesis of methyl orange, an azo dye, is shown in Figure 1.

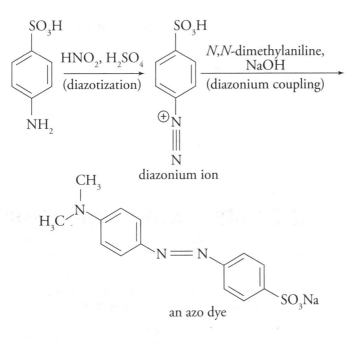

Figure 2 below represents the mechanism of the diazonium coupling reaction in the synthesis of methyl orange.

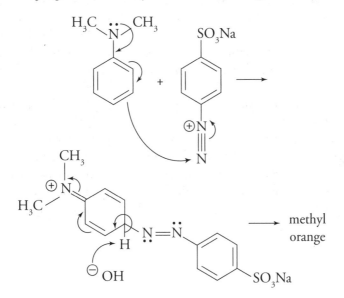

Figure 2 Mechanism of diazonium coupling

This is what you might jot down on your scratch paper for the passage above:

P1 – what dyes are and how they work
P2 – Definitions: mordant dye vs. direct dyes, fiber types dyed
P3 – Structure requirements for diazocoupling

17.5   ANALYZING FIGURES IN AN O-CHEM PASSAGE:

Passages don't always make it obvious what information you need in order to solve a problem, particularly since many important O-Chem passage details are found inside of figures or graphs.

In O-Chem passages, figures typically consist of molecular structures or reactions that are there to refer to and may or may not actually be required to solve a problem. Regardless, structures are almost always going to require scrutiny in order to understand, so the most time-effective way to approach structure-based figures is to acknowledge them when you first read the passage, noting the title, but then pay closer attention when a question references a particular structure. Often, simply reading the title of the figure is enough to understand its potential utility as you tackle the questions in the passage. This is when you'll put your ability to recognize differences in functional groups to the test to perhaps understand what reaction is being indicated or else to key in to an idea that relates several structures together. Often, when a series of structures are shown this is a cue to "look for the differences" between them. Spotting these differences is frequently the key to progressing in a solution. Zeroing in on the different functional groups will also help you to focus on what matters in most organic compounds, which are (sometimes large) biological or biochemical compounds that can intimidate even the most prepared test taker.

O-Chem passages may also present you with graphs, which appear infrequently, but always require interpretation since there won't necessarily be an accompanying description in the passage text. In these situations, you'll want to know what to look for so start by paying close attention to the axes on the graph. Almost all of the graphs that relate to O-Chem concepts will revolve around separation techniques so you'll frequently notice that the x-axis commonly measures time since all separation techniques take place over time. The separation technique you're most likely to encounter will be chromatography so the gas chromatogram, shown on the following page, is a reasonable example of a graph you may need to analyze in a passage.

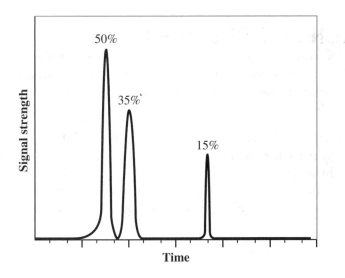

There are three main questions you need to ask when looking at a graph like this:

1. *How many peaks are there?*
   - Each peak indicates a different compound in a mixture.
   - In this example, there are 3 peaks so the mixture consists of 3 compounds.
2. *Which peak is earlier/later on the time axis?*
   - As time advances on the *x*-axis, each peak indicates a more retained compound.
   - In this example of a gas chromatogram, as time advances a compound is understood to have a higher boiling point (BP) so the leftmost peak is the compound with the lowest BP and the rightmost peak is the compound with the highest BP.
   - Note that this question is highly significant because it will change what it tells you based on the specific chromatographic technique employed.
3. *Which peak area is larger?* (This is typically indicated for you).
   - The peak area indicates the relative amounts of the compounds in a mixture.
   - In this example, percentage values are indicated above the peaks for the relative ratio of each of the three compounds in the mixture, thus, the first peak reflects the most abundant compound in the mixture.

By asking these three questions, you can uncover a substantial amount of information so be sure to know what to look for in order to know how to analyze a graph like this and be sure you know how question #2 above changes with each different chromatographic technique you're responsible for knowing.

17.6   TACKLING THE QUESTIONS

The Organic Chemistry passage-based questions are some of the most straightforward ones on the entire exam and, as a result, some of the quickest ones to answer. It may be a wise strategy to consider doing the O-Chem passages before the Biochemistry, General Chemistry, or Physics ones to help bank up some extra time to spend on the wordier, more involved passages.

However, you should also consider starting with the subject you feel the most comfortable with, saving your more difficult subject for last. Whatever subject you choose, do all of the passages in one subject first before switching. In addition, do the passages within a subject in the order with which you feel most comfortable, leaving the topic you struggle with most, or the passage that appears to be the most difficult, for last. Within the passages themselves, tackle the easier questions first, leaving the most time consuming ones for last.

17.7   O-CHEM QUESTION TYPES

Memory Questions

These questions can be answered directly from prior knowledge. You can often recognize this question type by the length of the answer choices; one- or two-word answer choices are a good indication that you have the answer to these questions in your head already. Freestanding questions are commonly Memory questions since there is no passage to refer to. In addition, O-Chem passages often have "hidden" FSQs associated with them. This is another good reason to get to the questions quickly, rather than getting stuck reading details within the passage text.

Here's an example of not only a "hidden" FSQ but also a Memory question from the passage above on alkenals:

If a chemist were to react (*E,E*)-2-4-octadienal with $NaBH_4$ in ethanol and monitor the reaction by TLC, the spot corresponding to the product would be expected to have an R_f value that is:

A)   less than that of the starting material.
B)   equal to that of the starting material.
C)   greater than that of the starting material.
D)   greater than 1.

While the passage shows the structure of the molecule described in the question, the suffix of the name is really all that is required to answer this question. By knowing that a reducing agent like $NaBH_4$ can be used to convert an aldehyde into an alcohol, and that alcohols are more polar than carbonyl compounds, giving them lower R_f values, you can deduce the correct answer (choice A) with no reference to the passage at all. Additionally, there is NO information in the passage, beyond the structure of the molecule, that could prove useful in answering this question.

Here is a true freestanding question that is also a Memory question:

Which of the following acetylating conditions will convert diethylamine into an amide at the fastest rate?

A) Acetic acid / HCl
B) Acetic anhydride
C) Acetyl chloride
D) Ethyl acetate

Your first step to attacking this question should be to consider what type of reaction is described. The conversion of an amine to an amide is a nucleophilic addition-elimination, where the amine acts as the nucleophile. Therefore, you're looking for the answer choice with the best electrophile, thereby increasing the reaction rate. Knowing the relative reactivities of carboxylic acids derivatives (amide < ester < anhydride < acid halide) allows you to eliminate choices B and D. In order to choose between the remaining answers that include a carboxylic acid and an acid derivative, rely on your fundamentals. Ask yourself: How would an amine be expected to behave under each set of conditions? When you consider that amines are not only nucleophilic but also basic, you can deduce that they will be protonated by both the HCl and the acetic acid to yield a non-nucleophilic conjugate acid under the conditions of choice A. The nucleophilic addition reaction is therefore faster with the acid chloride derivative, making choice C correct.

Explicit Questions

These questions have answers that are explicitly stated in the passage. To answer them correctly, for example, may just require finding a definition, reading a graph, or making a simple connection. Explicit questions are much more common in other sections of the test that rely more on reading comprehension. Since chemical structures are the most common source of referenced information in an O-Chem passage, Explicit questions in this section might ask you to identify the number of chiral centers in a given molecule, or to identify whether a particular functional group is present or not.

Here's an example of an Explicit question from the azo dye passage:

Mordant dyes are used in biological assays in addition to the textile industry. Which of the following biologically important molecules is most likely to be labeled by a mordant dye?

A) Glycogen
B) Chromatin
C) Cholesterol
D) Starch

You should recognize the term "mordant" as a new term you highlighted while reading the passage, so go back to the text to retrieve the important information. The passage states that mordants generally bind to protein-based fibers. Without this information, you might be able to eliminate choices A and D (glycogen and starch) since they are both carbohydrates, and as such, are not likely to be the answer. With the passage information at your disposal, however, this becomes a bit of a Memory question, and you need only determine which of your answer choices contain proteins. Cholesterol, a lipid, can be eliminated in addition to the two carbohydrates, leaving choice B as the correct answer (note that chromatin contains both proteins and DNA).

Implicit Questions

These questions require you to apply knowledge to a new situation or make a more complex connection; the answer is typically implied by the information in the passage. Answer choices are generally longer, and may come in two parts, where the second half provides an explanation for the first. As mentioned before, the relevant information in the passage is often a molecular structure, but the analysis required to answer the question is more involved than for Explicit questions that rely on structures. Implicit style questions are the most common type of O-Chem questions.

Here's an example of an Implicit question from the azo dye passage:

> The diazonium coupling reaction in Figure 2 is faster than most electrophilic substitutions of benzene. Which of the following statements best explains this fact?
>
> A) The diazonium ion is an electron withdrawing substituent, making its benzene ring a better electrophile than benzene.
> B) The diazonium ion is a good nucleophile.
> C) The dimethylamino group is an electron donating substituent, making its benzene ring a better electrophile than benzene.
> D) The dimethylamino group is an electron donating substituent, making its benzene ring a better nucleophile than benzene.

Since these answer choices are relatively long (and most have a second clause), try to use POE to eliminate choices based on obvious false statements in the first part of the answer. Remember, if any part of an answer choice is false, the entire statement can be eliminated. The first half of all the choices makes a statement about the inductive effects of substituents, or, in the case of choice B, the nucleophilicity of a compound. Refer to the structures in Figure 2. You should note that the diazonium ion is positively charged and therefore electron deficient. Since nucleophiles are by definition electron-rich, choice B can be eliminated. The first halves of the remaining answer choices are all valid statements, since a positively charged substituent will pull electron density toward it, while an amine with a lone pair of electrons on the nitrogen will push electron density toward the ring. This question requires a more critical approach to distinguish between answer choices.

✴ Half-wrong is all wrong!

You should identify this as an Implicit question since it asks you to compare a new reaction to one you might already be familiar with. Consider, then, what you already know about benzene. Since benzene has six pi electrons and is electron rich, it should behave as a nucleophile. This fundamental piece of information about the reactivity of benzene allows you to eliminate choices A and C. It does not matter whether the indicated substituents in Figure 2 make benzene a better or worse electrophile, since in the context of this reaction benzene behaves as a nucleophile. The remaining answer (choice D) is not only internally consistent but also answers the question.

Content Categories

O-Chem questions can be further classified from a content perspective into four main categories. Instead of trying to memorize a lot of detailed information, try to generalize as much as possible and focus on the fundamentals of structure and stability when approaching questions. Remember that the MCAT is more likely to ask you to apply fundamental concepts to novel situations rather than ask you to recall an exception to a rule and regurgitate trivia. Just about every O-Chem question can be put into one of the following five categories:

Structure

Questions are generally about functional groups, stereochemistry, isomers, electron density (nucleophiles vs. electrophiles), and nomenclature.

Stability

This generally refers to stability of products or reaction intermediates. These questions often ask about inductive effects, resonance, steric strain, torsional strain, ring strain, etc.

Laboratory practices

These questions may ask you to identify an appropriate separation technique (extraction, chromatography, distillation, etc.) for a given mixture of compounds, or ask you to interpret/predict the results of a separation procedure. You might also be asked to choose an appropriate spectroscopic technique (IR, NMR, mass spec, UV-vis, etc.) to identify a compound, or interpret spectroscopic data.

Predict the product

Given a starting material and reaction conditions, choose the major product of the reaction. This will only be a one step synthesis; no multi-step processes will be presented. These questions will generally be associated with a passage in which a reaction type is explained in detail rather than be a freestanding question.

17.8   ORGANIC CHEMISTRY QUESTION STRATEGIES

1. Remember that POE is paramount! The strikeout tool allows you to eliminate answer choices; this will improve your chances of guessing the correct answer if you are unable to narrow it down to one choice.

2. Answer the straightforward questions first. Leave questions that require analysis of experiments and graphs for later.

3. Make sure that the answer you choose actually answers the question and isn't just a true statement.

4. I-II-III questions: Always work between the I-II-III statements and the answer choices. Unfortunately, it is not possible to strike out the Roman numerals, but this is a great use for scratch paper notes. Once a statement is determined to be true (or false), strike out answer choices that do not contain (or do contain) that statement as appropriate.

5. Ranking questions: Look for an extreme in whatever is being ranked, then look at the answer choices. Use the strikeout feature to eliminate choices as you go. In some cases, you may immediately get the answer as only one choice lists the appropriate option as "least" or "greatest." Usually you will, at minimum, be able to strikeout two answer choices. Then just examine the remaining possibilities to determine which of the items at the other end of the ranking can be correct.

6. 2x2 style questions: These questions require you to know two pieces of information to get the correct answer, and they are easily identified by their answer choices, which commonly take the form A because X, B because X, A because Y, B because Y. Tackle one piece of information at a time, which should allow you to quickly eliminate two answer choices.

7. LEAST/EXCEPT/NOT questions: Don't get tricked by these questions that ask you to pick the answer that doesn't fit (the incorrect or false statement). It's often good to use your scratch paper and write a T or F next to answer choices A–D. The one that stands out as different is the correct answer!

8. If you read a question and do not know how to answer it, look to the passage for help. It is likely that the passage contains information pertinent to answering the question, either within the text or in the form of experimental data.

9. Math: Any questions that involve calculations should be left for last (there aren't many in O-Chem, but they happen). You should always round numbers and estimate while working out calculations on your scratch paper.

10. Don't ever leave a question blank since there is no penalty for guessing.

17.9   MCAT ORGANIC CHEMISTRY TOPIC LIST[1]

Structure

A.   Nomenclature
B.   Stereochemistry
  1.   Isomers
    a.   constitutional isomers
    b.   conformational isomers
    c.   stereoisomers
  2.   Polarization of light, specific rotation
  3.   Absolute and relative configuration (R and S, E and Z)
  4.   Racemic mixtures, separation of enantiomers

Stability

A.   Delocalized electrons and resonance
B.   Induction
C.   Ring strain
D.   Steric strain
E.   Acidity of classes of oxygen-containing compounds
F.   Effect of chain branching

Reaction Types

A.   Nucleophilic Substitutions (S_N1 and S_N2) of alcohols and alkyl halides
  1.   nucleophiles, electrophiles, leaving groups
  2.   mechanisms
  3.   stereochemistry
  4.   reaction rates/rate laws
  5.   alcohol protection (tosylation/mesylation)
B.   Reactivity and reactions of aldehydes and ketones
  1.   keto-enol tautomerism
    a.   enolate chemistry
  2.   acidity of α hydrogens
  3.   oxidations to carboxylic acids
  4.   Nucleophilic additions
    a.   alcohol formation
      I.   from hydride reduction
      II.   from organometallic reagents (Grignard reagents)
    b.   acetal, hemiacetal formation
    c.   imine, enamine formation
    d.   aldol condensation, retro-aldol
    e.   cyanohydrin formation
C.   Reactivity and reactions of carboxylic acids
  1.   physical properties, solubility, and hydrogen bonding
  2.   reduction to alcohols
  3.   decarboxylation (β-keto acids)
D.   Reactivity and reactions of carboxylic acid derivatives (acid chlorides, anhydrides, amides, esters)
  1.   relative reactivity of acid derivatives
  2.   addition-elimination reactions
    a.   preparation of acid derivatives
    b.   interconversions of acid derivatives
    c.   esterification/transesterification
    d.   hydrolysis of fats and glycerides (saponification)
    e.   formation and hydrolysis of amides

[1]   Adapted from *The Official Guide to the MCAT Exam (MCAT2015)*, 4th ed., © 2014 Association of American Medical Colleges.

Laboratory Techniques

A. Absorption Spectroscopy
  1. ^{1}H-NMR
  2. IR
  3. UV-vis
B. Mass Spectrometry
C. Separations and Purifications
  1. extractions
  2. distillation
  3. chromatography
     a. size-exclusion
     b. thin-layer
     c. column
     d. HPLC
     e. affinity
     f. ion-exchange
     g. gas
  4. gel electrophoresis

Biological Molecules

A. Carbohydrates
  1. nomenclature, classification
  2. absolute configurations
  3. epimers, anomers, cyclic structures
  4. reactions
B. Proteins
  1. absolute configurations
  2. amino acid classification (acid/base, hydrophobic/hydrophilic; 1- and 3-letter coding)
  3. amino acid synthesis (Strecker and Gabriel syntheses)
  4. primary, secondary structure
  5. reactions
C. Lipids
  1. structure (free fatty acids, triglycerides, phospholipids, terpenes, steroids)
D. Nucleic acids

Chapter 18
Organic Chemistry
Practice Section

FREESTANDING QUESTIONS

1. Reaction 1 takes exactly 45 minutes to go to completion and is measured to have bimolecular kinetics.

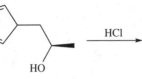

Reaction 1: HCl →

Reaction 2 proceeds through a similar mechanism as Reaction 1. Which of the following values for optical activity are expected at the beginning of Reaction 2 and after 60 minutes, respectively?

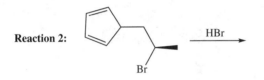

Reaction 2: HBr →

A) (+)-50°, (+)-50°
B) (+)-50°, 0°
C) (+)-50°, (–)-50°
D) 0°, (+)-50°

2. 0.54 mol of aminocyclopentane is dissolved into an Erlenmeyer flask filled with 25 mL of diethyl ether and 25 mL of 0.1 M $NaHCO_3$ (aq). These solvents are both immiscible. Addition of which of the following to the Erlenmeyer flask will result in a higher mole fraction of aminocyclopentane dissolved in the $NaHCO_3$ (aq) layer?

   I.   NaCl
   II. H_3O^+
  III. 1-pentanol

A) II only
B) III only
C) I and II only
D) I, II, and III

3. Which of the following will resolve a mixture of the two molecules shown below?

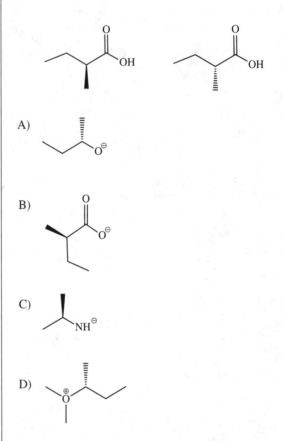

A)

B)

C)

D)

4. 1-Propanol is reacted with anhydrous PCC in an oxidation reaction and then purified. The compound is then added to a solution of deuterated methanol for seven days. ^1H-NMR spectroscopy is then performed on the purified compound. How many signals are expected to appear in the NMR spectrum of the purified compound?

A) 0
B) 1
C) 2
D) 3

5. What is the maximum number of sites that may be deuterated if the following compound is reacted with NaOD in D_2O?

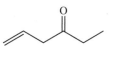

A) 2
B) 4
C) 6
D) 7

6. How many stereoisomeric products are expected for the reaction sequence shown below?

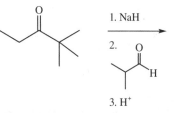

1. NaH

2.

3. H^+

A) 1
B) 2
C) 4
D) 8

7. Which one of the following molecules will react fastest with acetic acid?

A) $N(CH_3)_4^+$
B) $N(CH_3)_3$
C) $NH(CH_3)_2$
D) $PH(CH_3)_2$

8. Reacting the molecule below with which of the following will result in a saturated organic product that has the longest elution time in HPLC?

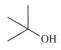

A) SH_3^+
B) HI
C) NH_4^+
D) HCl

9. The undecapeptide GNOWLLADNEK is placed in 6 M sulfuric acid (*aq*) for two days. Which of the following will be seen in the reaction mixture after this period of time?

  I.   Increased $[NH_4^+]$
  II. Increased amount of E residues
  III. Increased amount of D residues

A) III only
B) I and II only
C) I and III only
D) I, II, and III

10. An amide and a carboxylic acid, both with an equivalent number of carbons, are spotted in two different lanes on a TLC plate. After plate development, which will have the higher R_f value, and why?

A) Amide, because it is more polar
B) Amide, because it is less polar
C) Carboxylic acid, because it is more polar
D) Carboxylic acid, because it is less polar

11. Protease X possesses an active site lined with R residues known to assist with substrate binding and is known to preferentially cleave peptide bonds on the amino side of the residues it binds. After peptide Y is treated with protease X, the following three fragments are discovered: DYK, RLLC, EAK. Which of the following residues was located at the N-terminal of Peptide Y?

A) K
B) D
C) C
D) R

PRACTICE PASSAGE 1

Oligomer-based synthesis is vital to life processes, such as the synthesis of proteins. A peptide is a natural, biological polymer, however, scientists have created structurally unique synthetic biopolymers to mimic naturally occurring polymers.

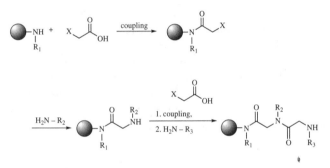

Figure 1 Structure comparison of natural and synthetic biopolymers

Peptoids and peptidines are a novel class of oligomeric scaffolds. Peptoids are peptidomimetics whose side chains are attached to the nitrogen atom of the peptide backbone instead of the α-carbon. Figure 2 illustrates how peptoids are typically synthesized on solid-support through a series of acylation reactions.

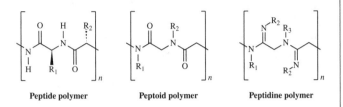

Figure 2 Synthesis of a peptoid on solid-support

Peptidines are different from peptides and peptoids because the scaffold can accommodate two substituents per monomeric unit, allowing for two sites of diversity per monomer. Peptidine synthesis consists of two separate, iterative synthetic steps. As shown in Figure 3, the first step (Reaction 1) is an amidation where a secondary amine reacts with an imidoyl chloride. The second (Reaction 2) is an amination step where a primary amine displaces a chloride.

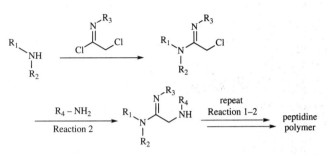

Figure 3 Preparation of a peptidine oligomer

The imidoyl chloride is a unique reagent and was synthesized in two steps from a primary amine, as shown in Figure 4.

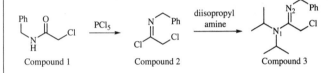

Figure 4 Synthesis and application of imidoyl chloride

Adapted from Vastl, J.; Kartika, R.; Park, K.; Cho, A. E.; Spiegel, D. A. *Chem. Sci.*, **2016**, *7*, 3317.

1. All are suitable electrophiles for the acylation shown in Figure 2 EXCEPT:

A)

B)

C)

D)

2. If the transformation from Compound 1 to Compound 2 was monitored by IR, what changes in the IR spectrum would be observed?

I.   Disappearance of a signal at 3050 cm^{-1}
II. Disappearance of a signal at 1650 cm^{-1}
III. Appearance of a signal at 1720 cm^{-1}

A) I only
B) II only
C) I and II only
D) I, II, and III

3. When treated with acid, which nitrogen in Compound 3 is most likely to be protonated?

A) N_1 because the sp^3-hybridized lone pair is more basic
B) N_2 because the sp^2-hybridized lone pair is more basic
C) N_1 because the positive charge would be resonance stabilized
D) N_2 because the positive charge would be resonance stabilized

4. How many doublets are present in the ^{1}H-NMR spectrum for the compound below:

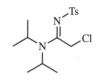

A) Two
B) Three
C) Four
D) Five

PRACTICE PASSAGE 2

Proteases are the largest and most important group of enzymes responsible for selectively catalyzing the hydrolysis of peptide bonds. Proteases can be divided into 4 major groups: aspartic, serine, cysteine, and metalloproteases. Proteases are involved in many biological functions but, if not controlled, can cause many disease states. As a consequence, protease inhibitors have been explored as a treatment for a variety of disease states.

Protease inhibitors can be segmented into 3 categories: irreversible, reversible, and transition state. Irreversible protease inhibitors form stable covalent bonds with the enzyme, often within the active site. Reversible inhibitors interact with enzymes through non-covalent interactions. The interactions may be weak individually, however, through several interactions, the collective interactions produce strong and specific binding. Transition state inhibitors possess a chemical structure that mimics the transition state of a substrate in enzyme-catalyzed reactions. For example, methylthioadenosine nucleosidases are enzymes that catalyze the deadenylation of methylthioadenosine via hydrolysis. The transition state for the hydrolysis can be defined as early or late depending on the stage of dissociation.

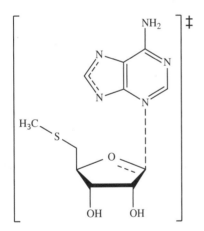

Figure 1 Transition state of the ionization of methylthioadenosine

Transition state inhibitors can also be irreversible, as is the case with chloromethyl ketones. Chloromethyl ketones can react with serine and histidine residues found in the active site. The first step involves nucleophilic addition of serine to generate a tetrahedral intermediate. This intermediate can react in an intramolecular manner to further generate an intermediate that facilitates alkylation of the imidazole of histidine.

1. Which of the following molecules is likely to be the strongest irreversible inhibitor of a protease with a serine in the protein active site?

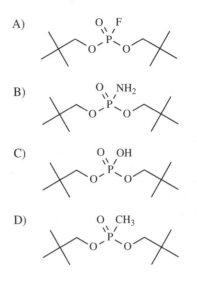

2. Which of the following analogs will most likely be a late-dissociation transition state inhibitor of methylthioadenosine nucleosidase?

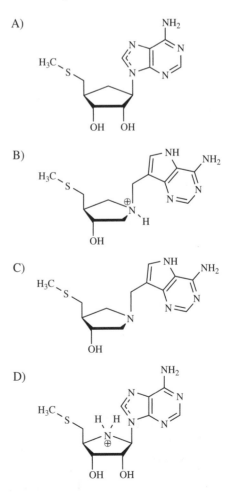

3. The following compounds are irreversible inhibitors EXCEPT:

A)

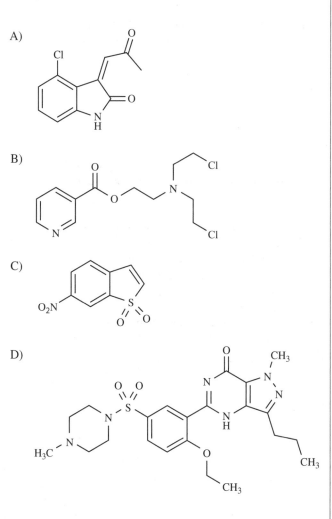

B)

C)

D)

4. Chloromethyl ketones are irreversible transition state inhibitors used to alkylate histidine. Which of the following intermediates is most likely to be involved in the mechanism?

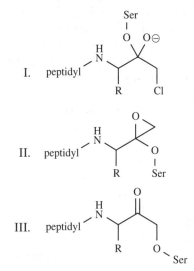

I.   peptidyl

II. peptidyl

III. peptidyl

A) I only
B) II only
C) I and II only
D) I, II, and III

PRACTICE PASSAGE 3

Selectively exploiting compounds with more than one reactive site is of interest to researchers wishing to build large molecular frameworks from simple core molecules. Studies have been carried out on the substitution chemistry of vinyl epoxides, since these compounds can be substituted with nucleophiles at either an epoxide carbon, in standard S_N2 fashion, or at the vinyl end the molecule through a related mechanism known as S_N2'. As shown in Figure 1, both substitution pathways result in ring opening of the epoxide.

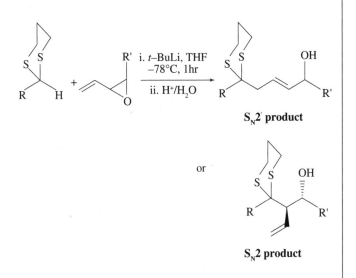

Figure 1 Substitution of a vinyl epoxide

In the S_N2' reaction a lithiated dithiane is formed by deprotonation of the initial dithiane using the very strong base *tert*-butyllithium. The new organolithium compound attacks the vinyl epoxide forming the final substitution products. It was found that the site of attack, and thus the final product, was controlled by the steric bulk of the dithiane near the deprotonated carbon. The table below details these results.

R	Ratio S_N2:S_N2'
H	100:0
phenyl	100:0
i-propyl	0:100
Si-(*i*-propyl)$_3$	0:100

Figure 2 Substituent effects on S_N2 and S_N2' pathways

1. A dithiane bearing which of the following R groups is *most* likely to give solely the S_N2' product?

A) Methyl
B) *t*-Butyl
C) Cyclohexyl
D) *n*-Propyl

2. *tert*-Butyllithium is extremely pyrophoric and dangerous to handle. What might be a complication in substituting *n*-butyllithium for *tert*-butyllithium?

A) *n*-Butyllithium isn't sufficiently basic to deprotonate the dithiane.
B) *n*-Butyllithium is unstable and undergoes dimerization reactions resulting in the formation of *n*-octane.
C) *n*-Butyllithium can deprotonate the vinyl epoxide leading to premature epoxide opening.
D) *n*-Butyllithium can act as a nucleophile and open the epoxide via substitution.

3. Another reaction, under the same conditions as shown in Figure 1 and utilizing –SiH(CH$_3$)$_2$ as the R group, went entirely though the S$_N$2 pathway despite having similar substitution to the case where R is *i*-propyl. Which of the following could explain these results?

A) The lower electronegativity of Si, compared to C, creates a strong nucleophile which favors the S$_N$2 mechanism.
B) The larger size of Si, compared to C, maintains a larger distance between the anionic carbon and the steric bulk of the methyl groups.
C) The hydrogen on the Si atom is acidic enough to hydrogen bond to the oxygen atom of the epoxide, aligning the anion for S$_N$2 attack on the epoxide carbons.
D) The larger size of the Si atom, compared to the C, provides steric shielding to the anionic carbon, favoring the S$_N$2 pathway.

4. The lack of ether products found in the reaction mixture indicates which of the following?

A) Oxyanions cannot open epoxides.
B) Nucleophilic attack by the lithiated dithiane is the fast step in the reaction.
C) Deprotonation of the dithiane is the fast step in the reaction.
D) Ethers are unstable to *tert*-butyllithium.

5. The reaction shown below is known as a 1,4-Brook rearrangement. It involves swapping an organosilicon moiety with a hydrogen atom of an alcohol group four atoms away.

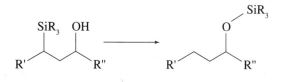

In trials of the reaction in Figure 1 with four silicon-containing R groups, only one of the following showed the Brook rearrangement product. Which was it?

A) -SiH(CH$_3$)$_2$
B) -Si(*i*-propyl)$_3$
C) -Si(*t*-butyl)(*i*-propyl)$_2$
D) -Si(*i*-propyl)(CH$_3$)$_2$

PRACTICE PASSAGE 4

A large polypeptide can be constructed by forming an amide bond between two smaller peptide fragments. This takes place when an alpha-amino group on one peptide nucleophilically attacks an activated carbonyl on the other. Reaction is often problematic for large peptides due to their low solubility, resulting in low reactant concentrations and slow reaction times. Generally, the reactivity between an amino group and an activated carbonyl are not high enough for acyl transfer to overcome the relatively low solubility of peptides.

In nature, peptide formation occurs via the transfer of a C-terminal acyl group to the 3′-hydroxyl end of a tRNA molecule. The C-terminal acyl group is only activated as an ester but the transfer is aided by the reactants being held in close proximity by the ribosome.

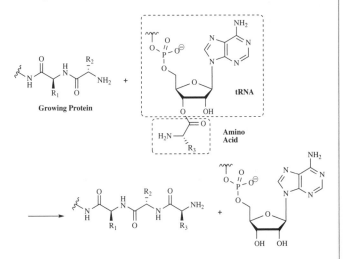

Figure 1 Peptide formation utilizing tRNA

New strategies have emerged that take advantage of proximity to couple peptides. These strategies provide practical and powerful means to assemble synthetic peptides, as the peptides can be protected or unprotected. In addition, coupling can occur in aqueous or organic solvents, in solution or on a solid support. Native chemical ligation is the most common method for the chemical synthesis of peptides. In native chemical ligation, the thiolate of an N-terminal cysteine residue of a peptide is critical in facilitating amide bond formation.

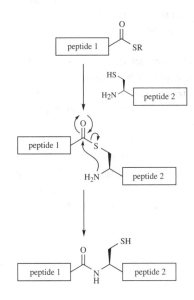

Figure 2 Native chemical ligation

Another approach to peptide ligation is the *in situ* generation of a cysteine thioester. In this method, as outlined in Figure 2, the C-terminal thioacid reacts with an electrophilic carbon on the N-terminal residue generating a thioester then undergoing an intramolecular native chemical ligation.

Adapted from Nilsson, B. L.; Soellner, M. B.; Raines, R. T. *Annu. Rev. Biophys. Biomol. Struc.* 2005, *34*, 91.

1. Which of the following atoms is analogous to sulfur in native chemical ligation?

A) Nitrogen
B) Selenium
C) Oxygen
D) Chlorine

2. Based on information in the passage, the addition of the amino acid onto the growing peptide is an example of what type of reaction?

    I.   Nucleophilic Addition
    II.   Nucleophilic Addition-Elimination
    III.   Acyl Transfer
    IV.   Hydrolysis

A) I only
B) II, III, and IV only
C) II and III only
D) III only

3. All of the following reagents could successfully perform the reaction below EXCEPT:

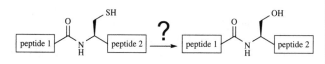

A)
```
1. CH₃I, NaH
─────────────→
2. H₂O, heat
```

B)
```
1. CH₃I, NaH
─────────────→
2. H₂O, heat
```

C)
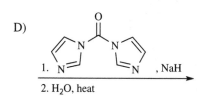
```
1.          , NaH
2. H₂O, heat
─────────────→
```

D)
```
1.          , NaH
2. H₂O, heat
─────────────→
```

4. Based on the information in the passage, which of the following would be LEAST likely to undergo *in situ* cysteine thioester formation?

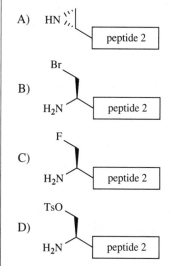

A) HN — peptide 2

B) H₂N, Br — peptide 2

C) H₂N, F — peptide 2

D) H₂N, TsO — peptide 2

PRACTICE PASSAGE 5

Sesterterpenes are a structurally diverse set of natural products found in a range of organisms including lichens, fungi, and various marine species, containing twenty-five carbon atoms in their primary skeletons. As a class, sesterterpenes are formed via the cyclization of geranylfarnesol (Figure 1) in enzymatic processes catalyzed by a range of cyclases. The structure of the active site of a cyclase largely determines the stereochemistry of the resultant sesterterpene through directing the conformational alignment of the rings undergoing cyclization.

Recent research into the natural products obtained from the herb *Aletris farinosa* (*A. farinosa*) has produced a number of new isolated tri- and tetracyclic sesterterpenes. Of the tricyclic varieties isolated, all showed identical stereochemistry in their tricyclic core, indicating that that their cyclization likely occurred in the same enzyme, and their differences were generated post-cyclization. Through sensitive NMR techniques coupled with computational quantum modeling, the stereochemistry of the products (**A**) were elucidated, and a likely intermediate proposed (Figure 1). Modeling indicated that in order to produce the observed stereochemistry, the cyclase aligned the three forming rings each in a chair conformation (chair-chair-chair cyclization).

Two tetracyclic sesterterpenes were isolated from *A. farinosa* with ring stereochemistries that ruled out formation via simple further cyclization of the intermediate in Figure 1. Computational modeling indicated that the difference between the cyclization process for the tricyclic compounds and the tetracyclic ones stemmed from the enzyme-stabilized cyclization conformation, which must be chair-boat-chair in order to achieve the different stereochemistries in **B** and **C**. Addition to the final double bond on one of its two faces led to the formation of compound **B**, which is completed by the removal of a proton from the carbon in the position adjacent to the carbocation (Figure 2a). If the other face of the double bond was accessed, a cascade reaction involving a sequence of seven methide/hydride shifts was induced, ending in molecule **C** (Figure 2b). An important feature of this cascade is that all methide/hydride shifts maintain groups on the same respective sides of the molecule.

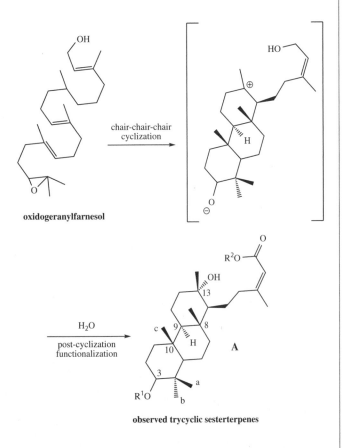

oxidogeranylfarnesol

chair-chair-chair cyclization

H_2O
post-cyclization functionalization

A

observed trycyclic sesterterpenes

Figure 1 Formation of tricyclic sesterterpenes from oxidogeranylfarnesol

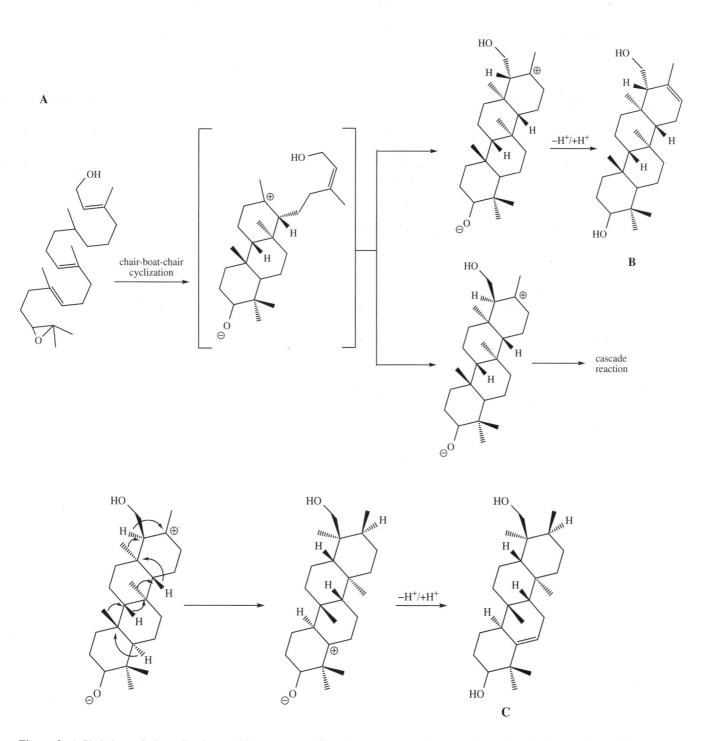

Figure 2 a) Chair-boat-chair cyclization to either compound **B** or the precursor to the cascade reaction; b) the cascade reaction ending in compound **C**.

Adapted from: De Voss et al., Chem. Sci. 2015, doi: 10.1039/c5sc02056e

1. Compounds **B** and **C** are isolated by HPLC and then examined by spectroscopic analysis using ¹H NMR. Which of the following ¹H NMR observations best distinguishes between the two separated compounds?

A) Compound **C** shows a close grouping of 5 three-proton singlets between 0 and 1 ppm, while **B** shows 5 three-proton singlets between 0 and 1 ppm and an additional three-proton singlet between 2 and 3 ppm.

B) Compound **C** shows a set of peaks between 6 and 7 ppm, while **B** shows no peaks in this region.

C) Compound **C** shows a one-proton triplet between 5 and 6 ppm, while **B** shows a similar one-proton triplet between 6 and 7 ppm.

D) Compound **C** shows two one-proton peaks between 4 and 5 ppm, while **B** shows one two-proton peak between 4 and 5 ppm.

2. If the intermediate in the cyclization shown in Figure 1 was quenched in heavy water ($D_2^{18}O$) and allowed to stir in the presence of heavy water for a number of hours, which would be the most prominent mass indicated by mass spectrometry.

A) 392 g/mol
B) 396 g/mol
C) 397 g/mol
D) 401 g/mol

3. If a sesterterpene of type A was identified in which carbon 3 was determined to have R stereochemistry, with the OR group occupying an axial position on the ring, which of the following must also be true?

A) Methyl groups b and c must be in axial ring positions, while a is in an equatorial position.
B) Methyl groups b and c are in equatorial positions, while a is in an axial position.
C) Methyl groups a and c are in equatorial positions, while b is in an axial position.
D) Methyl groups a and c must also be in axial ring positions, while b is in an equatorial position.

4. If a cyclase promotes the cascade reaction shown in Figure 2b, but rather than ending at compound C the overall reaction is terminated with fewer than seven hydride/methyl shifts, which of the following compounds might result if all stereochemistries are maintained?

A)

B)

C)

D)

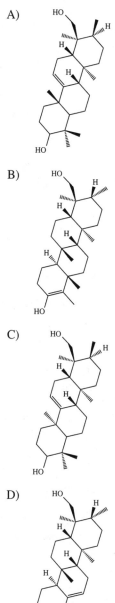

5. The thermodynamic driving force(s) for the cyclization reactions in Figures 1 and 2 are which of the following?

A) The opening of a strained epoxide and the formation of high-entropy polycyclic molecules.

B) The opening of a strained epoxide and the formation of σ-bonds from π-bonds.

C) The reaction-guiding influence of the cyclase being employed in each reaction.

D) The opening of a strained epoxide ring and the formation of a more soluble compound.

PRACTICE PASSAGE 6

The use of polymeric support (PS), or solid-phase, in organic synthesis is useful for three reasons: the procedures are simple (add reagent, then filter and rinse), the purification steps are circumvented, and high concentrations of reagents can be used to ensure full conversion of starting material. The polymeric support consists of 2 parts: resins and linkers. Resins are inert matrices that are passive to chemistry. Linkers are immobilized protecting groups that can be readily removed from the growing biomolecule. There are two types of linkers: integral and non-integral. As shown in Figure 1, an integral linker (the bolded portion of each structure) is one where the polymer support forms part or all of the linker.

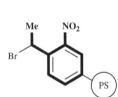
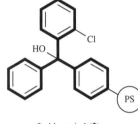
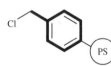
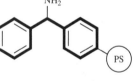

o-nitro (α-methyl) bromobenzyl (**1**)

2-chlorotrityl (**2**)

benzyl chloride (**3**)

benzhydrylamine (**4**)

Figure 1 Various types of integral linkers

As shown in Figure 2, a non-integral linker is one where the linker is attached to the resin core by an extension. The advantage of the non-integral linker is the synthesis is further away from the resin, thus eliminating sterics or electronic effects. These linkers can be loaded onto the resin then derivatized. The resin attachment is generally either an ether or amide functional group or a C—C bond.

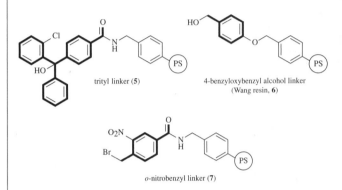

trityl linker (**5**)

4-benzyloxybenzyl alcohol linker
(Wang resin, **6**)

o-nitrobenzyl linker (**7**)

Figure 2 Various types of non-integral linkers

The original use of the solid phase methodology was for the synthesis of peptides. This methodology allowed for the linear synthesis of protected peptides without purification steps. The amino acid can react with the linker/resin by two approaches where the linker/resin is nucleophilic or electrophilic. In Figure 3, one approach is given where the electrophilic resin is attacked by the carboxylate of the amino acid. The amino acid behaves as the electrophile in the other approach by being activated for nucleophilic addition-elimination.

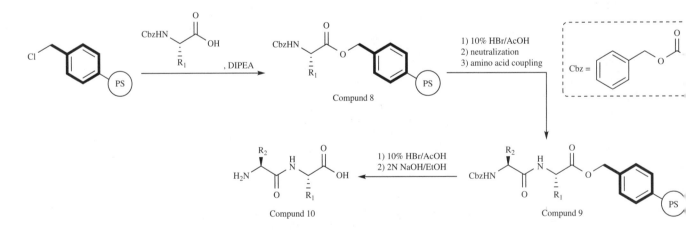

Compund 8

Compund 9

Compund 10

Figure 3 Example of a dipeptide synthesis.

Adapted from Guillier, F.; Orain, D.; Bradley, M. *Chem.* Rev. 2000, *100, 2091.*

1. Which of the following schemes accurately represents the preparation of a resin for solid-phase synthesis?

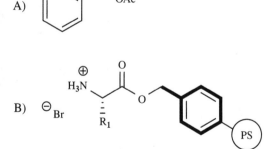

A) I only
B) I and II only
C) II and III only
D) I, II, and III

2. Which of the following integral linkers in Figure 1 would most likely attack an activated amino acid?

A) *o*-Nitro-(α-methyl)-bromobenzyl
B) 2-Chlorotrityl
C) Benzyl chloride
D) Benzhydrylamine

3. What is the unwanted by-product that forms when compound 8 is treated with 10% HBr/AcOH?

A)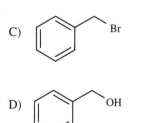

B)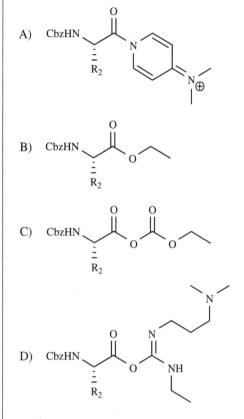

4. Which of the following amino acid derivatives is LEAST likely to undergo the amino acid coupling shown in Figure 3?

A) CbzHN ... R_2

B) CbzHN ... R_2

C) CbzHN ... R_2

D) CbzHN ... R_2

Chapter 19
Organic Chemistry
Practice Section
Solutions

SOLUTIONS TO FREESTANDING QUESTIONS

1. **B**   As given in the question, Reaction 1 is measured to have bimolecular kinetics, meaning that it proceeds through an S_N2 mechanism, thus Reaction 2 will also go through an S_N2 mechanism. Since the starting material for Reaction 2 is chiral (it has one chiral center), it is optically active so choice D can be eliminated. Recall that the resulting inversion of configuration observed in an S_N2 product will result in a new optically active compound. However, in Reaction 2 the nucleophile and the leaving group are both the same (Br$^-$), which means the S_N2 reaction occurs perpetually, inverting the configuration each time leading to a balanced mixture of both enantiomers—a racemic mixture—which shows no optical activity. After a period of time, this makes choice B correct (choices A and C can be eliminated).

2. **C**   In this solvent extraction, diethyl ether acts as a nonpolar solvent, while sodium bicarbonate is an aqueous solvent. Since H_3O^+ (Item II) is present in three of the four answer choices, determining if either Item I or Item III is correct first would allow you to eliminate more answer choices earlier. Adding NaCl (Item I) will cause ionization of the salt into the aqueous layer. The result of this is that the aqueous layer will become more polar due to the increased concentration of charge. Because aminocyclopentane is a polar molecule capable of H-bonding, it will dissolve more readily in the aqueous solvent that is now more polar (Item I is true; choices A and B can be eliminated). Because 1-pentanol will enter the non-polar diethyl ether phase, due to its carbon chain, it has no effect on the proportion of aminocyclopentane in the polar aqueous layer (Item III is false, choice C is correct, and choice D can be eliminated). Lastly, adding H_3O^+ to the flask will protonate aminocyclopentane, leaving it charged and causing more of it to enter the aqueous phase (Item II is true).

3. **A**   The two molecules given in the question are enantiomeric carboxylic acids so to best separate them they should be reacted with a chiral molecule in order to generate diastereomers (which are easier to separate). Recall that a carboxylic acid reacts through an addition-elimination mechanism and becomes a new carboxylic acid derivative. Reaction with a chiral alkoxide will lead to ester formation, which is a stable choice as an ester possesses an unfavorable leaving group (choice A is correct). Reaction with a chiral carboxylate nucleophile will form an anhydride, which is less stable than the reactant carboxylic acid due to its high leaving group tendency (choice B is wrong). Reaction with answer choices C and D are ineffective: choice C is not a chiral molecule and choice D is non-nucleophilic; thus both are incorrect.

4. **C**   1-Propanol is a primary alcohol, so oxidation with anhydrous PCC would yield an aldehyde functional group in the molecule, as shown below.

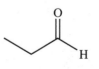

After placing this aldehyde in a deuteurated solvent, all alpha-hydrogens will be exchanged with deuterium, resulting in the molecule shown below.

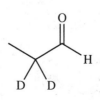

Deuterium atoms do not show up on ¹H-NMR spectroscopy. There will only be two signals, one from the aldehyde hydrogen and one from the terminal methyl group (choice C is correct).

5.   C   Reaction of the ketone starting material with a strong base (DO⁻) will result in the formation of two different enolates, as shown below:

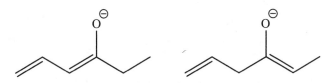

These enolates can then become deuterated at each of the alpha carbons, resulting in the following product.

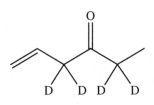

This deuterated compound can continue to react, reforming an enolate upon dedeuteration of the left alpha carbon. This enolate can then react as shown to deuterate the gamma carbon, as shown:

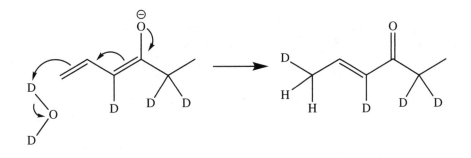

The gamma hydrogens can continue to be deprotonated as they are acidic due to resonance, leading to the formation of another enolate. This enolate can then be again deuterated at the gamma carbon, ultimately leading to the molecule shown below, which displays 6 deuterated sites (choice C is correct).

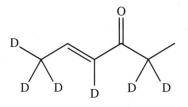

6. **C** Reacting this ketone with NaH will result in enolate formation, which then can undergo addition to the aldehyde reagent in step 2. Step 3 will result in protonation of the alkoxide product after step to form an alcohol, shown below:

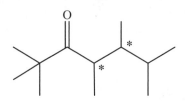

The atoms marked with asterisks are stereocenters so the absolute configuration of these carbons may be *R* or *S*. The presence of two stereocenters implies that the total number of possible stereoisomeric products is 4, as the number of possible stereoisomers is 2^n, where *n* = number of sterocenters (choice C is correct; choices A, B, and D are wrong).

7. **B** The answer choice option that reacts fastest with acetic acid will be the strongest base (note: this is an acid-base reaction). One factor that can increase an atom's basicity is the presence of electron-donating inductive groups, such as CH_3, resulting in an increased partial negative charge on the basic atom. Out of the answer choices, choice A has the most substitution, however, the nitrogen atom does not have a lone-pair, preventing it from deprotonating acetic acid (choice A is wrong). Comparing choices C and D, both have equal degrees of substitution, however, nitrogen is a more basic atom than phosphorus, as the electrons on phosphorus are more stable due to its larger relative size, decreasing its basicity (choice D can be eliminated). Between choices B and C, choice B has more substitution and therefore will be more basic.

8. **B** The stationary phase of in HPLC is nonpolar, thus the product that displays the longest elution time will be the most nonpolar. Reaction of the tertiary alcohol with any of the answer choices will result first in protonation of the alcohol, and then a subsequent S_N1 reaction, yielding the products shown below:

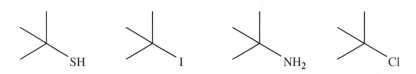

Out of these four options, the largest atom will be the most non-polar, as it has the greatest potential for hydrophobic forces such as London dispersion forces. The product with the largest atom is the one with iodine, which resulted from reaction with HI (choice B is correct).

9. **C** Placing a peptide in highly acidic conditions for a long period of time will result in complete hydrolysis of all peptide bonds. In addition to the peptide backbone being hydrolyzed, side chains with carboxylic acid derivatives will also be hydrolyzed. In the undecapeptide GNOWLLADNEK, N residues will be hydrolyzed into D residues via an addition-elimination mechanism (Item III is correct; choice B can be eliminated). Furthermore, the leaving group of the N residues will be an amine group which, under acidic conditions will become NH_4^+, increasing its concentration (Item I is true; choice A can be eliminated). E residues will not form unless Q residues were present in the peptide (Item II is false, choice C is correct, and choice D can be eliminated).

10. **D** This 2x2 question can be approached by first recalling that R_f value increases as the polarity of a molecule decreases. Thus, the molecule with the higher R_f will be the less polar choice (eliminate choices A and C because they are inconsistent with this notion). Between an amide and carboxylic acid, carboxylic acids are the less polar functional group (choice D is correct; choice B can be eliminated). This can be demonstrated by analyzing the resonance structures of each function group:

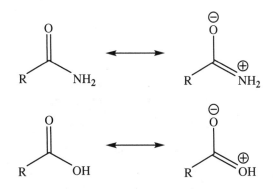

In the charged resonance structure for the amide, there is a positive charge on the nitrogen. Because nitrogen is more electropositive than oxygen, it can better stabilize the positive charge. Therefore, the charged amide resonance structure will contribute to a greater proportion of the resonance hybrid, making the amide overall more polar due to higher overall charge.

11. **D** The protease cleaves on the amino side of residues that most effectively bind to the R residues located in the active site. Because R residues are positively charged, negatively charged residues such as D or E will effectively bind. Since protease X cuts peptide Y on the amino side (to the left) of these D or E residues, any fragments with D or E had to have been inside the original sequence.

Peptide Y will have the following possible primary sequences, constructed from the three peptides:

1) RLLCDYKEAK

2) RLLCEAKDYK

Regardless of which of these possibilities is actually peptide Y, the N-terminus will be an R residue (choice D is correct).

SOLUTIONS TO PRACTICE PASSAGE 1

1. **B** Upon acylation, Figure 2 shows a primary amine (RNH_2) displacing a leaving group "X" from the portion of the attached acylating agent. Therefore, the acylating agent must bear a good leaving group in the "X" position. Eliminate choices A and C because they feature good leaving groups, as halide leaving groups (weak bases) are favored. Choice D is a resonance-stabilized tosylate group, which is also favored, and thus incorrect. The only choice that features a poor leaving group is choice B. A Bn group is a benzyl group ($-CH_2C_6H_5$), which means the –OBn leaving group in choice B is a strongly basic leaving group, making choice B the least suitable acylating agent.

2. **C** In the transformation of Compound 1 to Compound 2, the signals for both the C=O bond of the amide (Item II) and the N–H bond (Item I) disappear. No other relevant signals will appear, therefore Item I and II only, or choice C, is the correct answer.

3. **D** When Compound 3 is treated with acid, the acid will protonate the most basic nitrogen. sp^3-Hybridized lone pairs are more basic than sp^2-hybridized lone pairs (eliminate choice B). This is due to the electrons in an sp^3 orbital being less tightly held than in an sp^2 orbital due to the more elongated shape of the sp^3 orbital. As the lone pairs on N_1 are capable of delocalization, they are actually sp^2-hybridized, not sp^3 (eliminate choice A). As shown in the illustration below, when N_1 is protonated, the positive charge is NOT stabilized, however, the positive charge IS stabilized when N_2 is protonated. Thus, N_2 will get protonated when Compound 3 is treated with acid because the resulting positive charge is more stable.

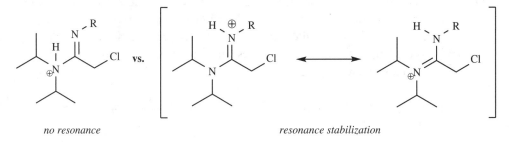

no resonance   *resonance stabilization*

4. **C** There will be three distinct doublets in the ^{1}H-NMR spectrum of Compound 3. Note: because of the *cis-trans* nature of amides, the methyl groups on the diisopropyl amine have distinct chemical environments, and will have distinct NMR shifts.

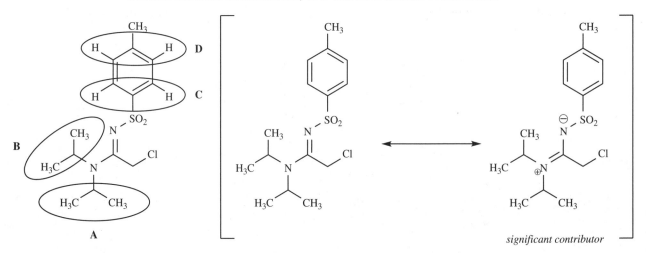

significant contributor

SOLUTIONS TO PRACTICE PASSAGE 2

1. A   As stated in the passage, irreversible inhibitors covalently bind to the enzyme disrupting its activity. Since the active site of this particular enzyme contains a nucleophilic serine residue, the best inhibitor will be the most electrophilic choice. Choice A is the correct answer due to the highly electronegative fluorine atom inducing a strong partial positive charge on the P atom. As shown below, when serine's nucleophilic hydroxyl attacks the electrophilic P atom on the inhibitor, a tetrahedral intermediate is generated. This intermediate will react in a similar fashion as in an addition-elimination reaction, thus it will reform the P=O bond while eliminating the fluoride leaving group. The other answer choices all feature inferior leaving groups, thus choice A will be the strongest irreversible inhibitor.

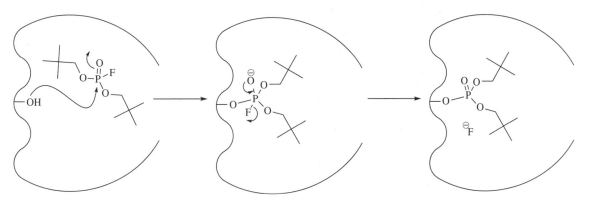

2. B   As specified in the passage, a transition state inhibitor possesses a chemical structure that mimics the transition state of a substrate. The transition state of the substrate for methylthioadenosine nucleosidase, namely methylthioadenosine, is given in Figure 1 of the passage. In Figure 1, and as shown below, a partial positive charge exists on the carbon atom of the five-membered ring possessing partial double bond character. When deadenylation breaks adenine away from this structure, a resonance contributor reveals a formal positive charge on this carbon.

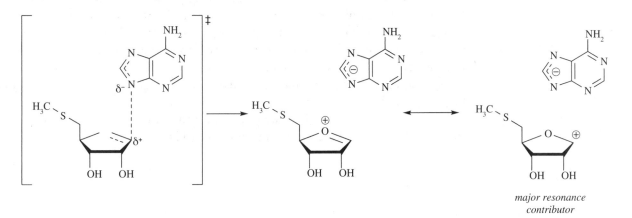

major resonance contributor

Therefore, choice B is the correct answer because this analog best resembles the transition state of methylthioadenosine by positioning a positive charge on the very same atom of its five-membered ring.

3. **D** Irreversible inhibitors form covalent bonds with a nucleophile within the active site of the enzyme. Choices A, B, and C are very electrophilic in that they possess a site with strong partial positive charge because of resonance (choices A and C) or they make very reactive intermediates (choice B). Choice D is the correct answer as it lacks a significantly electrophilic site on the molecules, thus choice D is likely to be a reversible inhibitor.

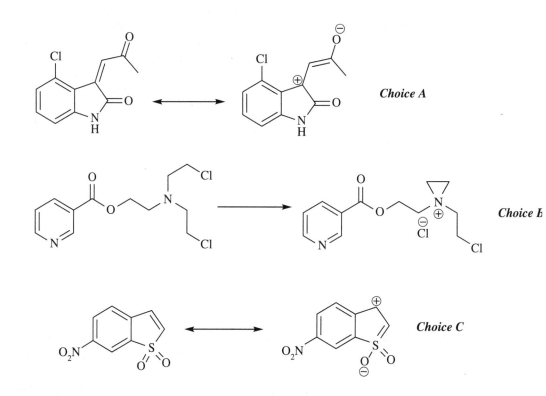

Choice A

Choice B

Choice C

4. **C** As given in the passage, chloromethyl ketones (transition state inhibitors) undergo nucleophilic addition with serine. In this reaction, the nucleophilic –OH in the serine side chain attacks the C=O of the chloromethyl ketone. An addition reaction to a ketone results in the C=O bond breaking, which is not observed in Item III as its C=O bond is still intact (Item III is incorrect; eliminate choice D). Note that Item III would result if serine performed an S_N2 substitution on the α-carbon bearing the Cl of the chloromethyl ketone. Item I presents a tetrahedral addition intermediate, showing the serine side chain correctly linking serine to the inhibitor (Item I is correct). The oxyanion shown in Item 1 may next attack the neighboring carbon in an intramolecular manner to give an epoxide, as indicated by the passage (Item II is correct). Recall that epoxides are highly strained and, when formed, are highly reactive, which will attract histidine for the alkylation mentioned in the passage. Thus, both Item I and II are correct, making choice C correct.

SOLUTIONS TO PRACTICE PASSAGE 3

1. **B** It is apparent that large, bulky R groups favor the S_N2' pathway. Thus, choices A and D can be eliminated as they are smaller than the other two choices. A *t*-butyl group is larger near the carbon where chemistry is happening than in the cyclohexyl group, and because the ring structure prohibits rotation it is in fact less sterically bulky than the *i*-propyl group at the carbon of interest. Choice B is the best option because it represents the largest steric bulk.

2. **D** Organometallic compounds, such as lithiated compounds or Grignard reagents, are very good nucleophiles. The use of *t*-butyllithium prevents nucleophilic chemistry thanks to the bulk of the *t*-butyl group around the anionic carbon. *n*-Butyllithium is just about as strong a base as *t*-butyllithium, so choice A can be eliminated. For this same reason, choice C can be eliminated; if deprotonation of the epoxide is an issue with *n*-butyllithium, it would have been a problem with *t*-butyllithium. Two anions cannot undergo dimerization reactions, so choice B can be eliminated.

3. **B** Silicon has a larger radius than does carbon. Thus, groups bound to the silicon atom will be, on average, at a greater distance to the anionic carbon than groups bound to a carbon. The silicon atom provides a "spacer" of sorts, between the carbon of interest and the steric bulk. Choice A is incorrect because it is the bulk of the nucleophile that plays the deciding role, and one silicon bearing reagent in the table is shown to go through only the S_N2' pathway. Choice C is incorrect because hydrogen is more electronegative than silicon, and as such all H atoms bound to silicon are hydritic, not acidic. Choice D is incorrect because, as the passage indicates, steric bulk near the carbanion favors S_N2'.

4. **C** Carbanions are better nucleophiles than oxyanions, so as long as the fast step is deprotonation of the dithiane, the only substitution present should be attack of the lithiated dithiane on the epoxide. If the attack by the lithiated dithiane is faster than the deprotonation of the dithiane, one might expect a buildup of oxyanion in solution (prior to the acidification step). You know that oxyanions *can* and *do* attack epoxides (choice A is incorrect), so any buildup of oxyanion in the absence of the better carbanion nucleophile would surely produce ethers. Choice D is incorrect due to the fact that if ethers were unstable to *t*-butyllithium the reaction could not be run in THF, nor could the ether-like epoxide ring survive.

5. **A** The 1,4-Brook rearrangement can only take place when the organosilicon group is three carbons away from the hydroxyl. This necessitates the S_N2 mechanism, which means that you seek the smallest of the four choices. The smallest is choice A.

SOLUTIONS TO PRACTICE PASSAGE 4

1. **B**   Within the mechanism of a native chemical ligation, a sulfur atom acts as a nucleophile and attacks an activated thioester to generate another thioester. Then an adjacent amine does a nucleophilic addition-elimination reaction to give the newly formed peptide. Selenium (choice B) would give an analogous mechanism since it is both a good nucleophile (eliminate choice D) and a good leaving group (eliminate choices A and C) which is necessary for the mechanism. Note that selenium belongs to the same family as oxygen and sulfur, thus it shares chemistry with these elements but its large size improves its nucleophilicity and leaving group ability.

2. **C**   The reaction in Figure 1 in an example of a nucleophilic addition-elimination reaction where the amino group from the growing peptide attacks the carbonyl of the tRNA activated ester, and the oxygen on the ribose sugar is the leaving group. In the reaction, the acyl function group on tRNA is transferred onto the amino group, thus the addition of the amino acid onto the growing peptide is an example of a nucleophilic addition-elimination AND acyl transfer.

3. **D**   As noted in the passage, thiols are capable of reacting with carbon electrophiles. Answer choices A, B, and C will generate a similar intermediate, a positively charged sulfonium ion.

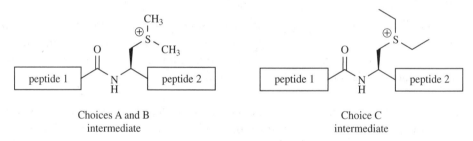

Choices A and B   Choice C
intermediate   intermediate

This sulfonium ion can undergo substitution with a water molecule when heated to generate an alcohol because it is a favorable leaving group. Choice D is different from the other reagents as the electrophilic carbon is an *acylating* reagent, not an alkylating reagent. The intermediate from choice D is:

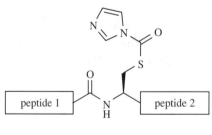

Choice D

The sulfur in this situation is a poorer leaving group relative to a sulfonium ion and in the presence of water will instead undergo an addition-elimination, as shown below, to generate an acid.

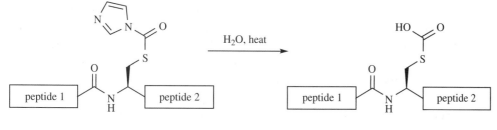

Choice D

Therefore, choice D is the correct answer.

4. **A** The passage states that the cysteine thioester can be formed *in situ* between a thioacid and an electrophile on the N-terminal peptide. Thus, the likelihood of making the thioester is based on the reactivity of the electrophile on the N-terminal peptide and its ability to release a good leaving group. Choices B and D are great electrophiles and they both have good leaving groups (eliminate choices B and D). Choices A and C are poor electrophiles, but choice A is the worst because the leaving group would be a negatively charged nitrogen. Therefore, choice A is the correct answer.

SOLUTIONS TO PRACTICE PASSAGE 5

1. **A** There are no aromatic protons on either of the compounds, so any choice indicating peaks between 6 and 7 ppm can be safely excluded (eliminate choices B and C). Choice D refers to the hydroxyl protons, on account of their relative deshielding; however, there is no reason to think that the hydroxyl protons should be exceptionally different for these two compounds, as they are in very similar environments, and there is no chemical equivalence. Choice A, indicating the existence of one methyl singlet peak in a slightly more deshielded environment than the others, is logical because compound **B** has an allylic methyl group (methyl adjacent to a double bond), which would give a three-proton singlet between 2 and 3 ppm. None of the methyl singlets in compound **C** are expected to exceed 2 ppm.

2. **C** The general formula of the molecule after quenching with regular water is shown below:

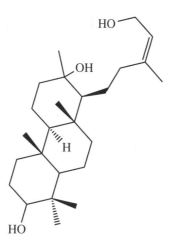

The passage states that these compounds, prior to post-cyclization modification, contain 25 carbon atoms. The three oxygen atoms are clear, so one must then count the hydrogen atoms. Doing so, one arrives at 44 hydrogens. Therefore, if quenched in normal water, the formula $C_{25}H_{44}O_3$ equates to $(25 \times 12) + 44 + (16 \times 3) = 392$ g/mol. This is the value given in choice A, which can be eliminated.

After quenching with $D_2{}^{18}O$, the compound will appear as follows:

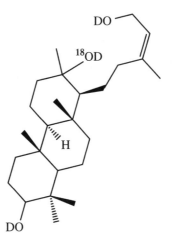

The hydrogen at the bottom of the molecule is quenched by heavy water, making it D instead of H (note: D is 1 g/mol heavier than H). The new hydroxyl is composed of ^{18}OD, as this comes from the heavy water as well (note: ^{18}O is 2 g/mol heavier than normal ^{16}O). The final D, at the top of the molecule, comes from H/D exchange, which happens readily to acidic protons, such as those in hydroxyl groups, in the presence of deuterated (protic) solvents for extended periods of time. The mass as drawn above is $392 + 5 = 397$ g/mol. Choice B neglects the final H/D exchange, and choice D assumes the swap of ^{18}O for all the oxygen atoms on the compound.

3. **D**   If compound *A*, as drawn, is to have *R* stereochemistry at position 3, it must be as such:

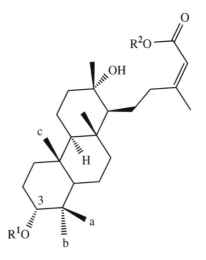

If the OR substituent on **C**-3 is in an axial (into-plane) orientation, then the methyl group a must be axial (out-of-plane) and c must likewise be axial (out-of-plane). The passage indicates that each of these rings is in a chair conformation, and in the chair conformation, the axial position on the ring alternates sides of the molecule. Methyl group b, being into the page immediately next to an axial group into the page, must be equatorial.

4. **A**   Choice B can be eliminated as this structure represents a process with more than the seven methide/hydride shifts required for the formation of **C**. Choice D may be eliminated as the initial hydride transfer in Figure 2b from the intermediate must take place on the same side of the molecule (an into-plane H is transferred to an out-of-plane H in choice D, which is incorrect). Choice C indicates a change in stereochemistry at a position that should not be affected if the carbocation migration is halted at the double bond. Choice A is a product wherein the reaction is halted prior to the end of the reaction in the passage, and all of the methide/hydride shifts that happen are carried out on their own respective sides of the molecule, as indicated in the cascade in Figure 2b and in the passage text.

5. **B**   Choice A is incorrect because compact polycyclic molecules have far fewer rotational degrees of freedom than linear compounds of the same formulae, meaning that they're more ordered and lower in entropy. Choice C can be ruled out as enzymes generally perform in a catalytic fashion—which explains rate enhancement—but is not a factor in the overall driving force of the reaction. Choice D may be excluded as the products and reactants will not have wildly different solubilities, as they contain the same number of electronegative hydrogen bonders and are overall significantly nonpolar. Choice B is correct as it includes both the opening of the strained epoxide ring, and the fact that σ-bonds (invariably stronger) are formed at the expense of π-bonds (invariably weaker). This means that the enthalpy change in cyclization is negative (in a spontaneous direction), driving the reaction forward despite the unfavorable entropic changes.

SOLUTIONS TO PRACTICE PASSAGE 6

1. **D**   Items I and II are very similar. The only difference is that in Item I the amino acid is bonded to the linker prior to being attached to the solid support. Both accurately represent the preparation of a resin as there is a linker between the template amino acid and the resin in addition the amino acid is available for peptide synthesis. The linker in Item I and II is a non-integral linker. The linker in Item III is an integral linker. In this case, the linker is not indicated because, as the passage states, the linker can be a part of the polymer support. Therefore, Item III is also an accurate representation on the preparation of a resin for solid-phase synthesis, making choice D the correct answer.

2. **D**   The passage states that an activated amino acid is an electrophile. Therefore, the most nucleophilic linker will be the correct answer. Choices A and C can be eliminated as they are electrophilic linkers. Choice D has the more nucleophilic functional group, an amine, thus is the correct answer.

MCAT ELITE: ADVANCED STRATEGIES FOR YOUR
HIGHEST SCORE

3. C   Cbz is a nitrogen protecting group that is commonly used in solid-support peptide synthesis. 10% Hydrobromic acid in acetic acid is a reagent that is used to remove the Cbz protecting group and reveal the desired nitrogen as the HBr-ammonium salt. Choice B can immediately be eliminated as that is the desired product. The mechanism for the reaction is outlined below:

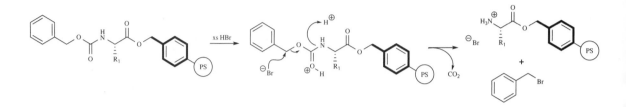

Bromide is the most nucleophilic atom in the reaction as it is negative. Choice A can be eliminated (it would be the product if acetic acid was the nucleophile) along with Choice D (it would be the product if water was the nucleophile).

4. B   The amino acid derivative that is least likely to undergo the coupling is the amino acid derivative that has the worst leaving group. Choice A can be eliminated as the leaving group would go from positive to neutral in charge, thus making it a good leaving group. Choice C and be eliminated as the leaving group would be a bicarbonate anion, which is resonance stabilized and very favorable as it would further decarboxylate to generate carbon dioxide. Choices B and D are similar in that they both have oxygens that would be negative upon leaving. However, the oxygen in choice D is resonance stabilized and forms a very stable functional group upon leaving (an urea). Therefore, choice B is the correct answer.

Chapter 20
Physics on the MCAT

Of all the sciences on the MCAT, Physics relies the least on information recall and the most on problem-solving and reading comprehension skills. This is in part because the subject matter lends itself to these kinds of problems. Perhaps more importantly, though, the subject content in Physics pertains less to the material you will ultimately study in medical school, whereas the critical thinking that Physics demands fits with what you will encounter (particularly during your clinical years). In many ways, your ability to formulate an "approach" to a tough problem is one of the most useful skills you can develop along the path to medicine.

The science sections of the MCAT have 10 passages and 15 freestanding questions. Physics makes up about 25% of the questions in the Chemical and Physical Foundations of Biological Systems section (Chem/Phys). The remaining 75% of the questions are divided up as General Chemistry (30%), Organic Chemistry (15%), Biochemistry (25%), and Biology (5%) questions.

20.1   TACKLING A PASSAGE

Passage Types as They Apply to Physics

Information/Situation Presentation

These passages tend to fall into two types for Physics. The first type consists of straightforward descriptions of phenomena you should already understand well, such as a passage comparing the function of a nerve cell to a DC circuit with a battery, a capacitor, a couple of switches, and a few resistors in parallel combinations. Common question types include solving unknown variables using memorized formulas, true-or-false questions about physical laws, and comparisons of the "real" to the "ideal."

The second type of passage consists of technical elaborations of phenomena you know something about, such as a passage about an electrocardiogram circuit with resistors, a capacitor, and a number of operational amplifiers (circuit elements that multiply input voltage) that provides equations for the time-dependent voltage input from the body and output by the device. Such technical passages are often marked by several new equations, italicized terminology defined in context, and possibly graphs, followed by paragraphs defining the variables and constants. Common question solving techniques for technical passages include algebraic manipulation, functional dependence or proportionality, and graph generation or interpretation.

Experiment or Research Presentation

These passages often include data tables or graphs with axes clearly labeled with numerical values; if there's a table, the passage probably covers an experiment or multiple experiments. The subject matter in experimental passages is typically familiar, though the concepts might be extended somewhat beyond basic knowledge, for example, measuring the viscosity in a fluid or the resistance of a conducting wire as a function of temperature. These passages tend *not* to push your understanding of content as much as the technical passages or heavily conceptual passages. Rather, the implicit questions found in experiment presentation passages are usually of the form, "If another trial were conducted changing [some set of parameters], then the resulting value of [another parameter] would be...." Such questions require you to read numbers from the tables and determine their functional dependence on the altered parameters. In other words, you need to write down an equation for the value of the parameter, and to check whether the altered variables affect that value and how.

Persuasive (Scientific) Reasoning

Persuasive Reasoning passages on the Physics portion of the MCAT are largely conceptual. They describe some particular phenomenon about which you most likely have no prior knowledge, offering one or more theories as to its causes and effects, and they do so almost entirely with words (as opposed to using figures, equations, and numbers). Any passage mentioning competing theories that might explain the phenomenon in question exemplifies this type. These are generally the hardest passages for most people, as they rely heavily on reading comprehension as well as the ability to recall and synthesize physics concepts and equations from different topics (e.g., atomic structure, magnetism, and standing waves). You can expect questions in which both the question text and the answer choices are themselves entirely in words. This means you must be comfortable translating sentences into proportions, ratios, or equations, and then translating them back into sentences. Moreover, it may not be enough to be a careful reader with a good memory for formulas: Conceptual passages will test whether you know the conditions under which equations apply (such as the conditions for an ideal fluid or when to hold Q or V constant in $Q = CV$).

Reading a Physics Passage

Don't let our heading here deceive you; "reading" in the sense we commonly use the word is seldom the best way to use physics passages effectively. A kind of "informed skimming" is usually the best strategy. A quick holistic scan of the passage, including reading its first sentence, should be enough to tell you its topic and type. This will help you to decide whether to do it now or to postpone it until you've tackled easier passages (for example, if you dislike circuits, or if a lot of reading comprehension slows you down, by all means leave those passages until later!). Once you decide to do a passage, use the following techniques to find what you need to know quickly.

1. Read the first sentence again carefully. It will probably define the main idea of the passage and might inform your answer to one of the questions directly. Similarly, if the passage describes a set of experimental procedures, read the first sentences in each subsection so that you understand precisely what is being done and why.

2. Look for the familiar Physics terms within the passage and highlight them. Remember that the questions on the MCAT can come directly from anything mentioned by the AAMC topics list, or they can come from a reading-comprehension topic in a passage. And in fact, many Physics passages may not seem to be about a particular Physics topic at first glance. For example, a passage about ultrasound scans may be about waves, or sound, or fluid dynamics, or all of those topics at the same time! If you can identify the relevant physics within the passage text, you can focus in on that text and topic rather than getting stuck on the paragraph about, say, the historical perspective of how we measure heart rate.

3. Look for any new terms. These are often italicized but not always, so scan for long unfamiliar phrases (phrases like "aeroelastic flutter" stick out in a paragraph even in plain type). Highlight them along with their definitions.

4. Find the equations and figures. The text immediately before or after them tends to define terms or provide numerical values (measurements in a diagram or values of constants in an equation). If the diagrams are basically complete or the equations make sense to you, *skip this text*: There's no good reason to read a paragraph describing the circuit diagram for a defibrillator if the picture already tells the whole story.

5. Look for numbers. These are sometimes worth highlighting or jotting down on your scratch paper and they are easy to find (however, if a passage gives you a whole pile of values, they're already easy to find so it's not important to highlight them). There are a couple of key things to remember about numbers:

    a. Numbers on the MCAT are always accompanied by their units, either immediately following the number, or in the heading of the table where the numbers appear. If there are no units, the number must be unitless.

    b. Highlighting can be done with a left-click and drag, then clicking the highlighting icon, but keep in mind that numbers in figures may not be in a format that allows for highlighting. In these cases, use scratch paper to note numbers.

6. Finally, for lengthy Persuasive (Scientific) Reasoning passages, you may need to spend time fruitfully highlighting the many new terms or names of theories in the text and dealing with complicated figures by redrawing a simplified version. The fact that this will take longer is a legitimate reason to leave conceptual passages for last, but don't make the common errors of thinking you have to understand everything you read or highlighting everything that "seems important" (or you'll end up highlighting everything)! This is a multiple-choice test, not an essay exam: You often don't need to understand this sort of question to be able to eliminate all but one answer choice.

Mapping a Physics Passage

Physics work should be done on paper; there are few answers on the test that can be found without writing something down. Thus, your scratch paper is your primary tool, whether solving FSQs or mapping a passage. As suggested above, there are a few specific reasons to use the highlighting tool, but apart from that you want to rely on your scratch paper. "Mapping" involves jotting down a schematic of the passage that will help you to answer the questions efficiently without having to fish for information. Here are some mapping strategies:

1. Label your scratch paper with the passage number and question numbers. Staying organized saves time and avoids errors.

2. Write down any given equations with space below to work on them. The chances that you will *not* end up using some equation given to you in a passage are low, so it's worth the time to prepare for the algebra and estimation the questions will require. Moreover, merely copying the equations helps you to understand them better than you would just looking at them.

3. If there are any simple diagrams, copy them down and label any values (some will be given in the text around the diagram and not labeled directly in the version on your screen). Again, you might resist this as a potential waste of time, but it is important to be able to manipulate the figures to answer the questions. For example, in a passage where forces are important (e.g., for most of mechanics, buoyancy in fluids, charges interacting with electric or magnetic fields, or simple harmonic oscillators), you should put the forces on your diagram *before* you do the questions. By doing so, you will probably anticipate the answers to one or more questions even before they are asked. Overall, this should both save you time and increase your percentage of right answers.

4. If the passage is conceptual or has conceptual parts to it, translate any mathematical statements written as sentences into symbols and treat those as you would equations given in a more technical passage. For example, if you were reading a passage on Poiseuille's Law applied to blood flow and came across the sentence, "Poiseuille's Law shows that the flow rate of a viscous fluid through a pipe with circular cross section is inversely proportional to the fourth power of its radius," you would jot down $f \propto 1/r^4$.

5. Especially for passages that don't include many diagrams or equations, write down the equations and basic ideas you recall about the passage topic. This will give you something tangible with which to tackle the questions. For example, a passage might describe how a cell membrane acts as a capacitor in some instances, and you might write down $Q = CV$ and "no battery present, Q is constant."

Practice all of these strategies with the passages in this book to see which work best for you; then make those strategies a part of your standard repertoire. Give yourself about 90 seconds to map a passage before you look at the questions. Many passage maps will take less time than this, a few might take longer. Don't worry that you're spending time not answering questions; practice will make you more efficient.

Another, more advanced study technique you might use once you feel more comfortable about your passage mapping is to map a couple of passages, including jotting down on paper any text you highlight. Put those maps aside for an hour or so while you do something else (practice FSQs), then go back to the passages, cover up their text, and try to do the questions with just your map. You shouldn't necessarily be able to answer all of the questions without referring to the passage, but if you find that you're unable to answer any but those that rely on memory of basic concepts, then you need to improve your mapping technique. Below is an example of these strategies applied to a passage.

Blood flow through the vascular system of the human body is controlled by several factors. The rate of flow, Q, is directly proportional to the pressure differential, ΔP, between any two points in the system and inversely proportional to the resistance, R, of the system:

$$Q = \Delta P / R$$

Equation 1

The resistance, R, is dependent on the length of the vessel, L, the viscosity of blood, η, and the vessel's radius, r according to the equation

$$R = \frac{8\eta L}{\pi r^4}$$

Equation 2

Under normal conditions, vessel length and blood viscosity do not vary significantly. However, certain conditions can cause changes in blood content, thereby altering viscosity. Veins are generally more compliant than arteries due to their less muscular nature. The flow of blood through the major arteries can be approximated by the equations of ideal flow.

The dynamics of fluid movement from capillaries to body tissue and back to capillaries is also driven by pressure differentials. The net filtration pressure is the difference between the hydrostatic pressure of the blood in the capillaries, P_c, and the hydrostatic pressure of tissue fluid outside the capillaries, P_i.

The oncotic pressure is the difference between the osmotic pressure of the capillaries, P_c (approximately 25 torr), and the osmotic pressure of the tissue fluids, P_i (negligible). Whether fluid moves into or out of the capillary network depends on the magnitudes of the net filtration and oncotic pressures. The direction of fluid movement can be determined by calculating the following pressure differential:

$$\Delta P = (P_c + \Pi_i) - (P_i + \Pi_c)$$

Equation 3

The sum in the first set of parentheses gives the pressure acting to move fluid out of the capillaries, while the sum in the second set of parentheses gives the pressure acting to move fluid into the capillaries.

Capillaries are porous, and the blood pressure on the arterial end of a capillary bed is enough to push fluid out of the capillaries and into the surrounding tissues. However, blood proteins and cells are too big to fit through the pores. Consequently, as the blood travels across the capillary bed, it becomes relatively more concentrated in proteins and cells; this leads to an osmotic influx of fluid on the venous side of the capillary bed. Note, however, that the volume of fluid lost to the tissues due to pressure is greater than the volume of fluid returned to the blood due to osmosis, so there is a net outward flow of fluid to the tissues. This excess fluid is recaptured and returned to the cardiovascular system via the lymphatic vessels.

Sample Passage Analysis and Mapping

Highlight the key phrase, "blood flow." Note that this passage is heavily laden with equations (three), has several potentially unfamiliar terms, and has no tabular data. This is best characterized as a technical Information Presentation passage, not as obscure as some if you understand the underlying Biology and Physics, but still challenging.

The overall lack of numbers is obvious, so just highlight the 25 torr for the osmotic pressure of the capillaries and be done with it. Some people might be more comfortable drawing a simple figure of blood moving from capillaries to tissues to capillaries and including pressures there, but that's up to you: This isn't a case in which a force diagram or simplified circuit will shed tremendous light on the phenomenon.

A few possibly unfamiliar terms like "net filtration pressure" and "oncotic pressure" appear and should be highlighted with their definitions. The definitions of some given variables are worth highlighting both because the symbols can be confusing (Q for flow rate, R for flow resistance) and in case you encounter a question that uses the words without the algebraic symbols. You should copy the three given equations on your scratch paper, noting mentally the difference between this flow rate equation and the one you know from memory ($f = Av$). Remember, a new equation in a passage is always more important than a memorized equation for any questions that deal explicitly with the phenomenon described in the passage. At this point it may also be worthwhile to write down the continuity equation ($A_1 v_1 = A_2 v_2$). You should have committed to memory the rules for ideal fluid flow (including negligible viscosity) and know therefore that Bernoulli's equation would not apply except to the case of "major arteries."

The third paragraph presents perhaps the greatest mapping challenge for this passage. You might be tempted to highlight the entire paragraph because it describes an unfamiliar phenomenon. However, highlighting is not the same as comprehension; further, none of the terminology here is specialized. Thus, it's better to skip highlighting the paragraph entirely or to follow the rule to highlight causal phrases (as shown). It's worth noting that the passage doesn't actually mention what "certain conditions" are, so this paragraph lacks the information necessary to answer Explicit questions.

Your scratch paper map should thus look something like this:

$$Q = \Delta P/R \qquad\qquad R = \frac{8\eta L}{\pi r^4} \qquad\qquad \Delta P = (P_c + \Pi_i) - (P_i + \Pi_c)$$

$$\Pi_c = 25 \text{ torr}, \Pi_i = 0.$$

20.2 PHYSICS QUESTION TYPES

As stated previously, the questions in this section of the MCAT fall into one of three main categories:

1. **Memory questions**: Answered from concepts and equations you know walking into the test with just brute facts from the questions or passage, such as numbers or vector directions.
2. **Explicit questions**: Answered from information stated explicitly in the passage. To answer them correctly may require finding a definition, reading a graph, or manipulating a given equation.
3. **Implicit questions**: Answered by applying outside knowledge to a new situation or making more complex connections than you know by rote. Often the answer is implied by the information in the passage but requires logical reasoning on your part.

Note that the way you categorize questions on the MCAT will depend on how much knowledge you bring to the test in the first place. The more confident you are about the basic material outlined in the list of Physics topics, the less you will have to rely on the passage and question text to answer questions. This will ultimately save you those few precious seconds that can be better used for answering the tougher questions. For example, a passage may explicitly state the formula for the relationship of potential difference to the electric field and physical parameters of a parallel plate capacitor (i.e., $V = Ed$), but if you already know this formula, you will not need your map of the passage to find it when you need it to answer a question. That changes the type of question for you from Explicit to Memory.

Physics Memory Questions

These questions are often the easiest to answer. They follow a format that is more familiar for most students; typical Physics course work requires the memorization of formulas and facts, as well as their applications. Since Memory questions rely minimally if at all on information from the passage, they are similar to the freestanding questions on the MCAT.

Consider a question about the flow speed of blood in the major arteries taken from the previous blood flow passage. The following is an example of a Memory question.

> The cross sectional area of the aorta is approximately
> 4 cm^2 and the total cross sectional area of the major
> arteries is 20 cm^2. If the speed of the blood in the aorta is
> 30 cm/sec, what is the average blood speed in the major
> arteries?
>
> A) 5 cm/sec
> B) 6 cm/sec
> C) 120 cm/sec
> D) 150 cm/sec

The equation to solve this question ($A_1 v_1 = A_2 v_2$) is not included in the passage.

Physics Explicit Questions

You need information directly from the passage in order to answer Explicit questions. It is critical to have a solid passage map so that information from the passage is easy to find and use. Even when you have inherent knowledge about the topic, it is important to read for information more specific to the precise situation in question.

Here's an example of an Explicit question from the blood flow passage:

> Blood flow to the various systems in the body is
> regulated by the dilation and constriction of the blood
> vessels. After a person has eaten a large meal, the blood
> vessels supplying the digestive system dilate, increasing
> their radii by 50%. As a result of this blood vessel
> dilation, the flow of blood to the digestive system will:
>
> A) increase to 500% of the original flow.
> B) increase to 225% of the original flow.
> C) increase to 150% of the original flow.
> D) decrease to 50% of the original flow.

The equation needed to answer this question is given in the passage (Equation 2) and should be one that you recorded in your map. Note that you will always have to include information from the passage for an Explicit question.

Sometimes Explicit questions require more basic facts or principles from memory. In order to get the correct answer, you need to merge information from the passage with information you already know. For example, the passage gives an equation for a familiar variable in a new situation, and that must be blended with an understanding of the significance of that variable generally, or of other equations featuring that variable. These questions can appear straightforward but may be deceptively difficult, and it would certainly be justifiable to think of them as Implicit questions in some cases (the lines between the types are sometimes blurry).

The following is an example of an Explicit question using the blend of passage information and a bit of knowledge from memory:

> At the venular end of skeletal muscle capillaries, the hydrostatic pressure of the capillary is 17 torr and the hydrostatic pressure of the surrounding tissue is 1 torr. Fluid movement is from:
>
> A) the capillary to the tissue, at a rate proportional to 7 torr.
> B) the tissue to the capillary, at a rate proportional to 7 torr.
> C) the capillary to the tissue, at a rate proportional to 9 torr.
> D) the tissue to the capillary, at a rate proportional to 9 torr.

This asks about the pressure differential and the direction of fluid flow. This requires remembering that fluids move from high to low pressure (or correctly interpreting the final paragraph), but it also requires using Equation 3 from the passage and the given values of osmotic pressures to solve for the numerical rate.

Physics Implicit Questions

This is generally the most difficult question type. Implicit questions often require information from memory, combined with information from the passage, and all applied to a new situation. They rely most heavily on critical reasoning skills, but also require a solid map, since information from the passage is usually needed. Most often, the answer choices for these questions contain a lot of words, but they can also sometimes be algebraic expressions or graphs. Note also that for many of these questions, you might be able to devise sound explanations that are not among the answer choices. However, there is always only *one* answer choice that *best* answers the question of all the options.

On Information and/or Situation passages, Implicit questions are often of the form "Which of the following best describes how [a parameter not mentioned in the passage] would change the [real world parameter described in the passage] from its present value?" The answers are verbal descriptions of increasing and decreasing values. Consider this example from the blood flow passage:

> Adaptation to life at high altitudes is characterized by polycythemia (high red blood cell count). Excluding other physiological compensations, what is the effect of this change on the flow of blood?
>
> A) Flow is decreased because viscosity is decreased.
> B) Flow is increased because viscosity is decreased.
> C) Flow is decreased because viscosity is increased.
> D) Flow is increased because viscosity is increased.

The correct answer would be selected by using background knowledge about viscosity and applying it to Equation 2, which describes the flow rate.

On Experiment/Research passages, Implicit questions are often of the form "Which of the following changes to the experiment would result in a change to [an experimental parameter]?" and are followed by verbal descriptions of changes to the apparatus, process, or mechanism of the experiment described in the passage. Suppose the following paragraph were added to the end of the Experiment/Research Presentation Passage example in Section 10.2.

> Confocal fluorescent microscopy relies on a light source of frequency tuned to the absorption frequencies of fluorescing compounds in the sample, focused through a pinhole using a converging mirror. This light illuminates the sample at specific focal planes, which are determined by a lens that focuses light both at the sample and eyepiece. Filters remove wavelengths other than those emitted by the fluorophores, and a semi-reflective mirror diverts the light to a pinhole, which is used in order to eliminate out-of-focus light from the image detector.

The following then is an example of an Implicit question in which the change to the apparatus is described in the answer choices:

> Which of the following changes if made without any additional changes would be LEAST LIKELY to affect the observed results of the experiments described in the passage?
>
> A) Using a fluorescing compound with a different wavelength dependence
> B) Changing the index of refraction of the lens without changing its curvature or position
> C) Decreasing the frequency of the light source from blue to yellow
> D) Rotating the sample 180°

This question requires recall of the principles of optics and properties of fluorescence, as well as some understanding of the apparatus described in the passage addendum.

Another common form of Implicit question in an Experiment or Research Presentation passage requires you to analyze the experimental apparatus depicted and described in the passage. Take for example a passage about the famous photoelectric experiment (see figure).

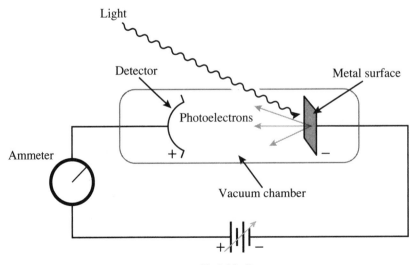

When you first see a figure like this, you should prepare yourself to answer three questions:

1. What is under the experimenter's direct control and what is a function of the phenomenon that is being observed? Another way of asking this question is to say "which variables are independent and which are dependent?"
2. Which inputs or outputs can be set arbitrarily within a range and which can have only set values, such as an input that requires putting the apparatus together differently or an observed value that is either on or off? Another way of asking this question is to say "which variables are continuous and which are discrete?"
3. Which outputs are directly observable and which are inferred or calculated?

In this particular example, the experiment involves a variable battery, in which the voltage can be changed with a dial and the polarity can be switched; a metal target plate connected to the battery and placed within an evacuated chamber for light to be shined upon it; a tunable laser light source; a detector plate connected to the opposite pole of the variable battery from the target plate, also placed within the evacuated chamber separated from the target plate; and an ammeter connected in series with the variable battery. The purpose of the experiment is to detect and determine the properties of the photoelectrons that scientists predict will be ejected from the metal target plate when light is shined on it. What can you deduce from the figure and the accompanying description?

First, it stands to reason that the variable battery and tunable laser are under the experimenter's control (that their values—voltage, intensity, and frequency—are independent variables) and that the metal target plate can be swapped out for another of a different metal. The most obvious dependent variable is the current measured by the ammeter: The purpose of any meter is to read a particular value passively, not to alter that value (you don't use an ammeter to control current).

Second, the use of the words "variable," "dial," and "tunable" suggest that the voltage of the battery and the intensity and frequency of the laser vary continuously. Thus, it makes sense also (drawing on your outside knowledge of circuits, such as $V = IR$) that current varies continuously. On the other hand, whatever property intrinsic to the metal plate that affects the experimental outcome would be discrete, depending upon swapping one plate for another (you can't "tune" between iron and zinc!).

Third, the settings on the variable battery and tunable laser can be directly observed, as can the reading on the ammeter. If the manufacturer or some reference has provided the value of the work function of the metal plate (the relevant intrinsic property to this experiment), then obviously it is a known constant in the experiment, but if the purpose of the experiment is to determine that value, then it must be calculated as a function of the directly observable values. Likewise, if the purpose of the experiment is to determine the conditions under which photoelectrons are ejected from the plate and what energies they have when leaving it, these values also must be inferred or calculated from the observed values: The scientist cannot directly see the electrons or measure their kinetic energies, for example.

The following is an Implicit question that could come in related to passage about the photoelectric effect.

Suppose you want to use the photoelectric experiment apparatus to determine the work function of an unknown metal. Which settings would you want to change and which output would you want to measure?

A) Vary light intensity and battery voltage, measure current
B) Vary light frequency and battery voltage, measure current
C) Vary light intensity and current, measure voltage
D) Vary light frequency and current, measure voltage

This question requires your quick ability to answer at least parts of the three questions previously detailed based upon some outside knowledge about the basic physics of circuits and light applied to the experimental apparatus described in the passage.

On Persuasive or Scientific Reasoning passages, Implicit questions are often of the form "Which of the following phenomena best exemplifies or analogizes to the [physics concept]?" and are followed by verbal descriptions of Physics phenomena. Often, selecting the right answer requires a combination of eliminating wrong answers by logical reasoning (or common sense) and revisiting the passage for the precise definition of the principle in question. Consider the blood flow passage: It's really more of a technical Information Presentation passage than a Persuasive or Scientific Reasoning passage, but this example suits either. An example of an Implicit question is

According to the following schematic diagram of systemic circulation, which of the following is true?

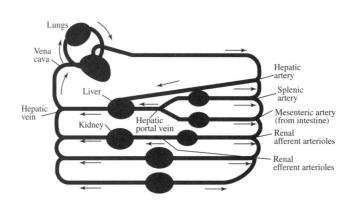

A) Vascular architecture of organs is in series so total peripheral resistance is greater than the resistance of individual organs.
B) Vascular architecture of organs is in parallel so total peripheral resistance is greater than the resistance of individual organs.
C) Vascular architecture of organs is in series so total peripheral resistance is less than the resistance of individual organs.
D) Vascular architecture of organs is in parallel so total peripheral resistance is less than the resistance of individual organs.

This question requires both understanding the analogy between resistance in blood flow and resistance in circuits and remembering the rules for adding resistors.

The Physics question types discussed so far categorize questions based on where to find the information for the answer. There is another way to categorize questions based on *how* you achieve the answer once you have the information.

Question Types by Technique

Algebraic Manipulation questions: These require use of one or several equation(s) to solve algebraically for a variable. Typically they have either numeric answer choices (e.g., "5 newtons") or algebraic equations for answer choices (i.e., "$F_c = F_G + F_N$"). Another twist on algebraic manipulation questions would be a question that asks for the units of an unfamiliar term (e.g., "What are the units for viscosity?") followed by answer choices with a variety of units of measure.

Approximation/Computation questions: Are there numerical answer choices? It's likely you need to do some computation/approximation with a given or memorized equation (though *not necessarily,* be on the lookout for numbers directly implied by the scenario, such as the work done by a magnetic field always being zero). Just remember when you start plugging in numbers to check for shortcuts. Do all the answer choices have the same coefficient multiplied by different powers of ten? Then focus on the powers of ten and assume the coefficient comes out as given! Is your calculation coming out at 100 − (something hard to estimate)? Then the answer is < 100 and all other choices can be eliminated.

Functional Dependence/Proportionality questions: These require the use of one or more equations, graphs, or data tables to calculate proportions and changes in variables or values. These can have numeric answer choices, algebraic answer choices (e.g., "$a_{car} = -2a_{truck}$"), or verbal answer choices (e.g., "The radius doubles," or "The range increases from launch angle of 0° to launch angle of 45°, then decreases from launch angle of 45° to launch angle of 90°.").

Graph Generation or Interpretation questions: These require use of one or more equations, proportions, other graphs, or data tables to create a graph of two variables; or they require you to locate points on a given curve, the slope of a curve, or the area under a curve.

Conceptual questions: Is the question a paragraph and are all of the answer choices sentences? Such questions often require you to narrow down your choices by eliminating choices that express nonphysical scenarios, like gravity having a horizontal component or a resistor dissipating more energy than was output by the only battery in its circuit.

20.3   SUMMARY OF THE APPROACH TO PHYSICS

As with all the science sections, when tackling the Chemical and Physical Foundations of Biological Systems section of the MCAT, it is best to do the easy questions first; typically, the freestanding questions are easier Memory questions, so when you get to them as you progress through the test the first time, do them all. As mentioned previously, the best strategy for tackling passages is probably to decide quickly whether each passage in sequence is a "Do Now" or a "Do Later." Skip the "Do Later" ones, note on your scratch paper the question numbers corresponding to that passage so you can be sure to come back to it, then come back to them once you've gotten to the end of the section. Within each passage, again, save especially difficult questions until last, and make sure to fill in answers for ALL the questions before moving to the next passage. If you find a question or two especially difficult, make your best guess and be sure to click the "Mark" button so that you can review the question later.

Since you will be skipping some questions within the test, it is important to keep your scratch paper organized. Clearly indicate the passage and question number beside the work that you do for that question. If you think you've made an error in calculation, do not waste time erasing, just draw a line through your work and start again.

Process of Elimination

Process of Elimination (POE) is paramount! Use the strikeout tool to indicate answer choices you have eliminated. Aggressively use POE to improve your chances of guessing a correct answer even if you are not able to narrow it down to one choice. Remember each of the following POE strategies:

1. Eliminate answer choices that are clearly false or that do not answer the question.
2. If you think an answer choice is correct, double-check the remaining choices to confirm that they are incorrect. There may be two true statements in the answer choices, but only one best answers the question; make sure the answer you choose addresses the issue in the question.
3. Remember that if two answer choices are essentially the same, neither can be correct, and both can be eliminated immediately.
4. Work backwards, trying each answer choice to see if it correctly answers the question. This is particularly useful for questions such as "An increase in which of the following results in an increase in [some parameter] except...." Track these on your scratch paper so you can see the work done for each answer choice tried.
5. If you have eliminated three answer choices, the fourth choice must be the correct choice. Don't waste time pondering why it is correct.

20.4   EXAMPLES OF STRATEGY IN USE

Below is an example of these strategies applied to the blood flow passage we mapped earlier.

1. The cross sectional area of the aorta is approximately 4 cm^2 and the total cross sectional area of the major arteries is 20 cm^2. If the speed of the blood in the aorta is 30 cm/sec, what is the average blood speed in the major arteries?

   A)   5 cm/sec
   B)   6 cm/sec
   C)   120 cm/sec
   D)   150 cm/sec

This is a memory computation question. Your initial reaction to the question might well be to check the given equations in the passage for a possible route, but you should quickly notice that none of them has a flow-speed term. The equation for flow speed in terms of area is the Continuity equation: $A_1v_1 = A_2v_2$. Solving for v_2 yields $\dfrac{A_1v_1}{A_2} = \dfrac{\left(4 \text{ cm}^2\right)\left(30 \text{ cm/s}\right)}{\left(20 \text{ cm}^2\right)} = 6$ cm/s. Nothing to it but plugging and chugging once you've identified that this might as well be a freestanding question. The correct answer is choice B.

2. Blood flow to the various systems in the body is regulated by the dilation and constriction of the blood vessels. After a person has eaten a large meal, the blood vessels supplying the digestive system dilate, increasing their radii by 50%. As a result of this blood vessel dilation, the flow of blood to the digestive system will:

   A)   increase to 500% of the original flow.
   B)   increase to 225% of the original flow.
   C)   increase to 150% of the original flow.
   D)   decrease to 50% of the original flow.

This is an explicit proportionality question. The question mentions a fractional change to the radius of the blood vessels and asks for a fractional change in blood flow rate (both expressed as percentages), which should immediately suggest to you that you want a proportion. Equations 1 and 2 combine to express just such a proportion, so directly under them on your mapping you can write $Q \propto 1/R$ and $R \propto 1/r^4$, thus $Q \propto r^4$. If r goes to 1.5 times its original value (immediately eliminating choice D), then Q goes to $(1.5)^4$ times its original value (eliminating choice C). Since $1.5^2 = 2.25$, choice B is eliminated, so the answer must be choice A.

3. Adaptation to life at high altitudes is characterized by
polycythemia (high red blood cell count). Excluding
other physiological compensations, what is the effect of
this change on the flow of blood?

A) Flow is decreased because viscosity is decreased.
B) Flow is increased because viscosity is decreased.
C) Flow is decreased because viscosity is increased.
D) Flow is increased because viscosity is increased.

This is an implicit functional-dependence question with a 2x2 answer choice pattern, that is, two variables vary between two possible values or trends (flow and viscosity are increasing or decreasing). With such questions, it is best to focus on one variable at a time. In this case, the question implies by stating that red blood cell count increases that viscosity will increase (eliminating choices A and B): This relies on commonsense reasoning (more stuff floating around in the fluid will make it more viscous) more than explicit knowledge of the passage or memory of a specific equation. On an Implicit question like this, you're being asked to rely on your intuition and logic when you have no specific equations or definitions to apply. If viscosity η increases, then according to Equations 1 and 2 combined (as with the previous question), Q will decrease (there's an inverse proportionality between flow rate and viscosity, $Q \propto 1/\eta$). Thus, choice C is correct.

4. At the venular end of skeletal muscle capillaries, the
hydrostatic pressure of the capillary is 17 torr and the
hydrostatic pressure of the surrounding tissue is 1 torr.
Fluid movement is from:

A) the capillary to the tissue, at a rate proportional to 7 torr.
B) the tissue to the capillary, at a rate proportional to 7 torr.
C) the capillary to the tissue, at a rate proportional to 9 torr.
D) the tissue to the capillary, at a rate proportional to 9 torr.

This is an Explicit computation question, with some dependence on basic outside knowledge. Like Question 3, it has a 2x2 pattern of answer choices. Applying Equation 3 (we recommend you do your work directly below where you wrote the equation on your mapping) with the numbers given in the question stem and the passage, you get $\Delta P = (17 + 0) - (1 + 25) = -9$ torr (eliminating choices A and B). If the pressure differential is negative, then there is greater pressure acting to move fluid into the capillaries (this is stated explicitly in the final paragraph, but you should also have basic knowledge that fluid naturally flows from high to low pressure). The correct answer is choice D.

5. According to the following schematic diagram of systemic circulation, which of the following is true?

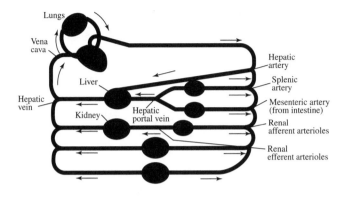

A) Vascular architecture of organs is in series so total peripheral resistance is greater than the resistance of individual organs.

B) Vascular architecture of organs is in parallel so total peripheral resistance is greater than the resistance of individual organs.

C) Vascular architecture of organs is in series so total peripheral resistance is less than the resistance of individual organs.

D) Vascular architecture of organs is in parallel so total peripheral resistance is less than the resistance of individual organs.

This is an Implicit Conceptual question. It requires you to make an analogy between fluid flow rate and current flow, an analogy justified by the similarity between Equation 1 and by Ohm's Law, $I = V/R$. The answer choices are once again in a 2x2 pattern, with the two variables being configuration (series or parallel) and total resistance (greater or less than the resistance of a single element, in this case an organ). Visual inspection of the provided diagram shows that the configuration (or "vascular architecture") is in parallel, because there are multiple paths the flow can take to get from and back to the heart. This eliminates choices A and C. At this point you must remember that resistors in parallel add reciprocally, so the total resistance is always less than any given resistive element. Choice D is correct.

20.5   MCAT PHYSICS TOPIC LIST[1]

Kinematics and Translational Motion

A.   Dimensions
B.   Vectors, components, addition and subtraction
C.   Speed, velocity, and acceleration

Force and Motion

A.   Translational Systems and Gravitation
    1.   Center of Mass
    2.   Concept of force and its units
        a.   Weight
        b.   Static and kinetic friction
    3.   Newton's laws
    4.   Analysis of forces acting on an object
        a.   Translational equilibrium
        b.   Inclined planes and pulley systems
B.   Rotational Systems
    1.   Uniform circular motion
    2.   Centripetal force
    3.   Torque and rotational equilibrium

Work and Energy

A.   Sign conventions and derived units (of work)
B.   Work done by a constant force
C.   Kinetic energy and its units
D.   Potential energy
    1.   gravitational, local, and general
    2.   elastic potential energy (spring)
E.   Conservation of energy
F.   Work-energy theorem
G.   Path-independence of work done in gravitational field
    1.   Conservative forces (gravity)
    2.   Non-conservative forces (friction)
H.   Power and its units
I.   Mechanical advantage

Thermodynamics

A.   Absolute temperature (kelvins)
B.   Pressure
C.   Temperature
D.   Heat capacity at constant volume and pressure
E.   Ideal gas
    1.   Ideal Gas Law
    2.   Temperature and kinetic energy
F.   First Law of Thermodynamics
G.   *PV* diagrams
H.   Second Law of Thermodynamics (entropy)
I.   Heat transfer mechanisms
J.   Thermal expansion

Fluids and Solids

A.   Fluids – Hydrostatics
    1.   Density, specific gravity
    2.   Buoyancy (Archimedes' principle)
    3.   Hydrostatic pressure and Pascal's Law
    4.   Surface tension
B.   Fluids – Hydrodynamics
    1.   Continuity equation
    2.   Poiseuille flow (viscosity)
    3.   Turbulence
    4.   Bernoulli's equation and principle

---

[1]   Adapted from *The Official Guide to the MCAT Exam (MCAT2015)*, 4th ed., © 2014 Association of American Medical Colleges.

Electrostatics

A. Charges, charge conversion
B. Insulators and conductors
C. Coulomb's Law and sign conventions
D. Electric fields
    1. Field lines
    2. Field due to a point charge and parallel planes of opposing charges
E. Potential differences and absolute potential
F. Equipotential lines
G. Electric dipoles
H. Electrostatic energy

Electricity and Magnetism

A. Circuit Elements
    1. Current, its units and sign conventions
    2. Batteries
    3. Resistance
    4. Capacitance and dielectrics
    5. Energy of a charged capacitor
    6. Resistors/capacitors in series and in parallel
    7. Theory of conductivity
    8. Voltmeters and ammeters
B. Magnetism
    1. Magnetic field
    2. Force on a charge moving in a magnetic field

Waves and Periodic Motion

A. Periodic Motion
    1. Amplitude, period, frequency, velocity, phase
    2. Simple harmonic motion in springs
    3. Potential energy of a spring system
B. Wave Characteristics
    1. Transverse and longitudinal waves
    2. Wavelength, frequency, wave speed
    3. Amplitude and intensity
    4. Superposition of waves, interference, wave addition
    5. Standing waves
    6. Harmonics

Sound

A. Production of sound
B. Relative speed of sound in different media
C. Sound intensity (decibels) and attenuation
D. Pitch
E. Doppler effect (and it's application to light)
F. Ultrasound
G. Shock waves

Light and Geometrical Optics

A. Electromagnetic Radiation (Light)
1. Properties of electromagnetic radiation
2. Classification of electromagnetic spectrum (radio, infrared, UV, X-rays, etc.)
3. Visual spectrum and color
4. Photon energy
5. Diffraction
6. Interference, Young's double-slit experiment
7. Polarization of light (linear and circular)

B. Geometrical Optics
1. Reflection from plane surface
2. Refraction and Snell's Law
3. Total internal reflection
4. Dispersion (change of index of refraction with wavelength)
5. Spherical mirrors
6. Thin lenses and combination of lenses
7. Optical instruments
8. Lens aberration

Atomic and Nuclear Structure[2]

A. Atomic Structure and Spectra
1. Emission spectrum of hydrogen (Bohr model)
2. Atomic energy levels

B. Atomic Nucleus
1. Atomic number and weight
2. Neutrons, protons, isotopes
3. Nuclear forces and binding energy
4. Radioactive decay
5. Mass spectrometer

---

[2] This information, even while listed by the AAMC as Physics topics, is also relevant to General Chemistry.

Chapter 21
Physics
Practice Section

FREESTANDING QUESTIONS

1. A train is starting its trip from Paris to Frankfurt with an acceleration of x m/s². What is the ratio of its displacement traveled during the 5th second from ($t = 4$ s to $t = 5$ s) compared with the 10th second from ($t = 9$ s to $t = 10$ s)?

   A) 7 : 17
   B) 8 : 18
   C) 9 : 19
   D) 10 : 20

2. A 1 m horizontal wooden plank with mass m is perfectly balanced by two masses x and y at the ends of the plank. Which of the following is the correct relationship between x and y if the pivot is located 25 cm from mass x?

   A) $x = m + 3y$
   B) $x = 3y$
   C) $y = m + 3x$
   D) $x = (m + y) / 3$

3. A yo-yo is being swung in a vertical circular motion by a constant tension force applied through the string. Which of the following correctly describes the yo-yo's motion?

   A) The yo-yo moves at a constant speed and the net acceleration points toward the center of the circular path.
   B) The yo-yo moves at a variable speed and the net acceleration points toward the center of the circular path.
   C) The yo-yo moves at a constant speed and the centripetal acceleration points toward the center of the circular path.
   D) The yo-yo moves at a variable speed and the centripetal acceleration points toward the center of the circular path.

4. As a person inhales, the lungs expand isothermally. Which of the following best describes the change in internal energy and the work done by the gas in the lungs?

   A) $\Delta E > 0$ and $W > 0$
   B) $\Delta E = 0$ and $W = 0$
   C) $\Delta E = 0$ and $W > 0$
   D) $\Delta E < 0$ and $W > 0$

5. A wooden cube of 8 cm length is partially submerged in a tank of canola oil with 2 cm of its length beneath the surface. If a hand suddenly pushes the cube so that the cube now has only 2 cm of its length above the surface, what is the magnitude of the new buoyant force compared to the previous one?

   A) ½ the previous magnitude
   B) Same as the previous magnitude
   C) 2 times the previous magnitude
   D) 3 times the previous magnitude

6. Two pipes of equal volume output per minute deliver water away from a water station to different areas of the city. Pipe A delivers the water to a mountain observatory, while Pipe B delivers the water to a university at ground level. Given equal pressures in the pipes, which of the following is true?

   A) The cross section area of Pipe A is larger than that of Pipe B.
   B) The cross section area of Pipe A is smaller than that of Pipe B.
   C) The flow rate of water in Pipe A is larger than that of Pipe B.
   D) The flow rate of water in Pipe A is smaller than that of Pipe B.

7. You have three resistors of 3 Ω, 6 Ω, and 8 Ω and a 50 V battery. You want to create a circuit where the current through the 8 Ω resistor is 5 A. How could you arrange the circuit?

A) All three resistors in parallel.
B) All three resistors in series.
C) The 3 Ω and 6 Ω resistors in parallel and the 8 Ω in series with it.
D) The 6 Ω and 8 Ω resistors in parallel and the 3 Ω in series with it.

8. If the time it takes for a proton to complete one circular revolution is T, what is the time needed for an alpha particle (helium nucleus) to complete one revolution in the same uniform magnetic field?

A) T
B) $2T$
C) $4T$
D) $8T$

9. The harmonic frequencies of a glass tube, which has one end closed off, are empirically measured using a note-emitting device. The beat frequency (f_{beat}), or absolute difference in frequencies, between the third and fourth harmonic is 680 Hz. What is second harmonic frequency and what is the length of the glass tube?

A) 1020 Hz, 20 cm
B) 1360 Hz, 20 cm
C) 1020 Hz, 25 cm
D) 1360 Hz, 25 cm

10. A single speaker produces music at an intensity level of 160 dB at 1 meter away from itself. A student stands 10 meters away from the speaker, and puts on a pair of noise canceling headphones, capable of reducing the intensity by 99.9%. What is the intensity level that is student hears?

A) 100 dB
B) 110 dB
C) 120 dB
D) 130 dB

11. A wind-chime made up of colored flat glass pieces is swaying in the sunlight. A physics student wants to measure the angles of light as they are refracted through the glass and back into the air. If the angle of incidence of the sunlight is 30° on the glass, which has an index of refraction of 1.50, at what angle does the ray emerge from the glass into the air at?

A) $\sin^{-1}(1/2)$
B) $\sin^{-1}(1/3)$
C) $\sin^{-1}(1/4)$
D) $\sin^{-1}(1/6)$

12. In diagnostic radiology, the photoelectric effect can be used to provide sharp images of bones. 200 keV X-ray photons eject photoelectrons from the innermost orbitals of calcium atoms with a binding energy of approximately 4 keV. An electron from an outer orbital then falls to the inner orbital to take the place of the ejected electron, releasing energy as a photon known as characteristic radiation. What can be said about the photon energy of the characteristic radiation?

A) $0\,keV < hf < 4\,keV$
B) $4\,keV < hf < 196\,keV$
C) $196 < hf < 200\,keV$
D) $hf > 200\,keV$

PRACTICE PASSAGE 1

Understanding the movements of multi-joint systems, like a human arm or leg, is a important problem for neurophysiology, kinesiology, and robotics. One approach to uncovering how the brain selects a particular motion among the infinite possibilities is to create a mathematical model focusing on one particular aspect of the motion, such as the trajectory of the hand, and to test whether and how well the predictions of that model match what is observed experimentally. The minimum jerk theory is one such experimentally verified mathematical model. Just as acceleration is the rate of change of velocity, jerk is the rate of change of acceleration, given by:

$$\mathbf{j} = \frac{\Delta \mathbf{a}}{\Delta t}$$

Equation 1

Jerk bears exactly the same relationship to acceleration as acceleration bears to velocity, and like acceleration, it is a vector.

In one set of experiments, experimenters observe the performance of simple tasks by healthy participants starting from a seated position in front of a table with hands set palm down on that table. The first task has the participant reaching out to grasp a cup, drinking from it, and returning the cup to the table. The second task involves eating food from a bowl with a spoon and setting the spoon down in its original position. The motions of twelve points on the trunk and active arm between the neck and hand are recorded on two planes: one parallel to the tabletop (the xy plane), the other the sagittal plane dividing the left and right sides of the body (the xz plane). These motions are then analyzed statistically in comparison to predictions made by minimum jerk theory. The figures below show some of the experimentally measured data compared against the predictions of the minimum jerk theory. Note in Figure 2 that the percentage of range is used because different participants took different amounts of time to reach out and grasp the cup.

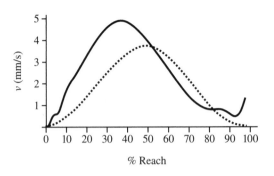

Figure 2 Averaged observed wrist velocity (solid line) and minimum jerk theory prediction (dashed line) for the reaching-to-cup portion of the drinking task

Adapted from Wisnesky, K. and Johnson, M, "Quantifying kinematics of purposeful movements to real, imagined, or absent functional objects: Implications for modeling trajectories for robot-assisted ADL tasks." *Journal of NeuroEngineering and Rehabilitation* 2007, 4:7.

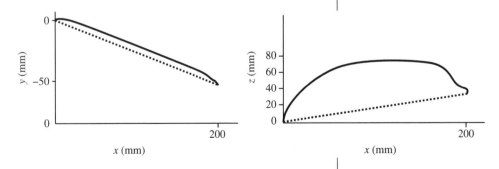

Figure 1 Averaged observed wrist trajectories (solid line) and minimum jerk theory predictions (dashed line) in the xy and xz planes for the reaching-to-cup portion of the drinking task

1. The purpose of the experiment is to inform robotic assisted therapies for stroke victims who have lost some degree of motor control. One concern with such therapies is ensuring that no potentially harmful torques are experienced by the patients. In observing the free movements of the healthy participants performing the two tasks, the experimenters might want to compute the torques at each of the following sensor points EXCEPT:

A) the shoulder.
B) the midpoint of the biceps.
C) the inner elbow.
D) the wrist.

2. During which range of percentages of the averaged experimental reaching task is it safest to assume that the jerk was equal to zero?

A) 0% to 10%
B) 20% to 30%
C) 35% to 45%
D) The jerk cannot possibly have been zero at any time during the experiment.

3. When the average participant's wrist was at its maximum distance from the surface of the table, approximately how far to the participant's right had it moved?

A) 5 mm
B) 30 mm
C) 75 mm
D) 110 mm

4. Which of the following are true about the averaged observed motion of the participants' wrists versus the motion predicted by minimum jerk theory during the reaching-to-cup portion of the drinking task?

   I. The maximum speed of the observed motion is greater than that of the predicted motion.
   II. The maximum acceleration of the observed motion is greater than that of the predicted motion.
   III. The total displacement of the observed motion is greater than that of the predicted motion.

A) I only
B) I and II only
C) II and III only
D) I, II, and III

5. Which of the following expressions could give displacement in terms of jerk, assuming zero initial velocity and acceleration?

A) $\frac{1}{6}jt^3$

B) $\frac{1}{3}jt^2$

C) $\frac{1}{2}jt^2$

D) $2j^2t^2$

6. Neglecting any frictional effects and assuming a cup of mass m, how much total work is done during the entirety of the first experimental task?

A) 0 J
B) 0.08 mg
C) mgh, where h is the height of the participant's mouth above the table
D) It cannot be determined from the information given.

PRACTICE PASSAGE 2

Wind chill tables were developed to indicate the subjective temperature a person perceives from wind at various air temperatures on exposed skin. Although in contact with air, skin temperature is not equal to bulk air temperature because of heat transfer between warm body tissue and skin, and between skin and bulk air.

Body core temperature is a constant 37° C, but at room temperature under windless conditions, exposed skin temperature is approximately 35° C. The latent heat of vaporization, ΔH_{vap}, for water is 2.4×10^6 J/kg, but for air temperatures less than about 4° C, evaporative cooling is a minor effect because skin is relatively dry. The main consequence of wind is to increase the efficiency of convection. If skin temperature is less than 0° C, frostbite may occur.

When immersed in a moving fluid, a solid object maintains a boundary layer of stagnant fluid at its surface. As distance from the surface increases, flow speed within the boundary layer increases until it is equal to the flow speed of the bulk fluid. The skin's boundary layer may be approximated as a thickness of still air that varies inversely with wind speed and affects the net thermal conductivity between skin and the environment.

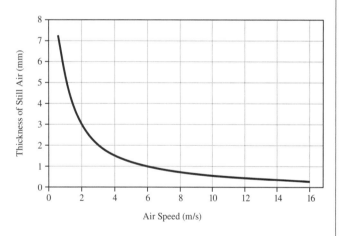

Figure 1 Thickness of the skin's still air layer vs. air speed

The heat transfer coefficient, h_c, of a thermally conductive layer is defined as

$$h_c = \frac{k}{t}$$

Equation 1

Here k is thermal conductivity (a material property) and t is the thickness of the layer. The thermal energy passing through this layer is the heat, Q, which depends on the temperature difference across the layer and is defined as

$$Q = h_c \Delta T$$

Equation 2

Air has a thermal conductivity of 0.026 W/m·K. The thermal insulation of clothing, I_{clu}, is measured in units of clo, with 1 clo = 0.155 m²·K/W. The heat transfer coefficient of clothing may therefore be expressed as

$$h_c = \frac{6.45}{I_{clu}}$$

Equation 3

The thermal insulation of multiple layers of clothing, excluding the effect of trapped air between the layers, is the sum of the clo values of each layer. In addition, at very low air speed clothing has a region of still air over it that is about 5 mm thick.

1. How does thermal energy flow through skin change if air at a temperature T changes from a wind speed of 2 m/s to a wind speed of 8 m/s?

   A) It increases by a factor of 2.
   B) It decreases by a factor of 4.
   C) It increases by a factor of 4.
   D) It cannot be determined without knowing the temperature difference across the skin.

2. Which statement is true about a block of steel that has been taken from a warm house and left outside on a cold, windy day?

   A) The temperature of the block falls more slowly than on a cold day without wind.
   B) After a long time the temperature of the block is the same as the outside air temperature.
   C) Wind chill reduces the temperature of the block to less than the outside air temperature.
   D) After a long time wind chill reduces the temperature of the block to a value between the house and outside air temperature.

3. A person wears a glove that traps a 5 mm thick layer of air next to his skin. Ignoring the effect of the glove's thermal insulation, what is the magnitude of the heat flux through the glove when the skin temperature is 30 °C and the air temperature is –10 °C on a windless day?

   A)   0.104 W/m²
   B)   10.4 W/m²
   C)   104 W/m²
   D)   208 W/m²

4. A single layer of cotton fabric has a thermal insulation of 0.02 clo. Ignoring the effect of trapped air between layers, what are the thermal conductivity, k, and heat transfer coefficient, h_c, of two layers of cotton fabric compared with a single layer.

   A) The thermal conductivity remains the same and the heat transfer coefficient doubles.
   B) The thermal conductivity reduces by one half and the heat transfer coefficient remains the same.
   C) The thermal conductivity doubles and the heat transfer coefficient reduces by one half.
   D) The thermal conductivity remains the same and the heat transfer coefficient reduces by one half.

5. Heat index tables indicate the subjective temperature a person perceives on a hot, windless day by accounting for the cooling effect of perspiration. The evaporative heat transfer coefficient, he, decreases as humidity increases, but convective heat transfer from skin to bulk air adds to the total cooling. Which of the following changes to her clothing should a person consider to improve her comfort on a very hot day?

   I.   Select clothes with higher permeability to water vapor
   II. Select clothes with looser weave
   III. Select clothes that absorb a lot of perspiration

   A) I only
   B) II only
   C) I and II only
   D) I and III only

6. How much heat does the evaporation of 10 grams of perspiration remove from the body?

   A) 2.4×10^4 J
   B) 2.4×10^5 J
   C) 2.4×10^7 J
   D) 2.4×10^8 J

PRACTICE PASSAGE 3

Arterial blood pressure, measured in mm of mercury, is measured at two moments within the circulatory cycle: one during the maximum thrust of the heart (*systolic* pressure, normally around 120 mm Hg), and one when the heart is relaxed (*diastolic* pressure, normally around 80 mm Hg). Systolic and diastolic blood pressures vary throughout the day. They can change in response to stress, exercise, change in diet, and other factors. Blood pressure decreases as blood moves through arteries, arterioles, capillaries and veins, as described by *Poiseuille's Law*:

$$\frac{\Delta P}{L} = \frac{8\eta f}{\pi R^4}$$

Equation 1

where $\Delta P/L$ is the pressure drop per length, η is the viscosity coefficient, f is the volume flow rate, and R is the radius of the artery.

One factor that affects blood pressure is the buildup of fatty deposits or plaque on the arterial walls. The effective diameter is decreased, which increases the speed of blood flow. The increase in speed, in turn, decreases the pressure inside that section of the artery.

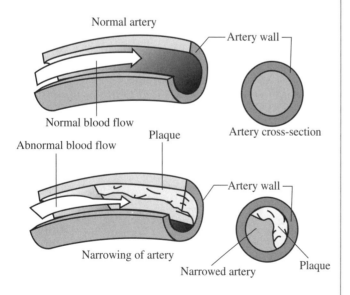

Figure 1

If the fluid pressure decreases too much, the artery will collapse on itself. Then, when the flow of blood has ceased, the artery opens up again. This process repeats in what is known as *vascular flutter*. This repetitive opening and closing of the

artery can act as a pump, which may dislodge the plaque and send it through the artery where it may potentially entirely block a down-stream vessel in the body.

While plaque decreases the fluid pressure along a section of artery, the average blood pressure in the body as a whole increases.

1. A bag contains a glucose solution with specific gravity 1.02. If the average gauge pressure of an artery is 1.33×10^4 Pa, what is the minimum height the bag needs to be placed to infuse the glucose solution into the artery?

    A) 1.30 m
    B) 1.36 m
    C) 13.0 m
    D) 13.6 m

2. Which of the following would increase the pressure drop per length as blood moves through an artery?

    I.   Using a blood thinner to decrease the viscosity
    II. Inserting a stent to widen the artery
    III. Increasing the blood flow rate

    A) I only
    B) II and III
    C) III only
    D) I, II, and III

3. During the systole, the heart produces a *vascular pressure wave*, which travels through the vessel walls to the peripheral arteries. These waves are reflected at the peripheral veins and interfere with the incoming waves, causing pressure readings that differ from the true aortic pressure. A high pressure reading would occur at:

A) a displacement node.
B) a displacement antinode.
C) halfway between a displacement node and antinode.
D) a pressure node.

4. A hypodermic syringe, positioned horizontally, contains medicine with specific gravity 1.0, initially at 1 atm. The barrel of the syringe has a cross-sectional area of 25 mm². A force of 5 N is exerted on the plunger. If the medicine leaves the needle at 1 atm, with what speed is it ejected? (Assume the needle cross-sectional area is much smaller than the barrel cross-sectional area.)

A) 2.0 cm/s
B) 63 cm/s
C) 20 m/s
D) 25 m/s

5. If blood traveling through a vessel encounters a region where plaque has decreased the effective diameter by one third its normal value, then the average speed of blood flow will increase by:

A) one third.
B) a factor of 3.
C) a factor of 9/4.
D) a factor of 9.

6. Certain foods, such as salt, can increase the amount of blood pumped out from the heart during each contraction. This would most likely:

A) decrease the frequency of flutter due to the increase in flow rate.
B) increase the frequency of flutter due to the increase in flow rate.
C) decrease the frequency of flutter due to the change in blood density.
D) increase the frequency of flutter due to the change in blood density.

PRACTICE PASSAGE 4

In flow cytometry, a heterogeneous sample of cells can be separated into subpopulations using electrostatic cell sorting. This techniques allows researchers to do targeted research on particular types of cells.

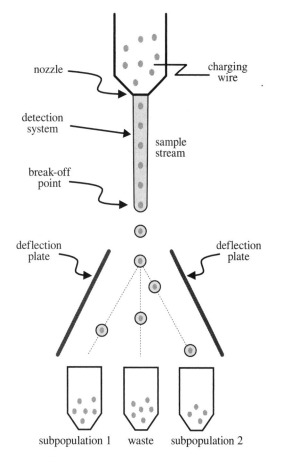

Figure 1 Schematic of flow cytometry

In flow cytometry systems, a sample cell suspension undergoes hydrodynamic focusing which causes the cells to flow out of the nozzle one at a time in a thin sample stream. This allows the cells to be analyzed individually at the interrogation point. Many systems analyze the cells optically using laser light that illuminates the cell at the interrogation point. A cell's scattering and/or fluorescent properties are used to identify the cell. The amount of laser light scattered in the forward direction (in the same direction that the laser light is travelling) is proportional to the size of the cell, whereas light scattered sideways (at 90°) is proportional to the internal complexity of the cell. To differentiate cells with similar size and complexity, fluorescent labels that bind to cell surface proteins can be used to mark cells of a desired population.

Once the cell has been interrogated, it continues down the stream to the break-off point. At the break-off point, an acoustic wave is used to break the stream into drops, each containing an individual cell. As the drop is being formed, it is charged according to the properties of the cell within. The charge of the drop is controlled by a charging wire upstream of the nozzle.

While there are no cells of interest in the sample stream, the wire remains neutral. When a cell of the desired subpopulation reaches the break-off point, a voltage is applied to the wire. The wire thus attracts ions of a particular charge from the entire stream. The ions move rapidly, leaving the rest of the steam, including the drop about to be formed, oppositely charged. The charge on the drop is proportional to its surface area. Once the charged drop is separated from the stream, the voltage of the charging wire is adjusted according to the next cell to arrive at the break-off point.

Once the drop breaks free of the stream, it passes through oppositely charged deflection plates. If the drop is uncharged, it drops straight down into a waste collection tube. Positively and negatively charged drops will be deflected in opposite directions, into sample collection tubes to either side of the waste collection tube. A typical voltage between the detection plates is 3000 V.

1. If the charging wire is brought to a positive voltage relative to the sample stream, what will the resulting charge of the drop released at the break-off point be?

A) Positive, because the current created in the sample stream will flow toward the charging wire
B) Positive, because the current created in the sample stream will flow away from the charging wire
C) Negative, because the current created in the sample stream will flow toward the charging wire
D) Negative, because the current created in the sample stream will flow away from the charging wire

2. Should it be possible to isolate purified samples of both T helper cells and T killer cells from a sample of whole blood using one run of a flow cytometer?

A) No, because all T-cells have approximately the same size and shape.
B) No, because these cells are not present in whole blood.
C) Yes, if the sample is prepared with an anti-CD_3 fluorescent antibody.
D) Yes, if the sample is prepared with both an anti-CD_4 and an anti-CD_8 fluorescent antibodies that fluoresce at different wavelengths.

3. If the mechanism that makes the drops is malfunctioning and produces drops that are too large, what happens to path of the large drop if the drop is approximately spherical?

A) The drop doesn't deflect as much as it should, possibly falling short of the sample collection container.
B) There is no effect on the path of the drop
C) The drop deflects more than it should, possibly overshooting the sample collection container.
D) Whether the path is affected depends on the magnitude of the electric field.

4. Successive drops are closely spaced. Consequently, how does a negatively charged drop leaving the break-off point affect the charge of the next drop if the voltage isn't adjusted to compensate?

A) The drop has no impact on the charge of the next drop since it is no longer connected to the sample stream.
B) The drop has no impact on the charge of the next drop since it is accelerating downward.
C) Residual negative ions from the formation of the negative drop cause the next drop to be slightly more negatively charged drop than would otherwise be formed.
D) The negative drop electrostatically attracts positive charges in the sample stream, causing the next drop to be slightly more positively charged drop than would otherwise be formed.

5. Why do RBCs and T-cells show similar side-scattering signals when illuminated by a laser?

A) They are about the same size.
B) They contain the same internal structures, so they have similar internal complexity.
C) The flat shape of a RBC increases the amount of light it scatters sideways compared to a sphere.
D) They are both significantly larger than the wavelength of the laser, so both cause equal amounts of diffraction.

6. If the electric field in the region between the deflection plates points to the right, which of the following could describe the charge of the deflection plates?

A) The plate on the right is positive and the plate on the left is negative because positive charges feel an electrostatic force in the same direction as the electric field, whereas negative charges feel a force in the opposite direction as the electric field.
B) The plate on the right is negative and the plate on the left is positive because positive charges feel an electrostatic force in the opposite direction as the electric field, whereas negative charges feel a force in the same direction as the electric field.
C) The plate on the left is positive and the plate on the right is negative because the electric field created by the charged plates will point away from the positive plate and toward the negative plate.
D) The plate on the left is negative and the plate on the right is positive because the electric field created by the charged plates will point away from the negative plate and toward the positive plate.

PRACTICE PASSAGE 5

Muscle-tendon units function as *damped oscillators* in response to certain perturbations. For example, under load (as when the knee is held at nearly complete extension supporting a weight at equilibrium), when jostled the muscle will contract and relax while the joint flexes and extends several times in rapid succession, returning to equilibrium in a few seconds. These oscillations provide clues to the stiffness of the muscle and other viscoelastic properties.

These muscle-tendon unit oscillators can be modeled as damped *harmonic oscillators*, such as a spring-block system with a damping force provided by drag (see Figure 1). Here the oscillating mass is attached by a rigid, low-mass rod to a rigid plate submerged in a tank filled with a low-viscosity liquid.

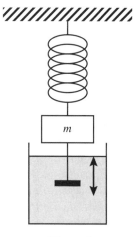

Figure 1

To a close approximation, the effect of the drag force on the oscillating submerged plate is directly proportional to its velocity, v. Thus, in place of Hooke's Law for the restoring force of ideal springs, we have the following force equation for damped harmonic motion:

$$F = -ky - bv$$

Equation 1

where **y** is the displacement from equilibrium of the spring-mass system, k is the stiffness of the spring, and b is a damping coefficient, a measure of the drag effect on the system due to the movement of the submerged plate through the fluid. Using Newton's Second Law and assuming a small value for b, one

finds the following solution for the position of the mass as a function of time:

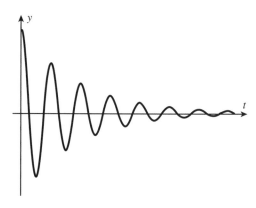

$$y = Ae^{-bt/2m} \cos\left(\left(\sqrt{\frac{k}{m} - \left(\frac{b}{2m}\right)^2}\right)t\right)$$

Equation 2

The graph of this equation is a sinusoidal curve whose amplitude is a decaying exponential, as shown below.

Figure 2

1. How does the frequency of oscillation of the damped harmonic oscillator change over time?

A) It is constant.
B) It decreases.
C) It increases.
D) It initially decreases, then becomes constant.

2. In one experiment, the subject is asked to flex her biceps muscle isometrically while holding a dumbbell in her hand, her elbow resting on a table and arm extended to 160°. The experimenter then pushes down suddenly on the subject's wrist and releases. The resultant vertical oscillations of her wrist are measured and plotted as a function of time (generating a curve similar to that in Figure 2). In order to determine the stiffness of her biceps muscle, each of the following data would be necessary EXCEPT:

A) the horizontal distance along the graph from peak to peak.
B) the height of the first peak on the graph.
C) the mass of the dumbbell.
D) none of the above is unnecessary.

3. What does the slope of the sinusoidal curve in Figure 2 represent?

A) The distance traveled by the oscillating mass
B) The velocity of the oscillating mass
C) The work done by gravity on the system
D) The decay rate of the amplitude of the oscillations

4. Which of the following would likely result from increasing the viscosity of the fluid in which the plate is submerged?

A) The amplitude of oscillations would decay more rapidly and their frequency would decrease.
B) The amplitude of oscillations would decay less rapidly and their frequency would decrease.
C) The amplitude of oscillations would decay more rapidly and their frequency would increase.
D) The amplitude of oscillations would decay more rapidly and their frequency would remain the same.

5. As the maximum amplitude of the oscillations decreases with time, so does the total mechanical energy of the system. At what time will this energy be one quarter its initial value?

A) $t = \dfrac{\pi}{2\sqrt{\dfrac{k}{m} - \left(\dfrac{b}{2m}\right)^2}}$

B) $t = \dfrac{2m\ln(4)}{b}$

C) $t = \dfrac{2m\ln(2)}{b}$

D) $t = \dfrac{2m}{b}$

6. Each of the following changes would affect the rate of decay of the amplitude of oscillations EXCEPT:

A) increasing the suspended mass.
B) changing the surface area of the submerged plate.
C) draining the liquid from the tank.
D) increasing the stiffness of the spring.

PRACTICE PASSAGE 6

Early in the 20th century, several crucial experiments established the dual wave-particle nature of light and the ways that electromagnetic radiation interacts with matter. In 1923, Arthur H. Compton conducted an important experiment showing how photons in the X-ray and gamma-ray portion of the spectrum interact with free electrons. Compton's experiment provided further verification of the photonic nature of electromagnetic phenomena.

Compton scattering occurs when incident photons strike electrons in inelastic collisions, imparting momentum and kinetic energy to the electrons and thereby reducing the momentum and energy of the scattered photons. The reduced energy of the photon implies a reduced frequency according to the photon energy equation $E = hf$, where h is *Planck's constant* ($h = 4.14 \times 10^{-15}$ eV·s). This change in frequency implies a corresponding change in wavelength; this shift in wavelength of Compton scattered photons is given by the Compton Shift equation:

$$\Delta\lambda = \frac{h}{m_e c}(1 - \cos\phi)$$

Equation 1

Here ϕ represents the *scattering angle*, or the angle between the photon's original path and its path after the collision, and m_e is the rest mass of the electron.

To study Compton scattering in the lab, a student conducts the following experiment. Using a radioactive source (Americium-241, a commonly manufactured radioactive isotope used in household smoke detectors with a peak gamma emission of 59.5 keV), a metallic target shaped into a circular arc, and an X-ray detector that converts incident X-ray photons into electric current by means of the *photoelectric effect*, the student counts the number of scattering events at various angles over set durations. So long as the source, detector, and target all lie on a circle on a flat surface, the student can be relatively assured of receiving only photons scattered at particular angles due to the geometric rule that inscribed angles in a circle are equal to half the intercepted arc. The experimental set-up is shown in Figure 1.

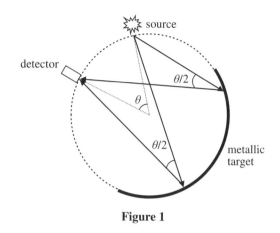

Figure 1

The student conducts experimental runs at four different scattering angles over four different durations. The following data record the scattered energy peaks in terms of scattering angle and photon counts (only the peak counts are included, not the entire energy spectrum for each scattering angle).

Scattering angle ϕ	Energy of peak	# of detections at peak energy	Duration of experimental run
60°	57.0 ± 0.4 keV	1242	4 hours
75°	55.2 ± 0.6 keV	989	4 hours
90°	53.5 ± 0.6 keV	1411	8 hours
120°	50.5 ± 0.5 keV	1206	8 hours

Table 1

1. What is the scattering angle ϕ in terms of the circular arc θ (see Figure 1)?

A) $\theta/2$
B) $90° - \theta/2$
C) $180° - \theta/2$
D) $180° - \theta$

2. The X-rays used in medical imaging are of high enough energy to experience Compton scattering with electrons in the body. Which of the following explains why Compton scattering can be problematic in diagnostic radiology?

   I. Scattered photons travel in all directions which can be detected on X-ray films
   II. Scattered photons can be a danger to nearby personnel.
   III. The scattered photons' wavelengths are larger than some skeletal structures in the human body.

A) I only
B) I and II only
C) II and III only
D) I, II, and III

3. What is the maximum change in wavelength of a Compton-scattered photon?

A) $\Delta\lambda_{max} = \dfrac{h}{m_e c}$

B) $\Delta\lambda_{max} = \dfrac{2h}{m_e c}$

C) $\Delta\lambda_{max} = \dfrac{h}{2m_e c}$

D) $\Delta\lambda_{max} = 0$

4. During experimental runs, the student places a thin sheet of lead directly between the Americium-241 source and the scintillation detector. Which of the following best explains the purpose of this measure?

A) It prevents electrons scattered in the air between the source and the detector from entering the detector and corrupting the data.
B) It ensures that photons scattered off the metallic target at angles different from the desired angle do not enter the detector.
C) It prevents high energy photons from cosmic radiation from entering the detector and corrupting the data.
D) It prevents photons emitted from the source from entering the detector directly without scattering off the target.

5. According to Table 1, for which scattering angle was the rate of detection events at the peak energy highest?

A) 60°
B) 75°
C) 90°
D) 120°

6. Suppose another trial of the experiment were conducted set up to record scatterings at an angle of 105°. If the experiment were allowed to run overnight (for a duration of 12 hours), which of the following would most likely correspond to the peak energy detected and the number of detections?

A) 51.8 ± 0.3 keV and 1320 detections
B) 51.8 ± 0.3 keV and 1935 detections
C) 54.3 ± 0.6 keV and 1320 detections
D) 54.3 ± 0.6 keV and 1935 detections

Chapter 22
Physics Practice
Section Solutions

SOLUTIONS TO FREESTANDING QUESTIONS

1. **C** The formula $d = v_0 t + \frac{1}{2} at^2$ is used to calculate the displacement traveled at the 5th second and at the 10th second. Express the displacement traveled at the 5th second, Δd_5, by finding the difference between the total displacement traveled in 5 seconds, d_5, by the total displacement traveled in 4 seconds, d_4. Thus, $\Delta d_5 = d_5 - d_4$. Applying the formula $d = v_0 t + \frac{1}{2} at^2$ with respect to d_5 and d_4, the equation becomes $\Delta d_5 = (v_0 t_5 + \frac{1}{2} at_5^2) - (v_0 t_4 + \frac{1}{2} at_4^2)$. Since the train was initially at rest, $v_0 = 0$. The acceleration, a, is a constant, and is equal to x,

$$\Delta d_5 = (\tfrac{1}{2} x(5)^2) - (\tfrac{1}{2} x(4)^2)$$
$$= (\tfrac{25}{2})x - (\tfrac{16}{2})x$$
$$= \frac{9x}{2}$$

Likewise, the equation for the displacement traveled at the 10th second, Δd_{10}, is as follows,

$$\Delta d_{10} = d_{10} - d_9$$
$$= (v_0 t_{10} + \tfrac{1}{2} at_{10}^2) - (v_0 t_9 + \tfrac{1}{2} at_9^2)$$

Since $v_0 = 0$, $a = x$,

$$\Delta d_5 = (\tfrac{1}{2} x(10)^2) - (\tfrac{1}{2} x(9)^2)$$
$$= (\tfrac{100}{2})x - (\tfrac{81}{2})x$$
$$= \frac{19x}{2}$$

The ratio $d_5 : d_{10}$ could be expressed as a fraction d_5 / d_{10},

$$\frac{d_5}{d_{10}} = \frac{\frac{9x}{2}}{\frac{19x}{2}}$$
$$= \frac{9x}{19x}$$
$$= \frac{9}{19}$$

and therefore, the ratio $d_5 : d_{10}$ is equal to 9:19.

2.   **A**   When calculating questions related to the center of mass, the center of mass of the plank is always taken into account unless assumed negligible. According to the scenario, mass y is 25 cm + 50 cm = 75 cm from the pivot point, whereas mass x is 25 cm on the opposite side. Therefore, if the pivot point is chosen as the origin, applying the formula for center of mass for point masses:

$$x_{cm} = \frac{(m_1 x_1 + m_2 x_2 + m_3 x_3)}{(m_1 + m_2 + m_3)}$$

$$0 = \frac{(-25x + 25m + 75y)}{(x + m + y)}$$

$$0 = \frac{25(-x + m + 3y)}{(x + m + y)}$$

Since the fraction must be equal to zero, this implies that the numerator must be equal to zero. That is, $-x + m + 3y = 0$. Solving for x, you get the equation $x = m + 3y$, which is choice A.

3.   **D**   This is another two-by-two question. In a vertical circular motion, the yo-yo is under the influence of both the tension force of the string, and the gravity of the yo-yo. Therefore, its speed is not constant and increases as the yo-yo swings down and decreases as it swings up. This eliminates choices A and C. In this scenario, the weight of the yo-yo could be split into a component force that is parallel to the tension of the string, and a force perpendicular to the tension force. The net force of the tension and the parallel component of the yo-yo's weight would be the centripetal acceleration. However, the perpendicular component of gravity introduces a tangential acceleration to the yo-yo. This results in a net acceleration that does not point toward the center of the circular path.

4.   **A**   Because the lungs are expanding, the work done by the gas in the lungs is positive, eliminating choice B. For a closed system, an isothermal process implies that there is no change in the internal energy, but the air in the lungs is not a closed system. It is an open system that takes in matter from the environment during inhalation and expels matter into the environment during exhalation. During inhalation, air molecules are being added to the system, while the temperature remains constant. An increase in the amount of material in the system, while the average energy per molecule (i.e., temperature) remains constant constitutes an increase in the internal energy of the system, making choice A the correct answer.

5.   **D**   This is an application of Archimedes' principle, in which the magnitude of the buoyant force is equal to the weight of the fluid displaced by the object. Choices A and B can be eliminated first because the more the object is submerged in the fluid, the larger the buoyant force. In the original scenario, the wooden cube, having a volume V, has a proportion of 2 cm / 8 cm = ¼ under the surface. The original buoyant force $F_1 = \rho\,¼Vg$. When pushed by the hand, the cube is now 8 cm − 2 cm = 6 cm submerged from the surface in length. This tells us that the new buoyant force is $F_2 = \rho\,¾Vg$, which is three times the original magnitude of the buoyant force.

6.   **A**   Since the pipes are delivering water at equal volume output per minute, the flow rate is the same in both pipes, eliminating choices C and D. According to Bernoulli's equation: $P_A + \frac{1}{2} \rho v_A^2 + \rho g y_A = P_B + \frac{1}{2} \rho v_B^2 + \rho g y_B$, and $P_A = P_B$, the equation becomes $\frac{1}{2} \rho v_A^2 + \rho g y_A = \frac{1}{2} \rho v_B^2 + \rho g y_B$. You know that $y_A > y_B$, so $v_A < v_B$. For a constant flow rate f, if $v_A < v_B$, that means that $A_A > A_B$, according to $f = Av$, which makes choice A the correct answer.

7.   **C**   If the current through the 8 Ω resistor is 5 A, then the voltage across it is 40 V. This eliminates choice A as the voltage across each of the resistors in parallel is the same. If all the resistors were in series, the total resistance would be 17 Ω, leading to a current across each resistor approximately 3 A, which eliminates choice B. If the 6 Ω and 3 Ω resistors are in parallel, then this gives an equivalent resistance of 2 Ω for the parallel set, and a total of 10 Ω for the circuit. The current across the 8 Ω resistor and the parallel resistor set would then be 5 A. Thus, the correct answer is choice C. A similar approach can be used to figure out choice D. If the 6 Ω and 8 Ω resistors are in parallel, this gives an equivalent resistance of 24/7 ≈ 3.5 Ω, and a total of 6.5 Ω for the circuit. In this case, the current across the 3 Ω resistor and the parallel resistor set would then be approximately 7.7 A, and splitting this current between the branches of the parallel circuit would give approximately 3.3 A across the 8 Ω resistor and 4.4 A across the 6 Ω resistor. This makes choice D incorrect.

8.   **B**   A charged particle that moves in a circle due to magnetic force will travel at a speed of $v = qBr/m$ (a formula which can be derived from $qvB = mv^2/r$). Since the particle must travel a distance $2\pi r$ in time T, you have $T = 2\pi m/qB$, where m is the mass of the particle, q is the charge of the particle, and B is the magnetic field strength. According to this formula, if m is the mass of the proton, and q is the charge of the proton, then the mass of the alpha particle will be $4m$, and its charge will be $2q$. If you substitute these variables into the formula, the cyclotron period of the alpha particle becomes $T_\alpha = 2\pi (4m)/2qB = 2(2\pi m/qB) = 2T$.

9.   **C**   The equation for beat frequency is given by $f_{beat} = |f_1 - f_2|$. In this example, f_1 is the fourth harmonic frequency and f_2 is the third harmonic frequency, due to how the fourth harmonic is greater than the third. For a pipe with one end closed off, the resonance frequencies are calculated using the equation $f_n = nv/4L$ ($n = 1, 3, 5...$). The fourth harmonic frequency has $n = 7$, while the third harmonic frequency has $n = 5$. With these equations in mind, Plug In:

$$f_{beat} = |f_{n2} - f_{n1}| = |f_7 - f_5|$$

$$f_{beat} = |[7v/4L] - [5v/4L]| = 2v/4L = v/2L$$

$$L = v/2f_{beat}$$

$$L = 340/(2 \times 680) = 0.25 \text{ m} = 25 \text{ cm}$$

Now that you have the length of the tube, you can use $f_n = nv / 4L$ ($n = 1, 3, 5...$) to find the second harmonic frequency. For a tube with one end closed, the second harmonic frequency has $n = 3$.

$$f_n = nv/4L, \text{ with } n = 3$$

$$f_3 = (3 \times 340)/(4 \times 0.25) = 1020 \text{ Hz}$$

10. **B** This question has two parts to it. In the first part, the intensity (I) is inversely proportional to the area over which the sound is produced ($I = W/m^2$). Sound travels from the speaker to the student in a spherical shape. When it reaches the student, its radius has increased ten times (from 1 meter to 10 meters). Since area is proportional to r^2, the area of the sphere increases $10^2 = 100$ times. A 100-fold increase in area translates to a 100-fold decrease in intensity ($I \propto 1/area$). Since intensity is decreased by a factor of 100, which is 10×10, then the intensity level must decrease by $10 + 10 = 20$ dB. Therefore, the intensity level before the sound enters the headphones is $160 - 20 = 140$ dB. In the second part, the headphones remove 99.9% of the intensity, or the intensity is 1/1000 of the original intensity. Therefore, the intensity is decreased by a factor of 10^3, meaning the intensity level is decreased by 30 dB. The intensity level before entry into the headphones is 140 dB, so the intensity level which is heard is 140 dB − 30 dB = 110 dB.

11. **A** This question relies on an understanding of Snell's Law. The light ray is first incident from the air onto the glass and then incident from the glass into the air. Since the index of refraction of the air does not change from one side of the glass to the other, the index of refraction of the glass does not change, and the angle that the light ray travels throughout the glass does not change, the angle at which the ray emerges into the air is unchanged from the angle at which it originally entered from the air. To see this proven mathematically, first take stock of the known information: The index of refraction of the air (n_1) is 1.00, the index of refraction of the glass (n_2) is 1.50, and the angle of incidence (θ_1) is 30°. Applying Snell's Law for the light incident on the piece of glass from the air,

$$n_1 \sin \theta_1 = n_2 \sin \theta_2$$
$$\sin \theta_2 = n_1 \sin \theta_1 / n_2$$
$$= 1.00(\sin 30°)/1.50$$
$$= 1/6$$

Applying Snell's Law for the light incident on the air from the piece of glass,

$$n_1 \sin \theta_1 = n_2 \sin \theta_2$$
$$\sin \theta_2 = n_1 \sin \theta_1 / n_2$$
$$= 1.00 \cdot (1/6)/1.50$$
$$\theta_2 = \sin^{-1} 0.5 = 30°$$

The angle of incidence for the ray emerging is now the reversed equation. Thus, the angle of the ray emerging from the glass into the air is the same as the angle of the ray entering the glass from the air.

12. **A** The characteristic radiation is produced from an electron falling from an outer to an inner orbital, so the photon emitted will have an energy equal to the difference in the orbital energies. The outer orbital must have a binding energy that is < 4 keV, so the photon emitted with have an energy between 0 keV and 4 keV, choice A. Note that the photoelectron will have a maximum kinetic energy equal to the energy difference between the X-ray photon and the binding energy of the innermost orbital, but the photoelectron is not the characteristic radiation.

SOLUTIONS TO PRACTICE PASSAGE 1

1. **B** If net torque about a point is not equal to zero, there will be a rotation about that point. In free movement of a human arm, only joints will experience rotational motion. This means the shoulder, elbow, or wrist could experience nonzero torques (eliminating choices A, C, and D), but the midpoint of the biceps will always experience zero net torque.

2. **B** The passage indicates (and you should recall) that acceleration is the rate of change of velocity and that jerk bears this same relationship to acceleration. This means graphically that acceleration is the slope of the velocity versus time graph, and that jerk is the slope of the acceleration versus time graph. Taking "percentage of reach" as analogous to time (see the last sentence of the passage), you're looking for a domain over which the slope is a constant. Between 20% and 30%, the curve appears straight, meaning the acceleration would be constant, which in turn means the jerk would be zero. Note that the slope is changing between 0% and 10% as well as between 35% and 45% (when the velocity curve is reaching its maximum and then decreasing), eliminating choices A and C.

3. **B** Answering this question correctly requires correctly interpreting both the description of how the data were taken of the graphs in Figure 1. First, note that since the plane of the tabletop is described as the xy-plane and the sagittal plane dividing the participant in half left and right is the xz-plane, the x direction must be toward and away from the participant. That makes the y direction to the participant's left and right, and the z direction up and down vertically. Thus, when the question asks about the maximum distance from the tabletop, it is referring to the maximum value of z. This occurs according to the right graph in Figure 1 at a value of about $x = 110$ mm (where $z = 80$ mm or so). However, this isn't the answer, because the question then asks for the distance at that point of the hand to the right of its starting point (left or right cannot be distinguished based upon the passage, but left or right must be a value of y). Reading the left graph in Figure 1, you can see that y is about -30 mm when $x = 110$ mm, so choice B is correct. Each of the other choices would be yielded by misinterpreting the significance of x, y, and z.

4. **D** In Figure 2, the peak of the averaged experimental velocity curve (the solid line) is higher than the theoretical curve (the dashed line), so Item I is true. This eliminates choice C. The area under the averaged experimental velocity curve is clearly greater than the area under the theoretical curve, and since the percent range axis is an analogue for time (as noted in the passages), this greater area corresponds to greater displacement. Alternatively, from Figure 1 you can tell that the average experimental participant's hand traveled further to its destination than the theoretical hand because the solid lines are longer. This means Item III is true, eliminating choices A and B. Thus, choice D is correct. Item II is also true, if less obviously so: The maximum slope of the averaged experimental velocity curve seems to be greater than that of the theoretical curve.

5. **A** Based upon units, only choice A can be correct for displacement. Jerk, as acceleration divided by time, has units of m/s^3. Choice A yields meters, choices B and C yield m/s, and choice D yields m^2/s^4.

6. **A** The passage defines the first task as grasping and lifting a cup, then setting it back on the table. Thus, the change in gravitational potential energy of the cup is zero, as is its change in kinetic energy. Thus, the total work must also be zero if other, nonconservative forces are neglected as indicated by the question stem. Note that choice B is the mistaken result of using the maximum vertical displacement of the wrist during the reaching part of the task (when the cup hasn't yet been grasped), and choice C neglects that the cup is set back down on the table.

SOLUTIONS TO PRACTICE PASSAGE 2

1. **C** The passage indicates that the thickness of the layer of still air is inversely proportional to wind speed. According to Equation 1, the heat transfer coefficient is inversely proportional to the thickness of the still air layer. According to Equation 2, heat flux is proportional to the heat transfer coefficient. Consequently, heat flux is proportional to wind speed. As wind speed increases from 2 m/s to 8 m/s, the thickness of the still air layer decreases by a factor of 4, in turn increasing both the heat transfer coefficient and the heat flux by a factor of 4.

2. **B** By the Zeroth Law of Thermodynamics, heat flows from warm regions to cold regions until thermal equilibrium is reached. The steel block has no internal source of heat, so its temperature eventually must equal the air temperature. Choice A is incorrect because wind increases convective cooling, which would increase the block's rate of cooling, not decrease it. Choice C is incorrect because, in the absence of the removal of additional heat energy by evaporation, the block's temperature cannot fall below the air temperature. Choice D is incorrect because after a long time the block must be in thermal equilibrium with the air and therefore must be at the same temperature as the air.

3. **C** Heat flux through the glove is the same as the heat flux through the total still air layer. The glove traps a layer of air that is 5 mm thick. On a windless day the glove has its own layer of still air that is 5 mm thick, for a total thickness of still air of 10 mm or 0.01 m. Ignoring the insulating effect of the glove itself, by Equations 2 and 3, the magnitude of the heat flux through the still air layer is $Q = (k_{air} / t_{air}) \Delta T = (0.026 \text{ W/m·K} / 0.01 \text{ m}) (30 \text{ °C} - (-10 \text{ °C}))$ = 104 W/m². Note that choices A and B can be eliminated without completing the final step of multiplying the coefficients of the terms because they are the wrong order of magnitude (power of ten).

4. **D** Thermal conductivity is a property of a material and does not depend on its thickness or geometry. According to Equation 1, the heat transfer coefficient is inversely proportional to thickness. Two layers of fabric doubles the total thickness of material and therefore reduces the heat transfer coefficient by one half.

5. **C** Item I increases comfort because clothes with higher permeability to water vapor allow greater evaporative cooling and removal of perspiration from the skin. This eliminates choice B. Item II increases comfort because clothes with looser weave allow more convective air flow, which the question stem indicates is another source of cooling. This eliminates choices A and D, so choice C must be correct. Indeed, Item III does not increase comfort because clothes that absorb and retain perspiration increase humidity near the skin, thus decreasing h_e and thus reduce evaporative cooling.

6. **A** The energy required to evaporate 10 grams of water is $\Delta H_{vap} \times m = (2.4 \times 10^6 \text{ J/kg}) (0.01 \text{ kg}) = 2.4 \times 10^4$ J. Though this is not an equation you need to remember, you should be able to derive it using unit analysis, as the question asks about heat (units of joules), the passage provides latent heat of vaporization in J/kg, and the question provides mass in grams (convert to kilograms), so the product of the two given quantities equals the units of the needed quantity.

SOLUTIONS TO PRACTICE PASSAGE 3

1. **A** For the glucose solution to enter the bloodstream, its gauge pressure must be at least as large as the gauge pressure within the artery. Hydrostatic gauge pressure is $\rho g d$, where ρ is the density of the fluid (which equals the specific gravity of the fluid times the density of water), g is acceleration due to gravity, and d is the depth of the fluid. Therefore, 1.33×10^4 Pa = $(1.02)(1000 \text{ kg/m}^3)(10 \text{ m/s}^2)(h)$. Solving for h you get approximately 1.30 m, which is choice A. Note that choices B and D can be eliminated as the answer is expected to be less than 1.33 times ten to the something. Also, as a practical matter, choices C and D could be eliminated since 13 m is very large.

2. **C** Item I is false: Equation 1 describes the pressure drop per length in an artery. It varies directly with viscosity, therefore, a decrease in viscosity would *decrease* the pressure drop per length (choices A and D can be eliminated). Item II is false: In a similar fashion, since R is in the denominator, widening the artery would also decrease $\Delta P/L$ (choice B can be eliminated). Item III is true: Increasing the flow rate also increases $\Delta P/L$ (choice C is correct).

3. **A** Choice C can be eliminated because you can expect the answer to be at an extreme location, a node or antinode. Choice D can be eliminated given that an increase in pressure indicates the individual pressure amplitudes must have added together, which corresponds to a pressure antinode. A pressure antinode occurs at a displacement node, which is choice A.

4. **C** The equation relating pressure and fluid speed is Bernoulli's equation. Since the syringe is horizontal, the potential energy term can be neglected: $P_{barrel} + (1/2)\rho(v_{barrel})^2 = P_{needle} + (1/2)\rho(v_{needle})^2$. Also, since the area of the barrel is so much larger than the area of the needle, then v_{barrel} is negligible (due to the continuity equation, $A_1 v_1 = A_2 v_2$). Therefore, $(1/2)\rho(v_{needle})^2 = P_{barrel} - P_{needle}$, which is equal to the force on the plunger divided by the area. So $(1/2)(1000 \text{ kg/m}^3)(v_{needle})^2 = (5 \text{ N})/(25 \times 10^{-6} \text{ m}^2)$. Thus, $v_{needle} = 20$ m/s, which is choice C.

5. **C** The continuity equation states that $A_1 v_1 = A_2 v_2$. If the diameter decreases by one-third its previous value, it is now 2/3 of its previous value. The area is therefore $(2/3)^2 = 4/9$ its previous value. Because A and v are inversely proportional, v is now 9/4 its previous value.

6. **B** The passage states that a blood vessel collapses when the pressure drops too low. It follows that the more rapidly pressure drops, the higher the frequency of collapse. Equation 1 shows which factors cause a drop in pressure. More blood being pumped from the heart increases the flow rate, which in turn increases the pressure drop per length, making choice B the correct answer. Choices C and D concern density, which does not appear in Equation 1.

SOLUTIONS TO PRACTICE PASSAGE 4

1. **B** There are two concepts tested in this question: the direction of current flow and the subsequent charge left on the drop. First, consider the current flow. Current is defined as the flow of positive charge, and thus will flow away from the positive voltage in the charging wire. This eliminates choices A and C. If current is flowing away from the charging wire, negative ions are flowing towards the charging wire and/or positive ions are flowing away from the charging wire. In either case, that would leave a positive charge at the break-off point, eliminating choice D. Thus, the correct answer is choice B.

2. **D.** Both types of T-cells are present in whole blood, which eliminates choice B. Although it is true that these types of T-cells have similar sizes and shapes, which would make them impossible to distinguish using scattered light, fluorescence could be used to differentiate between the two, eliminating choice A. Since the question asks about sorting out both T helper and T killer cells, two fluorescent antibodies are needed, making the correct answer choice D. (All T-cells are CD_3^+)

3. **A** The deflection of the drop in the x-direction is a result of the acceleration of the drop caused by the electric force $a = F/m = (qE)/m$. The size of the drop doesn't affect the external electric field, so the acceleration depends on the ratio q/m. (Note that the magnitude of the electric field determines the deflection of drop, but not how much it changes with a change in size, so choice D can be eliminated.) The passage indicates that charge is proportional to the surface area of the drop: $q \propto 4\pi r^2 \rightarrow q \propto r^2$. On the other hand, the mass of the drop is proportional to its volume, $m = \rho V \rightarrow m \propto (4/3) \pi r^3 \rightarrow m \propto r^3$. Therefore, $q/m \propto r^2/r^3 \rightarrow q/m \propto 1/r$. So for a larger r, the ratio q/m will be smaller, resulting in a lower acceleration. If the drop experiences less acceleration, it will not go as far in the x-direction, meaning that it will fall short of the sample container, choice A.

4. **D** If the drop is charged, it can affect the charge of the next drop through the electrostatic force. The electrostatic force is a force that acts at a distance, which eliminates choice A. The electrostatic force is independent of the acceleration of the drops as long as the acceleration isn't so great that the drops are very far from each other, and the question states that successive drops are closely spaced. This eliminates choice B. The passage states that the ions in the flow stream "move rapidly," which implies that residual charge from drop wouldn't linger too long in the break-off point once the charging wire voltage were changed, which eliminates choice C. Since the drop in this question is negatively charged, it will exert an attractive force to the positive ions in the flow stream, and that force will be strongest at the break-off point, which is closest to the drop. Thus, more positive ions will be in the next drop than there would be if the drop that just left the break-off point were neutral.

5. **C** The passage states that it is forward scattering, not side-scattering that is proportional to size, which eliminates choice A. Red blood cells do not contain nuclei, whereas T-cells do, which eliminates choice B. Because RBCs do not contain nuclei, they have less internal complexity than T-cells, which would suggest that they would have scatter less sideways than T-cells. Since the question tells us that the side-scattering is the same, something else must be increasing the side-scattering of the RBC. The difference in shape between the RBC and the T-cell is a possible candidate for that difference. Diffraction would only happen if the cells were about the size of the wavelength, not if they are larger, so that eliminates choice D. Thus, choice C is the answer.

6. **C** The deflection plates are creating the electric field which exerts electric forces on the charged droplets, so the answer can't be choices A or B because these answer choices describe what happens to charges feeling a force from the electric field, and they do not describe the charges creating the electric field. Electric fields created by source charges point away from positive source charges and toward negative source charges, which is described correctly in choice C.

SOLUTIONS TO PRACTICE PASSAGE 5

1. **A**   One should not typically rely on figures for precise answers, but Figure 2 does reveal that the period of oscillation is at least approximately constant. The key to this question is to notice that the term inside the argument of the cosine is of the form (ωt), or a constant (for any given set of values k, b, and m) times t, and thus the frequency of the cosine is itself constant ($\omega/2\pi$).

2. **B**   The easiest approach to this question is to write out the named and desired variables and then to consider the possible relations among them. The question stem asks for stiffness, which is k. Choices A though C specify period T (the distance from peak to peak along the time axis), the initial amplitude A, and the mass m. The argument of the cosine function in Equation 2 shows that m, k, and time T are all functionally related, whereas amplitude is absent (choice B is correct). Alternatively, recall the ideal case of the simple harmonic spring and mass oscillator, where period depends upon spring constant k and mass m but is independent of amplitude A.

3. **B**   As always, slope is rise over run, which in this case yields y/t. Taking the units of this quantity you find $[y]/[t]$ = m/s, which are of course the units of velocity.

4. **A**   This is a slight variation on the classic 2x2 POE question, because in this case the amplitude decays either more or less rapidly than in the experimental set up with a less viscous liquid, whereas the frequency can, among the choices, decrease, increase, or remain the same. The passage defines b, the *damping coefficient*, as "a measure of the frictional effects on the system due to the movement of the submerged plate through the fluid." Because a more viscous liquid has provides greater fluid friction, b should increase with increased viscosity. A larger b means a larger negative exponent in Equation 3, meaning a more rapid decrease in amplitude. It also means a smaller coefficient of t in the argument of the cosine function (because the term containing b is subtracted from k/m), which means a lower frequency of oscillation.

5. **C**   The total mechanical energy of a harmonic oscillator, the sum of its kinetic and potential energies at any time t, is equal to its maximum potential energy at that time t, or $\frac{1}{2}kA_t^2$ (this is just another way of saying that the energy in an oscillating system like a wave goes as the square of the amplitude). For the case of a simple harmonic oscillator, that energy is constant because amplitude is constant, but for this damped harmonic oscillator the amplitude varies as the exponential term in Equation 3. The question asks at what time the energy will be one-quarter its original value, which means you are looking for the time at which the amplitude will be half its original value (the square root of a quarter). Thus, you have

$$Ae^{-bt/2m} = \frac{1}{2}A \rightarrow \ln(e^{-bt/2m}) = \ln(\frac{1}{2}) = -\ln(2) \rightarrow \frac{bt}{2m} = \ln(2) \rightarrow t = \frac{2m\ln(2)}{b}.$$

Note that choice A corresponds to the time at which the oscillator first crosses its equilibrium length (that is, when cosine is zero).

6. **D**   The rate of decay of the amplitude of oscillations is determined by the exponential term, which contains b and m but not k. Thus, the stiffness of the spring has no effect on the amplitude. Choices B and C, changing the area of the plate or draining the liquid from the tank, would each alter the value of b.

SOLUTIONS TO PRACTICE PASSAGE 6

1. **C** The passage defines the scattering angle as "the angle between the photon's original path and its path after the collision." Drawing a continuation of any original path in the diagram shows that $\theta/2$ is the supplement of this angle. Therefore, $180° - \theta/2$, choice C, is correct.

2. **B** Since the scattered photon only loses a small portion of its energy to an electron, it is likely to still be an energetic X-ray photon. Since they are scattered in all directions, they can be detected on X-ray films as noise. This makes Item I true, eliminating choice C. For similar reasons, the scattered photons also pose a danger to nearby personnel who are at risk of being exposed to unknown amounts of scattered radiation. This makes Item II true, eliminating choice A. X-ray photons are higher in energy, and therefore higher in frequency than visible photons, which means that X-rays have shorter wavelengths than visible light. Since visible light has wavelengths in the 100s of nanometers, and the smallest bone in the body (the stapes) is a few millimeters, Item III is false, eliminating choice D. Thus, choice B is the answer.

3. **B** The maximum value of $\Delta\lambda$ will occur at the maximum value for $(1 - \cos\phi)$, as that is the term in Equation 1 subject to change for a given incident wavelength. Because cosine varies between 1 and –1 inclusive, the maximum value of this term is 2, hence the answer is twice the fractional coefficient. Choice B is correct.

4. **D** This problem can be solved using POE. Choice A is wrong because there is nothing in the passage to indicate that Compton scattering occurs with any regularity in the air (indeed there are far fewer free electrons in air than on the surface of a metal, making Compton scattering that much less likely). Moreover, the scintillation detector is designed to detect photons, not electrons. Choice B is wrong because the desired scattering angle is achieved by the experimental set up using the circular arced target. Choice C is wrong because cosmic rays would arrive at the detector from all directions above the experimental surface with equal probability, so placing the shield between the Am-241 source and the detector would not especially screen them out (if the problem had said that the lead shield formed a dome over the detector, choice C could be a viable choice). Choice D is correct because the experimenter desires not to allow photons leaving the Am-241 source to enter the detector directly without first scattering off the target.

5. **A** The rate of scattering events can be determined by taking the ratio of number of detections to the duration over which those detections occurred. The ratio of 1242:4 hours is greater than any of the remaining three ratios, so choice A is correct.

6. **B** This is a classic 2x2 MCAT question, in which the two differing options are the peak energy and the number of detections (the error factor is a trap—there is no information explicitly in the passage or table to indicate how it arises). Because the trend in peak energies is steadily decreasing as scattering angle increases, one should interpolate that the peak energy at 105° will fall between the peak energies at 90° and 120°, thus eliminating choices C and D. Determining the likely number of detections requires looking at the ratio between detection number and experimental duration. For a 12-hour run, one would expect about 1.5 times as many detections as in an 8 hour run at a scattering similar angle. Picking a number of detections between 1411 and 1206 (say around 1300) and multiplying that by 1.5 yields 1950, which is closest to 1935 (choice B is correct).

Chapter 23
Psychology and
Sociology on the MCAT

23.1 PSYCHOLOGY AND SOCIOLOGY ON THE MCAT

This section will test your content knowledge of psychological, biological, and sociological factors that shape human thought, perception, behavior, attitude, and learning. Furthermore, you will be expected to have a basic understanding of mental illness, social structure, and global disparities in health, health care, and social class. The MCAT will test your knowledge and application of these subjects at approximately the level that you would be expected to understand them in an introductory psychology class (one semester), introductory sociology class (one semester), and an introductory biology class (two semesters, though you should be prepared for more advanced physiology concepts, like you would see on the MCAT Biological and Biochemical Foundations of Living Systems section). The application of this material is potentially vast; passages can discuss anything from the specifics about a psychological research study to the complexities of studying population dynamics, to the nuances of an unusual neurological disease. Additionally, questions on the Psych/Soc section will require you to demonstrate your scientific inquiry, reasoning, and understanding of basic research and statistical methods as applied to concepts in the psychological, sociological, and biological sciences. Overall, this section is designed to test your knowledge and application of the behavioral, biological, and social determinants of health and wellness.

The science sections of the MCAT have 10 passages and 15 freestanding questions (FSQs). On the Psych/Soc section, introductory biology will comprise approximately 10% of the questions, introductory sociology concepts will comprise roughly 30% of the questions, and introductory psychology concepts will comprise about 60% of the questions.

23.2 TACKLING A PSYCH/SOC PASSAGE

In order to complete all of the passages and freestanding questions on the Psych/Soc section, it will be important to tackle this section strategically. An understanding about the types of passages you will encounter should help you accomplish this.

Experiment/Research Presentation

This type of passage on the Psych/Soc section will typically present some information about a relevant topic, and also present the details behind an experiment relating to that topic. Data will be presented in tables, graphs, and/or figures. These passages are challenging because they require an understanding of the reasoning and logic behind the experiment and research, the ability to analyze the results and form conclusions, and a basic understanding of statistics.

Information/Situation Presentation

This type of passage will generally present a basic concept with additional detail (that goes well beyond an introductory-level understanding) or a novel concept (like a rare neurological disease) that extrapolates information from more basic information. In order to tackle these passages, first, do not panic if you see information that you've never heard about! Rather, look for concepts that parallel what you *do* know about. For example, if you see a question about a rare neurological disorder, look for information that applies to your basic knowledge of the nervous system.

However, in order to answer passage questions and freestanding questions effectively and efficiently, you *will* need to know your basics. Don't waste time staring at a passage or question wondering, "Should I know this?" Instead, with a solid foundation in the basic core knowledge, you will be confident that you are *not* expected to know about this random, rare disease, and rather will find information in the passage and/or apply core concepts.

23.3   READING A PSYCH/SOC PASSAGE

The first thing to keep in mind about passages on the MCAT is that you can do the passages in any order you want to. There are no bonus points for taking the test in order. In fact you may lose points if there is in easy passage at the end and you either run out of time or have to rush through it. Therefore, tackle the passages that you are most comfortable with first, and save the harder ones for last.

Although tempting, try not to get too bogged down in reading all of the little details in a passage. While it is easy to get lost in the science or the glut of background information in a passage, it isn't necessary to read every nuance. In fact, try to spend no more than one or two minutes mapping a passage.

For Experiment/Research Presentation passages, you will need to read more closely/carefully. You will likely have questions concerning the experimental design and/or the data and results. Therefore, invest a little more time reading so you understand the experiment and the outcomes, but don't worry about completely absorbing the results until you see what types of questions are asked.

For Information/Situation Presentation passages, you will not need to read as closely or as carefully. These can be skimmed to get a general sense of where the information is located within the passage. Furthermore, these passages may contain a fair amount of detailed information that you may not need, so save your time—don't bother reading all of the details until you come to a question that asks about them, then go back and read more closely.

Advanced Reading Skills

To improve your ability to read and glean information from a passage, you need to practice. Be critical when you read the content; watch for vague areas or holes in the passage that aren't explained clearly. Remember that information about new topics will be woven throughout the passage; you may need to piece together information from several paragraphs and a figure to get the whole picture.

After you've read, highlighted, and mapped a passage (more on this in a bit) stop and ask yourself the following questions:

- What was this passage about? What was the conclusion or main point?
- Was there a paragraph that was mostly background?
- Were there paragraphs or figures that seemed useless?
- What information was found in each paragraph? Why was that paragraph there?
- Are there any holes in the story?

- What extra information could I have pulled out of the passage? What inferences or conclusions could I make?
- If something unique was explained or mentioned, what might be its purpose?
- What am I *not* being told?
- Can I summarize the purpose and/or results of the experiment in a few sentences?
- Were there any comparisons in the passage?

This takes a while at first, but eventually becomes second nature and you will start doing it as you read a passage. If you have a study group you are working with, consider doing this as an exercise with your study partners. Take turns asking and answering the questions above. Having to explain something to someone else not only solidifies your own knowledge, but helps you see where you might be weak.

23.4   MAPPING A PSYCH/SOC PASSAGE

Mapping a Psych/Soc passage is a combination of highlighting and scratch paper notes that can help you organize and understand the passage information. First, determine whether it is an experiment/research or information/situation passage. How you highlight will vary slightly depending on the type of passage.

Resist the temptation to highlight everything (everyone has done this: You're reading a psychology textbook with a highlighter, and then look back and realize that the whole page is yellow!). For Information/Situation passages, restrict your highlighting to the following:

- the main theme of a paragraph
- an unusual or unfamiliar term that is defined specifically for that passage (e.g., something that is italicized)
- statements that either support the main theme or contradict the main theme
- list topics: sometimes lists appear in paragraph form within a passage; highlight the general topic of the list
- key words that are topics or definitions you learned during class
- transition words like "however," "although," and "therefore"

For Experiment/Research passages, you will want to highlight the above and also include the most important details about the study:

- What did the researchers hypothesize?
- What methods did they use?
- What were the results?

To keep highlighting minimal, highlight only the words you need that tell you where to look for the details of the study. Look for key words that tell you where to look, not entire sentences. Highlighting phrases like "the study found," "the researchers predicted," or "participants were drawn from" lets you know where important information about the study is located without turning your screen into a bright yellow mess.

Scratch paper should be organized. Make sure the passage number and the range of questions for that passage appear at the top of your scratch paper notes. For each paragraph, note "P1," "P2," etc., on the scratch paper, and jot down a few notes about that paragraph. Try to translate science-y jargon into your own words using everyday language (this is particularly useful for experiments). Also, make sure to jot down simple relationships (e.g., the relationship between two variables).

Pay attention to figures and tables to see what type of information they contain. Don't spend a lot of time analyzing at this point, but do jot down on your scratch paper "Fig 1" and a brief summary of the data. Also, if you've discovered a list in the passage, note its topic and location down on your scratch paper.

Let's take a look at how we might highlight and map a practice passage:

Psychotic disorders—most notably schizophrenia and bipolar disorder with psychotic features—affect approximately 2% of Americans. These disorders are extremely manageable with psychotropic medications—to relieve symptoms such as hallucinations and delusions—and behavioral therapy, such as social skills training and hygiene maintenance.

However, individuals with psychotic disorders have the lowest level of medication compliance, as compared to individuals with mood or anxiety disorders. Antipsychotic medications can have extremely negative side effects, including uncontrollable twitching of the face or limbs, blurred vision, and weight gain, among others. They also must be taken frequently, and at high doses, in order to be effective. While relatively little is known about the reasons for noncompliance, studies do suggest that in schizophrenia, age of diagnosis and medication compliance is positively correlated. Evidence also suggests that medication noncompliance is disproportionally prevalent in individuals of a low socioeconomic status (SES) due to issues such as homelessness, lack of insurance benefits, and lack of familial or social support.

Researchers were interested to see how drug education might affect compliance or noncompliance with psychotropic medications based on patient socioeconomic status. In a study of 1200 mentally ill individuals in the Los Angeles metro area, researchers measured baseline psychotropic medication compliance, then provided patients with a free educational seminar on drug therapy, and then measured psychotropic medication compliance six months later. The one-day, 8-hour seminar included information on positive effects of psychotropic medication, side effects of psychotropic medication, psychotropic medication interactions with other substances such as alcohol and non-prescribed drugs, and information on accessing MediCare benefits. Compliance was measured by number of doses of prescribed psychotropic medication that the patients took in a week, over the course of 12 weeks, as compared with the number of doctor-recommended doses per week. Compliance was measured using a self-report questionnaire.

Results indicated that post-seminar, mentally ill patients from middle or upper class backgrounds (Upper and Middle SES) were significantly more compliant with their psychotropic medication regimens than prior to the seminar. However, no significant differences were found in patients at or below the poverty level (Lower SES). Table 1 displays psychotropic medication compliance by SES and disorder.

Disorder	SES	Pre-Seminar Compliance	Post-Seminar Compliance
Bipolar I	Upper	60%	73%
	Middle	57%	61%
	Lower	25%	27%
Schizophrenia	Upper	53%	65%
	Middle	51%	62%
	Lower	22%	26%

Table 1 Psychotropic Medication Compliance by Socioeconomic Status (SES) and Disorder

Analysis and Passage Map

This passage is an Experiment/Research Presentation passage and starts with an introduction to the topic, psychotic disorders (specifically schizophrenia and bipolar disorder). This is primarily a background information paragraph and can be skimmed quickly, with a few specific words/phrases highlighted.

The second paragraph starts with "however" indicating a change in direction. The first paragraph said that schizophrenia is easily managed with drugs and therapy, but the second paragraph indicates that that isn't the whole story—in fact, the main topic of the passage is presented—medication noncompliance, particularly in low socioeconomic (SES) individuals.

The third paragraph presents relevant information about the study conducted to determine the impact of drug education on medication noncompliance in various SES groups. It is important to highlight the key features of the study here—what is it looking at and how is data collected. You do not necessarily need to highlight every single detail, but understand the basic premise of the study.

The final paragraph describes the results of the study, and it presents the data in Table 1. The paragraph provides you with the significant finding that is demonstrated by the data in the table—while upper and middle SES individuals demonstrated an increased medication compliance after the drug education treatment, low SES individuals did not.

Here is what your scratch paper should look like:

P1—psychotic disorders are manageable with medication and therapy
P2—but medication compliance is a big problem, especially for low SES
P3—STUDY: medication compliance by SES before and after a drug education seminar
P4—RESULTS: medication compliance increases for upper and middle SES, no improvement for low SES
Table 1—medication compliance by SES for schizophrenia and bipolar I

Table Analysis

The previous passage, like most passages on the MCAT, included a table, graph, or figure. To maximize your score, it is important to develop table analysis skills. Often, tables will include much more information than is needed to answer any given question on the passage.

Don't try to understand every piece of information in a table or figure the first time through. This will take valuable time away from attacking the question and POE, which is where you stand to pick up the most points.

Here is what you should look for the first time through a passage:
- Read the caption that describes the table or graph. It is short and contains most of the info you need to understand the results. If you get a question about the data, you will know where to look.
- Is there an indicator for significant results? Often stars are used to indicate that results reach a significance criteria set out in the study. Questions like to play around with significance and noticing this can help you avoid trap answers and add points to your raw total.
- For graphs, does it contain a key? Make a mental note if it does.
- For tables, what are the different categories? Most tables contain only about 3–5 rows and columns, so take a quick moment to scan how the table is broken down.

Most figures on the Psychology and Sociology section are relatively straightforward: simple bar graphs and tables are the most common. You are unlikely to see complex conceptual layouts that you might find in an O-Chem or Biology passage. Other simple figures like line graphs may also appear but this is less likely. This is more reason to get through the figure as quickly as possible. Many passages with figures don't even contain questions that require you to look back to the figure!

For the figure above, notice that it is a table. Read the caption for background. Make note of the categories in the columns (SES, Pre-Seminar Compliance, and Post-Seminar Compliance) and rows (Bipolar I and Schizophrenia). Finally, notice that there is no marker for significance and that's it, you're off to the passages. Do not spend too much time on figures during the first pass on the Psyc Soc section. Save in depth analysis (and time) for the questions!

23.5   TACKLING THE QUESTIONS

Questions on the Psych/Soc section mimic the three typical science question types: Memory, Explicit, and Implicit.

Memory Questions in the Psych/Soc Section

Memory questions are exactly what they sound like: They test your knowledge of some specific fact or concept. While Memory questions are typically found as freestanding questions, they can also be tucked into a passage. The questions, aside from requiring memorization, do not generally cause problems for students because they are similar to the types of questions that would appear on a typical college psychology or sociology exam. Below are two examples of Memory questions, taken from the passage above:

1. What is one "positive" symptom of schizophrenia?

   A) Catatonia
   B) Weight gain
   C) Flattened affect
   D) Auditory or visual hallucinations

2. Bipolar disorder involves periods of mania and depression, and for some, episodes of hypomania. Hypomania, a state that is less severe than mania, is characterized by "feeling good/high" and increased well-being and productiveness. Which of the mechanisms is most likely involved with the hypomanic episodes experienced by individuals diagnosed with bipolar disorder?

   A) Increased dopamine in the brain
   B) Decreased stimulation of the enteric plexus
   C) Increased activation of the posterior pituitary
   D) Decreased serotonin in the central nervous system

These are Memory questions because, even though they are associated with the passage, you could have answered them (and should be able to answer them) without reading the passage. It is important that you recognize them as a Memory questions so you don't go back to the passage and waste time looking for answers that are not there! There is no specific "trick" to answering Memory questions; either you know the correct answer or you don't.

If you find that you are missing a fair number of Memory questions, it is a sure sign that you do not know the content well enough. Go back and review.

Solutions for the questions above are:

1. **D** A "positive" symptom of schizophrenia is an addition to, excess of, or distortion of normal functions; auditory or visual hallucinations are positive symptoms of the illness (choice D is correct). A "negative" symptom of schizophrenia is a diminishment or absence of normal function; catatonia (lack or responsiveness to stimuli) and flattened affect (lack of emotion) are both negative symptoms (choice A and choice C are wrong). Weight gain is often a side effect of psychotropic medications, not a symptom of schizophrenia (choice B is wrong).

2. **A** Dopamine is the primary neurotransmitter involved with the "reward centers" of the brain; since hypomania is characterized by "feeling good/high," it can reasonably be concluded that an increase of dopamine in the brain could produce this effect (choice A is correct). The enteric plexus or enteric nervous system is a portion of the autonomic nervous system that controls the gastrointestinal tract; decreased stimulation of the enteric nervous system would not produce any of the characteristics of hypomania described (choice B is wrong). The posterior pituitary is responsible for producing oxytocin, a hormone that controls lactation and uterine contractions, and vasopressin, a hormone that controls how much water the kidneys resorb; therefore, increased activation of the posterior pituitary would not produce any of the characteristics of hypomania described (choice C is wrong). Serotonin is a neurotransmitter with widespread effects in the brain; a decrease of serotonin in the brain has been shown to produce symptoms of depression, not hypomania (choice D is wrong).

Explicit Questions in the Psych/Soc section

A purely Explicit question can be answered with only information in the passage. Below is an example of a pure Explicit question from the passage above:

3. What is the incidence of psychotic disorders in the American population?

    A) 1%
    B) 2%
    C) 4%
    D) Unknown

Referring back to the first paragraph of the passage, it clearly states that "Psychotic disorders—most notably schizophrenia and bipolar disorder with psychotic features—affect approximately 2% of Americans;" therefore, choice B is correct.

True, pure Explicit questions are rare in the Psych/Soc section. More often on the Psych/Soc section, Explicit questions are more of a blend of Explicit and Memory; they require not only retrieval of passage information, but also recall of some relevant information. They usually do not require in-depth analysis or connections. Here is an example of a common type of Explicit question:

4. Based on the design of the study described in the passage, what limits the researchers' abilities to draw conclusions about the causal relationship between socioeconomic status and psychotropic medication compliance?

A) Age at first diagnosis was not measured.
B) Participants were not randomly assigned to socioeconomic status.
C) The sample contained only Los Angeles metro area residents.
D) Severity of symptoms were not measured.

To answer this question, you first need to retrieve information from the passage about the study's experimental design (from paragraph 3). You also need to recall some information about experimental design, and what sort of factors limit a researcher's ability to infer a causal relationship.

Here is the solution to the question above:

4. **B** Causation is extremely difficult to determine when experimenting with humans, particularly because all of the variables in a given experiment must by controlled by the researcher, and subjects must be randomly assigned to experimental and control groups. Therefore, random assignment of subjects to a group (in this case, a socioeconomic status group) is one of the many variables that should have been controlled for in order to determine a causal relationship between socioeconomic status and psychotropic medication compliance (choice B is correct). While age at first diagnosis and symptom severity are important variables that could have been measured, neither specifically limits the researchers' abilities to draw conclusions about the causal relationship between socioeconomic status and psychotropic medication compliance (choices A and D are wrong). The fact that the sample only contained participants from the Los Angeles metro area limits the researchers' ability to draw conclusions about how their results might apply to the general population, not about causality (choice C is wrong).

A final subgroup in the Explicit question category are graph or data interpretation questions. These questions will either ask you to take graphical information from the passage and convert it into a text answer, or will ask you to take text from the passage and convert it into a graph. Below is an example from the passage above:

5. Which of the following graphs would best illustrate the relationship between age of schizophrenia diagnosis and medication compliance described in the passage?

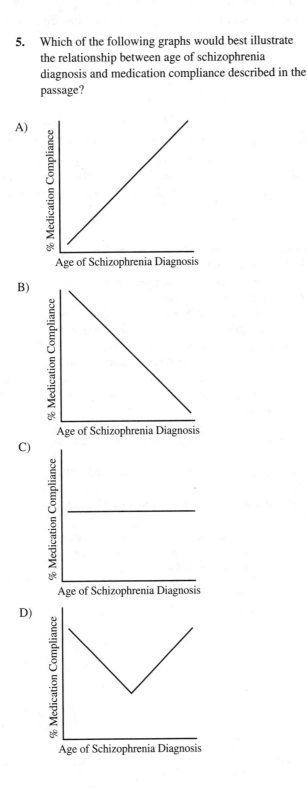

The passage states, in the second paragraph, that "...studies do suggest that in schizophrenia, age of diagnosis and medication compliance is positively correlated." Therefore, as age of diagnosis increases, so does compliance. Therefore, a graphical representation should look like the figure in choice A.

If you find you are missing Explicit questions, practice your passage mapping. Make sure you aren't missing the critical items in the passage that lead you to the right answer. Slow down a little; take an extra 15 to 30 seconds per passage to read or think about it more carefully.

Implicit Questions

Implicit questions require the most thought. These require recall not only of Psych/Soc content information, but also information gleaned from the passage, and a more in-depth analysis of how the two relate. Implicit questions require more analysis and connections to be made than Explicit questions. Often they take the form "If...then...." Below is an example of a classic Implicit question, based on the passage above:

6. If the experiment described in the passage were repeated, but instead of testing how drug education affects compliance, researchers measured how incentives affect compliance in low SES schizophrenics. The low SES schizophrenia group was broken into two groups. Group A received an incentive every time they took their medication for seven consecutive days, while Group B received an incentive every two weeks, regardless of compliance level. Based on operant conditioning principles, what results should the researchers see?

A) There is no difference in compliance levels from the first study.
B) Group A's compliance should be higher than Group B's compliance.
C) Group B's compliance should be higher than Group A's compliance.
D) Both groups should demonstrate increased compliance from the first study, but it is impossible to tell which group's compliance is expected to be higher.

To answer this question, conclusions have to be drawn about the experiment described in the passage, and the new experiment described in the question stem, and then applied to your content knowledge about reward schedules in operant conditioning. Many, many more connections need to be made than when answering an Explicit question. A detailed explanation for this question is below:

6. **B** According to the question, Group A is receiving an incentive on a fixed-ratio schedule (after every seven consecutive days of medication compliance) and Group B is receiving an incentive on a fixed-interval schedule (every two weeks, regardless of compliance). According to operant conditioning principles, a fixed-ratio schedule should produce a high rate of desired behavior (in this case, medication compliance), while a fixed-interval schedule produces a steady rate of response that tends to increase closer to the reward, but is not nearly as frequent as what is expected from a fixed-ratio reward schedule (choice B is correct; choice C is wrong). Based on operant conditioning principles, rewarding desired behavior should increase behavior (choice A is wrong), and applying a fixed-ratio and fixed-interval reward schedule should increase behavior in predictable ways (choice D is wrong).

If you find that you are missing a lot of Implicit questions, first of all, make sure that you are using POE aggressively. Second, go back and review the explanations for the correct answer, to figure out where your logic went awry. Did you miss an important fact in the passage? Did you forget the relevant Psych/Soc content? Did you follow the logical train of thought to the right answer? Once you figure out where you made your mistake, you will know how to correct it.

23.6 SUMMARY OF THE APPROACH TO PSYCHOLOGY AND SOCIOLOGY

How to Map the Passage and Use Scratch Paper

1) The passage should not be read like textbook material, with the intent of learning something from every sentence (science majors especially will be tempted to read this way). Passages should be read to get a feel for the type of questions that will follow, and to get a general idea of the location of information within the passage.

2) Highlighting—Use this tool sparingly, or you will end up with a passage that is completely covered in yellow highlighter! Highlighting in a Psych/Soc passage should be used to draw attention to a few words that demonstrate one of the following:
   - the main theme of a paragraph
   - an unusual or unfamiliar term that is defined specifically for that passage (e.g., something that is italicized)
   - statements that either support the main theme or counteract the main theme
   - list topics (see below)
   - relationships

3) Pay brief attention to figures and experiments, noting only what information they deal with. Do not spend a lot of time analyzing at this point.

4) For each passage, start by noting the passage number, the general topic, and the range of questions on your scratch paper. You can then work between your scratch paper and the review screen to easily get to the questions you want (see Chapter 1).

5) For each paragraph, note "P1," "P2," etc. on the scratch paper and jot down a few notes about that paragraph. Try to translate psych/soc jargon into your own words using everyday language. Especially note down simple relationships (e.g., the relationship between two variables).

6) Lists—Whenever a list appears in paragraph form, jot down on the scratch paper the paragraph and the general topic of the list. It will make returning to the passage more efficient and help to organize your thoughts.

7) Scratch paper is only useful if it is kept organized! Make sure that your notes for each passage are clearly delineated and marked with the passage number and question range. This will allow you to easily read your notes when you come back to review a marked question. Resist the temptation to write in the first available blank space as this makes it much more difficult to refer back to your work.

Psych/Soc Question Strategies

1) Remember that the content in Psychology and Sociology is broad but not necessarily super deep, so don't panic if something seems completely unfamiliar. Understand the basic content well, find the basics in the unfamiliar topic, and apply them to the question.

2) POE is paramount! The strikeout tool allows you to eliminate answer choices; this will improve your chances of guessing the correct answer if you are unable to narrow it down to one choice.

3) Answer the straightforward questions first (typically the Memory questions). Leave questions that require analysis of experiments and graphs for later. Take the test in the order YOU want. Make sure to use your scratch paper to indicate questions you've skipped.

4) Make sure that the answer you choose actually answers the question, and isn't just a true statement.

5) Try to avoid answer choices with extreme words such as "always," "never," etc. In Psych/Soc, there is almost always an exception and answers are rarely black-and-white.

6) I-II-III questions: Always work between the I-II-III statements and the answer choices. Unfortunately, it is not possible to strike out the Roman numerals, but this is a great use for scratch paper notes. Once a statement is determined to be true (or false), strike out answer choices that do not contain (or do contain) that statement.

7) LEAST/EXCEPT/NOT questions: Don't get tricked by these questions that ask you to pick that answer that doesn't fit (the incorrect or false statement). It's often good to use your scratch paper and write a T or F next to answer choices A–D. The one that stands out as different is the correct answer!

8) Again, don't leave any question blank.

23.7   MCAT PSYCHOLOGY AND SOCIOLOGY TOPIC LIST[1]

Sociology

A. Social Theories
1. micro vs. macro sociology
2. functionalism
3. conflict theory
4. symbolic interactionism
5. social constructionism
6. rational choice/social exchange
7. feminist theory

B. Social Institutions
1. education
2. health and medicine
3. family/religion
4. government/economy

C. Culture
1. statuses, roles, groups
2. material vs. nonmaterial (symbolic) culture
3. transmission/diffusion of culture
4. culture lag/culture shock
5. assimilation and multiculturalism
6. dominant culture, subcultures/ countercultures

D. Demographics
1. age, gender
2. race/ethnicity, immigration
3. sexual orientation
4. shifts and social change (population changes, social movements, globalization, urbanization)

E. Social Inequality
1. spatial (residential, environmental, global)
2. social class/stratification (class, status, power, cultural/social capital, privilege/ prestige)
3. intersection with race, gender, age
4. social mobility (inter/intragenerational, downward/upward, meritocracy)
5. poverty (absolute/relative)
6. health and healthcare disparities

F. Self-Identity
1. types of identities (race/ethnicity, age/ gender, class, sexual orientation)
1. self-efficacy, self-esteem, locus of control
2. identity development theories (gender, moral, social, etc.)
3. effect of social factors on identity formation (individual/groups)
4. effect of culture/socialization on identify formation

G. Social Interaction
1. attribution (theory, fundamental error, effect of culture)
2. prejudice/bias
3. stereotypes, self-fulfilling prophecy, stereotype threat
4. stigma
5. facilitations/hindrances
6. impression management, dramaturgical approach
7. message processing (verbal/nonverbal communication, roles of gender/ culture etc.)
8. persuasion and compliance
9. social behavior (attraction, aggression, attachment, altruism)
10. discrimination
11. effects of others on individual behavior (social facilitation, social loafing, bystander effect, peer pressure, conformity, etc.)
12. group dynamics (polarization, groupthink)
13. social norms/social deviance
14. collective behavior
15. socialization agents (peers, family, media, coworkers/workplace)

---

[1]   Adapted from *The Official Guide to the MCAT Exam (MCAT2015)*, 4th ed., © 2014 Association of American Medical Colleges.

Psychology

A. Personality
1. psychoanalytic perspective
2. humanistic perspective
3. behaviorist/social cognitive perspective
4. trait/biological perspectives

B. Attitude
1. affect, behavior, cognition
2. attitudes predict behavior
3. cognitive dissonance

C. Motivation
1. major elements (drive, needs, instinct, etc.)
2. drive-reduction theory
3. incentive theory
4. levels of need (Maslow's hierarchy)
5. biological drives

D. Emotion
1. components (behavioral, physiological, cognitive)
2. six universal emotions
3. adaptive role of emotion
4. James-Lange Theory
5. Cannon-Bard Theory
6. Schachter-Singer Theory
7. biological role of emotion (brain regions, limbic system, autonomic nervous system, physiological markers)

E. Stress
1. appraisal
2. types of stressors
3. physiological, behavioral, emotional effects
4. managing stress

F. Disorders
1. classification/rates
2. types of disorders (personality, anxiety, obsessive-compulsive, bipolar, depressive, dissociative, schizophrenic, somatic, trauma-related)
3. biological basis (Alzheimer's, Parkinson's, schizophrenia, depression)
4. sleep and sleep disorders

G. Consciousness
1. alert/sleep
2. drugs that alter consciousness (types and effects)
3. drug addiction/reward pathway

H. Attention and Cognition
1. selective vs. divided attention
2. cognitive development (Piaget, cognitive changes, culture, heredity, environment, biological factors)
3. problem solving (types, shortcuts, barriers)
4. theories of intelligence

I. Language Development
1. theories
2. brain areas that control language

J. Learning and Memory
1. nonassociative learning
2. classical conditioning (Pavlov)
3. acquisition, extinction, recovery
4. operant conditioning (Skinner)
5. positive/negative reinforcement, positive/negative punishment
6. four major reinforcement schedules and learning rate
7. insight/latent learning
8. observational learning, modeling, mirror neurons
9. stages of memory (encoding/storage, retrieval)
10. short-term/long-term memory, working memory
11. memory effects (primacy, recency, etc.)
12. recall vs. recognition
13. spreading activation
14. memory failure and dysfunction (forgetting, Alzheimer's, etc.)
15. neural processes underlying memory

Biological Psychology

A.   The Nervous and Endocrine Systems
1.   neurons and neurotransmitters
2.   CNS/PNS
3.   components of endocrine system

B.   Behavioral Genetics
1.   genes and heredity
2.   twin/adoption studies
3.   heredity and environment
4.   influence of genes on behavior

C.   Sensory Perception
1.   types of receptors
2.   threshold stimulus
3.   difference thresholds (Weber's Law)
4.   sensory adaptation
5.   bottom-up/top-down processing
6.   Gestalt principles
7.   pain perception

D.   Special Senses
1.   vision (eye structure/function, visual processing)
2.   hearing (ear structure/function, auditory processing)
3.   taste (chemoreceptors)
4.   smell (chemoreceptors, pheromones)
5.   balance
6.   touch

E.   Physiological Development
1.   prenatal development
2.   changes in adolescence

Chapter 24
Psychology and Sociology Practice Section

FREESTANDING QUESTIONS

1. When Patrick first began working as a waiter in order to save money for medical school, he worked very hard throughout his shifts in order to impress his manager. However, he soon noticed that his manager only came out of her office to observe employees at the height of dinner service, around 7 pm. As a result, Patrick has begun slacking off at the beginning of his shift, becoming a relatively inefficient worker. As 7 pm draws closer, his efficiency picks up in anticipation of potentially receiving praise from his boss. After his boss returns to her office, Patrick's performance dwindles once again. Which of the following intermittent reinforcement schedules is demonstrated?

    A) Fixed-interval schedule
    B) Fixed-ratio schedule
    C) Variable-interval schedule
    D) Variable-ratio schedule

2. Validity is an important component of experimentation. In testing the effectiveness of a new drug, a team of researchers forgot to control for confounding variables. This error would directly affect which of the following?

    I. Construct validity
    II. External validity
    III. Internal validity

    A) II only
    B) III only
    C) I and III only
    D) I, II, and III

3. Kristina is very passionate about conservation and protecting nature, so she joins a local organization aimed at conserving the environment. According to Etzioni, this organization could be classified as a(n)

    A) coercive organization.
    B) informal organization.
    C) normative organization.
    D) utilitarian organization.

4. Which of the following is the strongest predictor of friendship?

    A) Appearance
    B) Attraction
    C) Proximity
    D) Similarity

5. Language consists of five main components: phonemes, morphemes, lexemes, syntax, and context. Which of the following represents the correct definitions of each?

    A) Phonemes are the smallest sonic building blocks of language, morphemes are the smallest units that have a specific meaning, lexemes are all the forms of a single word, syntax are the rules for forming sentences, and context is how the elements of language work together to form particular meanings.
    B) Phonemes are the smallest sonic building blocks of language, morphemes are the smallest units that have a specific meaning, lexemes are combinations of morphemes and phonemes but may not actually form real words, syntax is the choice of words, and context is how all the lexemes fit together syntactically.
    C) Morphemes are the smallest sonic building blocks of language, lexemes are the smallest units that have meaning, phonemes are the words we form with morphemes and lexemes, syntax is the order of the phonemes, and context is the meaning of those phonemes in order.
    D) Phonemes are the smallest sonic building blocks of language, lexemes are the smallest units that have meaning, morphemes shape those phonemes and lexemes into words, syntax orders the morphemes, and context gives a particular meaning to the morphemes.

6. A girl drops out of school to have a baby and raises the child in poverty since she can't get a job that requires even a high school diploma. If that child then drops out of school to parent a child, what social phenomenon has been described?

    A) Social reproduction, which is consistent with the functionalist theory of society
    B) Social stratification, which is consistent with the social exchange theory of society
    C) Social reproduction, which is consistent with the conflict theory of society
    D) Social stratification, which is consistent with the conflict theory of society

7. Which of the following is NOT an example of socialization?

A) Parents punish their child for writing on the walls in order to teach the child that writing on the walls is not an appropriate way to behave.
B) Parents punish their child for not eating their broccoli for dinner while reminding them that there are children starving all over the world.
C) A teacher give gold stars to every kindergartener who sits quietly during story time.
D) A teacher speaks to a child's parents after noticing the child is often absent from class.

8. Religion has been famously described as "the opiate of the masses" since it keeps poorer members of societies from attaining class consciousness. This concept is most consistent with:

A) rational choice theory.
B) structural functionalism.
C) conflict theory.
D) symbolic interactionism.

9. A woman is told a friend's phone number but does not have a pen to write it down. She rehearses the number internally, breaking the 10 digit number up into three groups (xxx - xxx - xxxx) until she has it memorized. Why is this strategy useful for encoding the information from short term to long term memory?

I. Short term memory has a short decay time. If the phone number has not been encoded yet, it will decay after about 30 seconds unless it is rehearsed.
II. Short term memory has unlimited capacity, but retrieving the phone number from short term memory at a later date may prove difficult.
III. Short term memory has a limited capacity. If more than 5 to 9 distinct pieces of information are held in short term memory at once, they may be displaced.

A) I only
B) II and III
C) I and III
D) I, II and III

10. Albert Bandura broke from B.F. Skinner's traditional behaviorist perspective of learning by proposing a new type of learning that was cognitive, instead of solely behavioral. Which type of learning did Bandura introduce?

A) Operant conditioning
B) Classical conditioning
C) Non-associative learning
D) Social learning

11. A KKK member is defended from an angry mob by an African American woman. The KKK member is thankful for the stranger's help, but her behavior does not influence his overall prejudice against her. He assumes her behavior is more of "the exception than the rule." Which attributional bias most accurately describes the KKK member's response?

A) The ultimate attribution error
B) The fundamental attribution error
C) Self-serving bias
D) Just world belief

12. After a car accident a man is temporarily blinded in one eye. His doctors warn that his depth perception may be affected until he regains vision in both eyes. Which components of depth perception will be impaired?

A) Binocular cues, such as relative size and linear perspective
B) Binocular cues, such as retinal disparity and convergence
C) Monocular cues, such as relative size and linear perspective
D) Monocular cues, such as retinal disparity and convergence

13. Many behavioral psychologists test addiction in rats by placing rats in isolated cages with two or more available water bottles. At least one water bottle is spiked with morphine, or some other addictive drug. The researchers then measure the rats' consumption of the various water sources over time to determine how addictive the drug is. More recent research suggests that socially isolated rats are more susceptible to addiction than rats that are not held in the isolated laboratory environments common in behavioral research. Which of the following suggestions might improve external validity of future research on addiction?

A) Replicating the addiction experiment with rats that are not socially isolated

B) Replicating the addiction experiment with one group of rats that is socially isolated, and one group of rats that is not socially isolated

C) Examining the existing data from the original experiment to determine if social isolation is a confounding variable

D) The external validity does not need to be improved, now that it is known that social isolation affects addiction in rats

14. A patient suffering from social anxiety disorder has been referred to two different therapists with different approaches. The first therapist uses the psychoanalytic approach, while the second therapist uses a cognitive-behavioral approach. Which answer choice most accurately reflects the beliefs and goals of these two therapists, respectively?

A) The first therapist will focus his efforts on analyzing and interpreting the patient's behaviors and interactions, with the end goal of helping his patient reach insight into their unconscious desires. The second therapist will focus on identifying and subsequently replacing her patient's learned behaviors with new, healthier behaviors.

B) The first therapist will focus on identifying and subsequently replacing his patient's unhealthy habits and cognitive processes. The second therapist will focus her efforts on analyzing and interpreting the patient's behaviors and interactions, with the end goal of helping her patient reach insight into their unconscious desires.

C) The first therapist will focus his efforts on analyzing and interpreting the patient's behaviors and interactions, with the end goal of helping his patient reach insight into their unconscious desires. The second therapist will focus on identifying and subsequently replacing her patient's unhealthy habits and distorted cognitive processes.

D) The first therapist will focus his efforts on exploring his patient's childhood experiences, in an attempt to uncover any psychosexual fixation that they may have developed. The second therapist will focus on showing her patients unconditional positive regard and helping them remove barriers towards self-actualization.

PRACTICE PASSAGE 1

During the latter half of the 20th century, Americans lost an average of 1.5 hours of sleep per night. While individuals vary, the recommended number of hours of sleep per night ranges between 7 and 9 hours. However, sleep researchers estimate that the average number of hours is less than 7 per night. Concurrent increases in insulin-resistant diabetes, obesity, and psychiatric pathology have also been well-documented.

In fact, an estimated 2/3 of the American population is overweight and 1/3 have pre-diabetic or diabetic hemoglobin A1c. Citing wide-ranging effects of sleep deprivation on energy expenditure and endocrinologic function, sleep researchers have proposed the schematic matrix of interactions shown in Figure 1.

Multifactorial interactions among psychological, endocrinologic, and metabolic functions in which sleep and energy expenditure are reduced while insulin resistance, appetite, and body weight increase form a "vicious cycle" which results in the degradation of lifestyle decisions, worsening of depression, and increase in chronic stress which further reinforces the cycle. In conjunction with these findings, clinicians continue to implement interventions to help patients interrupt this cycle and resume the arduous climb toward a sustainable physiologic steady-state.

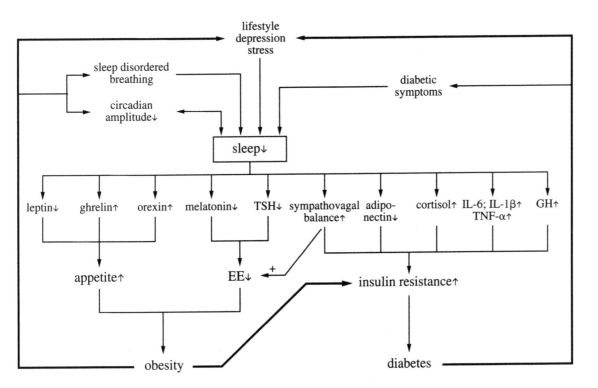

Figure 1 Proposed schematic of interactions among sleep an numerous endocrinologic functions; EE: energy expenditure; TSH: thyroid stimulating hormone; GH: growth hormone

One simple, potentially useful means for mitigating the "vicious cycle" is melatonin supplementation. Synthesized in the pineal gland located behind the thalamus, melatonin has numerous theorized functions including sleep induction. One proposed mechanism for its function is that melatonin binds to the MT1 receptor in the suprachiasmatic nucleus (SCN), inhibiting SCN activity, as well as the MT2 receptor in the same nucleus, inducing sleep by an unknown mechanism. It is known that the SCN receives optic input and that exposure to light—particularly blue light in the range of 446–447 nm—diminishes levels of endogenous melatonin and is associated with diminished feelings of sleepiness. Researchers demonstrated the influence of light color by measuring salivary melatonin levels as a proxy for serum levels:

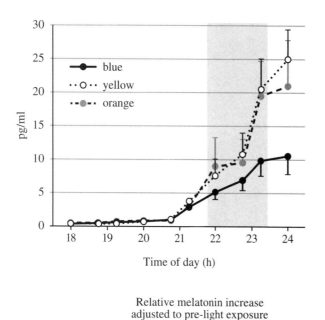

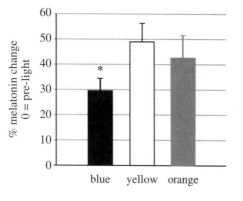

Figure 2 Salivary melatonin levels measured throughout the day with light exposure (above) and groups coded by color of light (below)

The same researchers also demonstrated the following effect on response time in a simple "go-nogo" task during later nighttime hours:

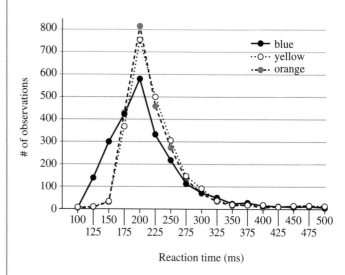

Figure 3 Response time distribution in Go/NoGo task after exposure to different wavelengths of light

Adapted from Lucassen, E.A., Rother, K.I., and Cizza, G. "Interacting epidemics? Sleep curtailment, insulin resistance, and obesity," 2012, and Chellappa, S.L, et al. "Non-visual effects of light on melatonin, alertness, and cognitive performance: can blue-enriched light keep us alert?", 2011.

PSYCHOLOGY AND SOCIOLOGY
PRACTICE SECTION

1. In patients who experience a decrease in average sleep time each night, the amount of which of the following stages is most likely to be reduced with respect to the others?

A) Stage 1
B) Stage 2
C) Stage 3
D) Stage 4

2. Which of the following psychiatric disorders is most likely associated with the "vicious cycle" described in the passage?

A) Bipolar disorder
B) Major depressive disorder
C) Generalized anxiety disorder
D) Post-traumatic stress disorder

3. Which of the following is the most likely daily trend of serum melatonin levels in a health individual?

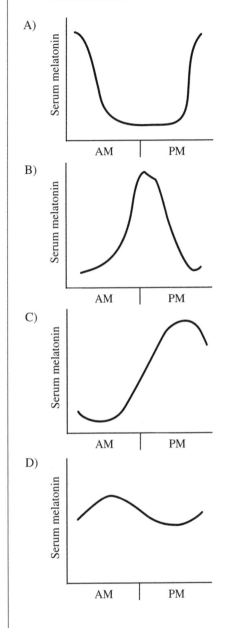

4. A lesion in which part of the brain would be most likely result in the disintegration of the body's circadian rhythm?

A) Retina
B) Cerebral cortex
C) Thalamus
D) Hypothalamus

PRACTICE PASSAGE 2

Several specialists set out to determine the impact eye disease and vision impairment may have on quality of life. Researchers collected data from a sample of 4,000 Mexican-Americans living in the American Southwest. Participants, all of whom were aged 45 or older, were given ophthalmic exams and then a questionnaire developed by a prestigious institution. The types of eye disease prevalent in the study were cataracts, diabetic retinopathy (RD), and glaucoma. Some participants had only one condition, while others had a combination of two or three of these conditions. About 85% of the sample did not have eye disease. Some persons with uncorrected refractive error, whereby the difference between best-corrected and presenting acuity was greater than 2 lines, were also included in the investigation.

Researchers adjusted for potential confounding variables such as age, education level, gender income level, and insurance coverage. A total of 25 domains regarding quality of life were included in the survey. A sample of the results pertaining to seven of those domains is included in Figure 1. This cross-sectional study found that subjects with better-eye acuity and monocular impairment tended to report lower scores in domains associated with quality of life. Participants affected by cataracts, DR, glaucoma, or uncorrected refractive error had more decrements in quality of life than those participants who did not suffer from any eye diseases.

	Glaucoma	DR	Cataract	Uncorrected Refractive Error
	Est.	Est.	Est.	Est.
General Health	−1.72	−14.77*	−.07	.055
General Vision	−6.22*	−5.23*	−3.03*	−2.44*
Driving	−15.01*	.66*	−5*	−3.46*
Role Difficulties	−9.44*	−9.44*	−4.22*	−5.23*
Dependency	−12.74*	−9.01*	−3*	−3.44*
Social Functioning	−7*	−4.44*	−1.22	−2*
Mental Health	−11.11*	−9.16*	−3.22*	−4.99*

* Indicates a significant estimate

Figure 1 Sample of data regarding effect of eye disease on quality of life

Adapted from A. T. Broman, B. Munoz, J. Rodriguez, R. Sanchez, H. A. Quigley, R. Klein, R. Snyder, & S. K. West. "The impact of visual impairment and eye disease on vision-related quality of life in a Mexican-American population: Proyecto VER." *Investigative Ophthalmology & Visual Science.* © 2002 Association for Research in Vision and Ophthalmology.

1. In which of Piaget's four developmental stages do children generally develop the coordination of vision and touch, or hand-eye coordination?

A) The sensorimotor stage
B) The preoperational stage
C) The concrete operational stage
D) The formal operational stage

2. Research into diabetes, which in some cases can lead to diabetic retinopathy, as mentioned in the passage, suggests that both environmental and genetic factors affect prevalence rates. In particular, a handful of studies have shown that social isolation can lead to increased rates of diabetes while feelings of ingroup identification with a dominant culture can lead to improved outcomes. Based on this research we would expect the highest rates of diabetes in:

A) Hispanics.
B) Asian Americans.
C) African Americans.
D) Native Americans.

3. John is conducting a capstone project for his graduate program. He is a strong advocate of an alternative treatment of glaucoma and decides to complete his research on this topic. John chooses to read only information that supports the effectiveness of the treatment and takes little time to explore contradictory research. He ultimately concludes that the alternative treatment must be effective in reducing, even eliminating, the problems associated with glaucoma. John is exhibiting which of the following?

A) Confirmation bias
B) Self-serving bias
C) Pre-screening bias
D) Optimism bias

4. Suppose the researchers would like to test the effectiveness of a new treatment for glaucoma. Subjects affected with the disease are divided into two groups, and only one of the groups is administered treatment. Considering that scientists are aware of which participants are receiving the treatment and participants are observed over the course of several months, which of the following types of studies is being conducted?

A) Double-blind randomized controlled trial
B) Randomized controlled trial
C) Case-control study
D) Cross-sectional study

5. Based on the passage and the figure, which of the following statements is NOT true?

A) Persons with cataracts did not have significantly lower scores in most domains.
B) Persons with uncorrected refractive error had significantly lower scores in most domains.
C) Persons with glaucoma had significantly lower scores in most domains.
D) Persons with DR had significantly higher scores in no domains.

PRACTICE PASSAGE 3

The term *arbovirus* is used to describe the hundreds of predominantly RNA viruses that are transmitted by mosquitoes and other arthropods. One of these, Zika virus, was first discovered in Uganda in 1947. For many years, the virus was found predominantly in primates and was restricted to a thin, equatorial belt running from Africa through Asia. Only in the second decade of the 21st century did a Zika pandemic spread to the West.

The symptoms of Zika, which is related to dengue but displays milder symptoms, include eye pain, fever, maculopapular rash, muscle aches, and prostration. Zika is also believed to sometimes carry complications. In Brazil, the incidence of microcephaly increased about 20-fold from 2014 to 2015; many public health officials believe the condition is linked to a significantly increased incidence of Zika among pregnant mothers in the region. Although a causal relationship between Zika in pregnant women and microcephaly was not definitively established, pregnant women and women planning to become pregnant were advised to refrain from travelling to areas in which the virus is apparent.

Some of the best preventive measures include applying insect repellent as well as wearing long pants and shirts. Other precautions that may be taken are using screens, mosquito nets, and air-conditioning as well as eliminating debris and still water that provide conditions for mosquito-breeding. Access to these items can be limited in developing regions, and this partially explains the prevalence of the disease in countries with less robust economies. Also, Zika is classified as a diseases of poverty, disease that are endemic to poor regions with underdeveloped public health systems that can allow diseases to spread unchecked. Confronting these diseases in regions where the capacity of public health officials to respond in a systematic and orchestrated way is limited is an ongoing challenge for health policy officials and governments.

Adapted from A.S. Fauci & D.M. Morens. "Zika virus in the Americas—Yet another arbovirus threat." *The New England Journal of Medicine.* © 2016 Massachusetts Medical Society.

1. Ana lives in a small village in Latin America. Her parents, like many other parents in the area, have always struggled to provide food and clean water for their five children. When Anna becomes sick with Zika, she does not have access to healthcare and must suffer the symptoms with no reprieve or definitive diagnosis. This situation demonstrates:

A) absolute poverty.
B) cyclical poverty.
C) relative poverty.
D) situational poverty.

2. Considering that Zika affects some of the poorest populations in the world, which of the following is most likely true regarding persons living in regions affected by the virus?

A) Many people are unable to take precautionary measures, such as staying indoors in air-conditioned buildings, but the majority of them have access to reliable healthcare should they become infected with the virus.
B) Most people have access to reliable healthcare and are easily able to remove waste and debris that may attract mosquitoes.
C) Many people cannot afford screens, air-conditioning, or other luxuries to protect themselves from mosquitoes, and their access to good healthcare is limited.
D) Few people are aware of the implications of Zika because they lack access to media outlets and information on the disease.

3. A team of researchers is testing an intravenous vaccine to prevent the spread of Zika. One hundred participants are divided into two groups. Members of the first group are given glucose fluid intravenously, while members of the second group are given the vaccine. Which of the following is true in this study?

A) The independent variable is vaccine efficacy, and the dependent variable is health outcomes.
B) The independent variable is type of fluid, and the dependent variable is health outcomes.
C) The independent variable is the vaccine, and the dependent variable is vaccine efficacy.
D) The independent variable the vaccine, and the dependent variable is vaccine efficacy.

4. A non-profit organization wants to raise awareness about the dangers of Zika as well as convince people of the importance of taking precautions to avoid being bitten by mosquitoes. The organization decides to run a 30-second television ad that will be aired in households across the Western Hemisphere. However, the ad was run during high ratings sporting match with short breaks. It was also administered in markets where few individuals understood nuances of health outcomes and outbreak prevention. Which of the following types of ads would be most likely to encourage viewers to initiate short term measures to reduce being bitten?

A) A short clip of statistics showing how specific measures can reduce risk of infection
B) An expert using statistics and up to date research to delineate best practices and risk mitigation
C) A member of one of the sports teams in the match indicating use of a specific regimen to avoid mosquito bites
D) An attractive model reciting the most effective measures depending on region

PRACTICE PASSAGE 4

Optimism is a social construct that refers to the expectation or hope that good things will occur. There are many external factors that can influence one's levels of optimism, including but not limited to age, education level, gender, income level, and socioeconomic status. The activities in which individuals engage in their daily lives can also impact their overall levels of optimism.

Researchers decided to evaluate optimism levels among collegiate athletes and non-athletes. In doing so, they administered questionnaires to 207 first-year and final-year athletes and non-athletes in New England. The sample included 100 athletes and 107 non-athletes. Participants were divided into four groups: first-year non-athletes ($n = 50$), final-year non-athletes ($n = 57$), first-year athletes ($n = 54$), and final-year athletes ($n = 46$). Among the student athletes, twelve different sports were represented.

Results showed that there was no significant difference in optimism levels between first-year athletes and first-year non-athletes. However, there was a significant difference in optimism levels between first-year and final-year athletes. That is, final-year athletes demonstrated significantly higher levels of optimism than their first-year athlete peers. Final-year athletes also had greater optimism levels than all non-athletes.

Researchers hypothesized that the increased levels of optimism among athletes might be attributed to mastery challenges and self-efficacy that arise as a result of athletic participation. There was no significant difference in the optimism levels of first-year and final-year non-athletes. Investigators speculated that the lack of increase in optimism levels among non-athletes might be the result of fewer opportunities for challenges involving mastery among members of this population.

Adapted from S. A. Venne, P. Laguna, S. Walk, & K. Ravizza. "Optimism levels among collegiate athletes and non-athletes." *International Journal of Sport and Exercise Psychology.* ©2006.

1. Imagine one of the final-year athletes is confident in his abilities to not only succeed as a basketball player but also to excel in the classroom. The athlete's perceptions of his own competence is a reflection of which of the following?

A) Self-esteem
B) Self-actualization
C) Self-consciousness
D) Self-efficacy

2. A social scientist would like to examine how sports reflect class relations as well as how sports can be used to sustain the interests of society's wealthy and powerful. Which of the following theories would be most useful in addressing the topics of the investigation?

A) Symbolic interactionism
B) Functionalism
C) Conflict theory
D) Social constructionism

3. Athletes, just like non-athletes, may experience both intrapersonal and interpersonal problems in their daily lives. Which of the following is an example of situational attribution?

A) Sharon just finished softball practice and is ready to go home. However, when she reaches the parking lot, she realizes that a car has parked behind her, blocking her vehicle in. "What an inconsiderate person!" she thinks.
B) Jason is having a rough day at soccer practice, having trouble performing his duties as a goalie. Jason's coach scoffs at him, assuming that the player is being lazy.
C) Alex is on the range. He swings and misses the ball. He later hits the ball backwards, to which his coach responds by calling him a vulgar name.
D) Jane has not made contact with the ball all morning during tennis practice. Her teammates notice her irregular performance and assume she must be struggling with personal issues at home.

4. The results of the study described in the passage suggest which of the following?

A) There is a possible relationship between athletic participation, income level, and self-efficacy.
B) There is a possible relationship between optimism levels, gender, and athletic participation.
C) There is a possible relationship between athletic participation, year, and optimism levels.
D) There is a possible relationship between optimism levels, self-efficacy, and athletic participation.

5. Christina is a dancer working on a new, complicated routine. The day after she first choreographed the dance, her trainer and her mother come to her studio to watch her practice it. In their presence, Christina flounders and makes many mistakes. This is an example of:

A) social facilitation effect.
B) normative social influence.
C) social loafing.
D) social dysfunction.

PRACTICE PASSAGE 5

Sociologists and social psychologists have discovered many factors that lead to dysfunctional decision making by groups. When the desire for unity and harmony among group members outweighs the perceived importance of critical thinking, the result is *groupthink,* a phenomenon where pertinent information and crucial considerations are not adequately explored in favor of reaching consensus. A critical predisposing factor for groupthink is group cohesiveness, which may lead to the suppression of dissenting opinions and facts that contradict the consensus.

In addition to self-censorship, *mindguarding* occurs, in which members shield the group from potentially divisive material, often by actively censoring other members. Groupthink is more likely to occur when the group is dealing with a moral dilemma, faces serious external threats, or lacks impartial leadership. Some purported historical examples of groupthink-induced fiascoes include the Bay of Pigs invasion of Cuba, the misconduct underlying the Watergate scandal and attempts to cover it up, and the failure to take adequate precautions to prevent the Japanese attack on Pearl Harbor.

A prominent psychologist noted for his work in the area of groupthink conducted a study in which 11 groups of junior executives at a large corporation had their discussions filmed. The discussions occurred during at regularly scheduled meetings) for a five-week period, and all were deemed by senior executives to involve "decisions resulting in significant consequences" to the company and its employees. The groups ranged in size from 8 to 15 members and were each recorded between 3 and 5 times, for a total of 42 discussions. The participants were simply told that a few of their discussions would be recorded via hidden camera "for educational purposes."

After the recordings were made, but prior to any analysis of them, the 7 senior executives at the company rated each group on a 10-point Likert-type scale on 9 traits thought to be associated with cohesiveness (e.g., intragroup loyalty, frequency of member interactions, degree of amicability among members). The senior executives also rated the various decisions ultimately rendered by the groups as "good," "bad," or "neither good nor bad." The researcher then reviewed the recordings in light of these ratings, finding that instances of mindguarding were significantly more prevalent in groups rated high in cohesiveness ($p < .01$). Analysis of the data further revealed that those groups that were high in cohesiveness (i.e., who received a score of 7 or above on the scale) were significantly more likely ($p < .05$) to render bad decisions as determined by senior executive ratings.

1. Which one of the following is a problem with the study described in paragraph 3?

A) Demand characteristics
B) A lack of external validity
C) Improper inference of causality from correlational data
D) Experimenter bias

2. "D" is a teenager who participated in a violent attack upon a classmate that resulted from a groupthink process. "D" is appalled at what he saw as the cruelty and callousness of his fellow perpetrators, believing that he himself only participated because of intense peer pressure. "D"'s beliefs are suggestive of:

A) in-group bias.
B) bystander effect.
C) actor-observer bias.
D) just-world hypothesis.

3. Which of the following research designs would be the LEAST effective method by which to study groupthink?

A) A controlled laboratory experiment
B) A meta-analysis of self-reported measures
C) Naturalistic observation
D) A case study

4. Suppose that "J" was a participant in one of the discussions described in paragraph 2 who initially expressed an opinion in opposition to the consensus. Every time that "J" voiced his dissenting opinion the other members sharply criticized him, while they praised him profusely whenever he conceded a minor point to the majority until he eventually sided with the group. The methods that the group used to influence "J" are best described as, respectively:

A) negative reinforcement and positive reinforcement.
B) positive punishment and negative punishment.
C) negative reinforcement and shaping.
D) positive punishment and shaping.

PRACTICE PASSAGE 6

The availability heuristic states that situations encountered more frequently are judged as likelier to happen, irrespective of the probability of the event. *Perceived risk* is related in that it is a subjective measure of the probability of a negative event. Risk is perceived to be greater when the event in question is more vivid, more dramatic, and more easily comes to mind.

Decision Psychologists and heuristics researchers initially believed that mass media portrayal of risky events would lead people to conclude that the probability of an event is higher than it actually is. However, recent studies on availability tell a more complex story. A recent study looking at the anniversary of the Chernobyl nuclear disaster in April 1986, accompanied by heavy media coverage, did not seem to raise the perceived fear of nuclear risk to any significant levels. The researchers concluded that two principles are at work here: (1) the salience effect, which is essentially the availability heuristic, and (2) the effect of new information. When the Chernobyl disaster happened in 1986, it was largely unexpected and new, and thus created fear of nuclear disaster. In the years following, new knowledge about nuclear energy and the reminder of this event did nothing to add to the perceived risk.

Researchers interested in this question decided to look at the effect entertainment movies have on perceived salience and risk. The researchers used five films to study viewers' risk perception. They showed two films about risk in the experimental condition: The China Syndrome (1978), about a nuclear disaster, and The Towering Inferno (1974), about a fire in a high-rise building. The three control films were Alien (1979), The Party (1968), and A Jungle Tale (1957), inducing negative affect, positive affect, and neutral affect, respectively.

The researchers hypothesized that there will be specific risk perception effects, related to the theme of the films, because the films would make specific risks more salient. In other words, nuclear disaster and the power of fire would stimulate more perceived risk. The researchers showed the movies to 200 participants, ranging in age from 16–75. Each participant was randomly assigned to a movie theater showing one of the five movies. Participants filled out questionnaires before and after the screenings, measuring mood and risk perception, including their feelings about what risks are likelier for them as well as how they enjoyed the movie. Ten days later, they filled out a third questionnaire.

Results showed when the specific fire risk was analyzed for the group that saw Towering Inferno, a repeated measures ANOVA gave no significant effect, neither for personal. Similarly, repeated ANOVA measures showed so significant effect for The China Syndrome, disproving the researchers' hypothesis. When the researchers looked at participants' moods after the movies, they found that with The China Syndrome and Towering Inferno, mood correlated negatively with the mean risk ratings; see Figure 1.

Film	Happi-ness		Activity Level		Relax-ation	
	Personal Risk	General Risk	Personal Risk	General Risk	Personal Risk	General Risk
China Syndrome	−0.26	−0.32*	−0.05	−0.14	−0.04	−0.26
Towering Inferno	−0.41**	−0.37**	−0.42*	−0.32*	−0.35*	−0.30

Note: * $p < 0.05$; ** $p < 0.01$

Figure 1 Correlations between mood after seeing a film and overall well-being and risk perception

Adapted from Sjoberg, L. and Engelberg, E. (2010) Risk Perception and Movies: A Study of Availability as a Factor in Risk Perception Risk Analysis, (30) 1, doi: 10.1111/j.1539-6924.2009.01335.x

1. If a person walked into an arena for an event, and saw a person with a big mustache, that person would be most likely to assume that the person was a man because of the principles of the:

A) availability heuristic.
B) confirmation bias.
C) mental set.
D) representative heuristic.

2. How would the numbers in Table 1 change if the researchers' hypothesis were correct and that these movies did increase participants' sense of risk perception?

A) The numbers for all risk categories would stay negative, but different numbers would be statistically significant.

B) The numbers for all risk categories would stay negative, but all figures would be statistically significant.

C) The numbers for all risk categories would be positive rather than negative.

D) The numbers for personal risk would increase, but the numbers for general risk would decrease.

3. The biological structures most associated with cognitive skills such as using heuristics in problem-solving are:

A. sensory information in the occipital and temporal lobes and the prefrontal cortex.

B) sensory information in occipital, temporal, and parietal lobes; the frontal lobes, the hippocampus, and the amygdala.

C) sensory information in occipital, temporal, and parietal lobes, the hippocampus, and the amygdala.

D) the prefrontal cortex, involved in executive function, and the hippocampus, involved in memory consolidation.

4. Which of the following statistical measurements in Figure 1 is the most statistically significant?

A) General risk for the Towering Inferno

B) General risk to relaxation for the China Syndrome

C) Personal risk to activity level for the Towering Inferno

D) General risk to relaxation for the Towering Inferno

5. Perceived risk often stimulates negative emotions such as fear or anger. Which of the following correctly describes the three components of emotion based on the scenario in the passage?

A) As participants watch the scary parts of the movie, their heart rates increase, they begin to sweat, and they recognize their emotion as fear.

B) As participants watch the scary parts of the movie, they recognize the danger in which the characters find themselves, their respiration increases, and they scream.

C) After a scary part of the movie, the participants find themselves breathing harder, sweating, and they also feel their pulses pounding.

D) After a scary part of the movie, the participants recognize that they interpreted the situation that the characters were in as danger, and find themselves screaming and crying.

Chapter 25
Psychology and
Sociology Practice
Section Solutions

SOLUTIONS TO FREESTANDING QUESTIONS

1. **A** A fixed-interval schedule indicates that reinforcement (in this case, praise from the boss) is provided after a set, constant period of time. The boss emerges from her office at approximately 7PM, the set period of time, at which point she may provide Patrick with praise for his work (choice A is correct). A fixed-ratio schedule exists when reinforcement is provided after a set number of instances that a certain behavior is performed. There is no indication that Patrick only receives praise after a set number of observations (choice B is wrong). A variable-interval schedule indicates inconsistency in the times at which one is reinforced. Patrick knows that his boss observes employees at the height of dinner service, so the opportunity for reinforcement is consistent (choice C is wrong). A variable-ratio schedule signifies that reinforcement is provided after an unknown number of occurrences. The question stem does not indicate this type of reinforcement schedule (choice D is wrong).

2. **C** Construct validity is the degree to which relationships between constructs such as variables or test instruments is correctly established. Introducing a confounding variable would affect the proposed relationship between the independent and dependent variables (Item I is true and Choices A and B can be eliminated). External validity refers to how generalizable studies are to real-world populations or situations (Item II is false). Internal validity refers to the extent to which a causal relationship can be determined between the independent and dependent variables (Item III is true, choice C is correct, and choice D is wrong).

3. **C** A normative organization is one that people join voluntarily. Its members share common goals or values that they consider worthwhile. Kristina has joined the environmental group on her own accord, and it can be inferred that other members share her goals of conservation (choice C is correct). A coercive group is one that people are forced to join; Kristina was not forced to join her group (choice A is wrong). An informal organization may form within a formal organization, and it does not rely on the formal rules and regulations of a formal organization. The local organization Kristina joins would be considered a formal organization. Etzioni is associated with defining three types of formal organizations: coercive, normative, and utilitarian (choice B is wrong). A utilitarian organization, such as a job, is one that people join in an attempt of obtaining material rewards. The question stem does not indicate that Kristina is seeking some sort of material reward (choice D is wrong).

4. **C** Proximity, or geographical nearness, is the strongest predictor of friendship. This idea is rooted in the mere exposure effect, which holds that individuals prefer repeated exposure to the same stimuli. Thus, generally, familiarity can lead to trust and friendship (choice C is correct). Appearance greatly affects attraction, which is a social behavior (choice A is wrong). In fact, there are three features of attraction: physical attractiveness, proximity, and similarity. While attraction can explain some aspects of friendship, it is not a predictor in and of itself (choice B is wrong). Similarity impacts attraction, but proximity is a far greater predictor of friendship (choice D is wrong).

5. **A** Phonemes are the smallest sonic building blocks of language (choice B is wrong), morphemes are the smallest units of language that have a particular meaning, such as the suffix "-ed" that indicates past tense (choices C and D are wrong), lexemes are all the forms of a single word, syntax are the rules for forming sentences, and context is how all these elements combine to create meaning (choice A is correct).

6. **C** This question is best answered with the 2x2 method. The situation characterized in the question stem is an example of social reproduction, where cycles of economic inequality are repeated over generations, not social stratification, which basically describes the way society is divided into different classes (choices B and D can be eliminated). This idea is consistent with the sociological theory of conflict theory, which states that individuals and groups are constantly vying for limited resources and cycles of inequality are often perpetuated by the dominant group in its attempt to remain dominant, while the theory of functionalism describes how structures work together to maintain the dynamic equilibrium of the whole society (choice A can be eliminated; choice C is correct).

7. **D** Socialization refers to the process through which people learn the values, beliefs, behaviors, and moral precepts of their societies. In choice A, the parents are trying to teach the child how to behave correctly, which is an example of socialization (choice A can be eliminated). In choice B, the parents are trying to teach the child the value of food, another example of socialization (choice B can be eliminated). In choice C, the teacher is rewarding the value of good behavior when others are speaking, which is another example of socialization (choice C can be eliminated). In choice D, the teacher is speaking directly to the child's parents, and is not directly influencing the child's norms or beliefs (choice D is correct).

8. **C** Karl Marx, one of the founders of modern sociology, said that religion was "the opiate of the masses." This statement is most consistent with Conflict Theory, as he saw the state's use of religion to ensure the continued inequality of the system (choice C is correct). Rational Choice Theory asserts that people use cost-benefit analyses in order to choose which action will be most beneficial to them (choice A can be eliminated). Structural Functionalism says that there are individual structures in society that all work together for the good of the whole—for dynamic equilibrium. Religion is one of these structures (choice B can be eliminated). Symbolic Interactionism is a micro-level theory that says that people use language express what objects mean individually to them. While Marx might be expressing his own symbolic understanding of religion, the quote itself refers not to an individual interpretation on the micro-level, but rather to how the larger society uses religion as a tool (choice D can be eliminated).

9. **C** Item I is true: Short term memory has a decay time between 30 seconds to 1 minute (choice B can be eliminated). Item II is false: Long term memory is thought to have theoretically unlimited capacity, but short term memory is not. Additionally, information is generally retrieved from long term memory, not short term memory (choice D can be eliminated). Item III is true: Short term memory has a capacity of between 5 to 9 distinct memories. Attempting to memorize each individual digit separately would exceed the woman's short term memory capacity, but lumping the digits together into three distinct (but larger) numbers will make it easier to keep the information in short term memory. This strategy is known as "chunking" (choice A can be eliminated; choice C is correct).

10. **D** B.F. Skinner was famous for his research on operant conditioning (choice A is incorrect). Behaviorists such as Skinner also acknowledged classical conditioning and nonassociative learning. All three of these types of learning can be explained purely in terms of the behavior the animal or human (choices B and C are incorrect). Bandura's social learning on the other hand is driven by a social cognitive mechanism, rather than a strictly behavioral mechanism (choice D is correct).

11. **A** According to the ultimate attribution error, attribution is influenced by the ingroup or outgroup status of the observed person (the African American Woman) in relationship to the observer (the KKK member). Positive actions from members of the ingroup are more likely to be attributed internally, while positive actions from members of the outgroup are more likely to be attributed externally. The KKK member would not view an African American woman as a member of his ingroup (choice A is correct). The fundamental attribution error states that observes generally tend to over-attribute the behavior of others to internal causes (choice B is incorrect). In the self-serving bias, an individual tends to attribute their successes to internal factors, but their failures to external factors (choice C is incorrect). Someone with a just world belief will attribute any negative events in a person's life as a consequence of previous immoral behavior, and any positive events as a consequence of previous moral behavior (choice D is incorrect).

12. **B** Binocular cues are visual cues used in depth perception that depend on both eyes for accuracy, while monocular cues require only one eye for accuracy (choices C and D are incorrect). Relative size and linear perspective are examples of monocular cues: In relative size, if two objects are assumed to have the same actual size, the one that casts the smaller image on the retina will appear as more distant. In linear perspective, parallel lines appear to converge as distance increases. The greater the convergence, the greater the perceived distance (choice A is incorrect). Retinal disparity and convergence are examples of binocular cues. In Retinal disparity, the two images cast onto the two retina are compared; the greater the difference in the images, the shorter the distance. In convergence, the two eyes turn more inward (increasing the angle of convergence) when an object is closer (choice B is correct).

13. **A** External validity measures the ability to be generalize the results of a study to other situations. The original study would have low external validity in respect to "natural" rat behavior, because rats generally are not socially isolated in their natural habitats. Using rats that are not socially increases the external validity (choice A is correct). Replicating the study with a socially isolated, and a not socially isolated group might determine if social isolation is a confounding variable. In other words, to see if social isolation is a variable that influences addiction rates in the rats. Although these would be useful results to have, they do not increase the external validity. The passage implies that social isolation is already known to be a confounding variable (choices B and D are incorrect). Discovering a confounding variable does not replace the need for increasing external validity. In fact, discovering a confounding variable often prompts new study designs (choice C is incorrect).

14. **C** In choice C, the first therapist focuses on uncovering unconscious desires, which is consistent with the psychoanalytic method, and the second therapist is concerned with correcting maladaptive patterns, consistent with the cognitive behavioral method. In choice A, the second therapist does not seem to focus on any cognitive influences. Based on the description, the second therapist is taking a behavioral approach, not a cognitive-behavioral approach (choice A is incorrect). In choice B, the approach of the first therapist is consistent with cognitive-behavioral therapy, and the second therapist's approach is consistent with psychoanalytic therapy. This is the opposite of the question stem (choice B is incorrect). In choice D, the first therapist's goals are consistent with psychoanalysis, but the the second therapist is using a humanist perspective, rather than cognitive behavioral therapy (choice D is incorrect).

SOLUTIONS TO PRACTICE PASSAGE 1

1. **A** Among the other sleep stages, stage 1 sleep comprises about 10% of total sleep architecture and is known to take place with higher relative frequency and duration later in the night. This stage would show the greatest proportional decrease with respect to the others (choice A is correct). Stage 2 comprises about 50% of normal and complete sleep architecture and is more evenly distributed across the entire period of sleep and its proportion would respond less to a decreased period of sleep (choice B is wrong). Stages 3 and 4 are known to decrease in frequency throughout the full period of sleep and, thus, curtailing the period of sleep would have a minimal effect on its proportion (choices C and D are wrong).

2. **B** As depicted in Figure 1, the psychological and physiologic changes associated with a pathologic decrease in sleep feeds back into lifestyle degradation as well as depression; diagnostic criteria for major depressive disorder also includes a sleep disturbance often characterized by insomnia (choice B is correct). The complex interaction of psychological and physiologic abnormalities shown in Figure 1 is typically a chronic process; though bipolar disorder is often characterized by extended depressive episodes, it is more specifically defined by the incidence of manic or hypomanic episodes which drive a decreased need for sleep whereas depression inhibits the ability to sleep (choice A is wrong). Though stress is often associated with increasing anxiety about any number of matters, generalized anxiety is often more driven by long run genetic and environmental factors and not short term stress exposure (choice C is wrong). As stress continues to increase over time, it is possible for patients to exhibit signs consistent with PTSD; however, the defining characteristic of this diagnosis is past historical trauma which results in stress-related changes in behavior and physiologic functioning (choice D is wrong).

3. **A** The passage links blood melatonin levels with exposure to light, in particular blue light; thus, it would be expected that normal physiologic and environmental conditions would result in a sharp increase in melatonin levels at night and a decrease during the day (choice A is correct). High levels in the midday and low levels at night would be the exact opposite trend expected in normal serum melatonin levels (choice B is wrong). Though some increase in melatonin levels might be expected in the late afternoon and evening, an increase beginning in the late morning and peaking in the evening is too early (choice C is wrong). Melatonin levels are expected to be quite high during night time and quite low during the midday; indeed, there is no reason to expect elevated levels in the midday even if relatively lower than at night (choice D is wrong).

4. **D** With visual input from the retinas conveyed by the optic nerves, the suprachiasmatic nucleus located in the hypothalamus is primarily responsible for regulating the body's circadian rhythm; a lesion of the SCN would be most likely to disrupt the circadian rhythm (choice D is correct). Though a lesion in the retina could result in a decrease in visual input to the SCN, a lesion to the retina destroying all function would be unlikely and there are two retinae to compensate should one of them suffer injury (choice A is wrong). The cerebral cortex is not directly implicated in regulation of the circadian rhythm (choice B is wrong). Though a thalamic lesion could be associated with pineal gland dysfunction, the thalamus is not primarily implicated in circadian rhythm regulation (choice C is wrong).

SOLUTIONS TO PRACTICE PASSAGE 2

1. **A** During the sensorimotor stage, which occurs from about birth until the age of two, babies and infants become acquainted with their senses. As they explore their environments through looking, grasping, and touching, they also tend to develop hand-eye coordination (choice A is correct). The preoperational, concrete operational, and formal operational stages occur after hand-eye coordination has developed (choices B, C, and D are wrong).

2. **D** Among the racial groups listed, Native Americans in the United States are most likely to experience social isolation and a sense of disillusionment with the dominant culture due to historical factors like systemic oppression and demographic factors such as low population and residence in rural areas (choice D is correct). Asian Americans, on the other hand, are known to form tight-knit communities and assimilate well relative to other racial demographics. They are also frequently associated through positive stereotyping with favorable traits such as high intelligence and dependability (choice B is wrong). Hispanic Americans and African Americans, although they frequently experience systemic oppression and institutional racism, are known to have tight-knit families and a stronger sense of belonging to the dominant culture than Native Americans (choices A and C are wrong).

3. **A** Confirmation bias refers to the idea that researchers may be inclined to look for data that conforms to their a priori assumptions or preconceived ideas rather than considering various perspectives. In the scenario described in the question stem, John is looking for information to support his own preconceived ideas and beliefs (choice A is correct). The self-serving bias involves the individual attributing his or her failures to the the external environment or other people (choice B is wrong). Pre-screening bias, also known as advertising bias, occurs commonly in medical research. However, this bias arises when researcher screen participants or recruit participants in such a way that methods skew who is included in the sample (choice C is wrong). Optimism bias denotes the idea that bad things will happen to other people but not to oneself (choice D is wrong).

4. **B** In randomized controlled trials, there is a treatment group and a control group. The former receives a treatment, while the latter does not. The trial described in the question stem fulfills the basic requirements of a randomized controlled study (choice B is correct). A double-blind randomized controlled trial is different from a randomized controlled trial in that in the former, investigators are unaware of who is receiving the treatment (choice A is wrong). In a case-control study, there are two groups—members one group have a certain disease or condition while members of the other do not. In the study described in the question stem, all participants have glaucoma (choice C is wrong). Cross-sectional study was the type of study described in the passage. This observational method involves collecting information from participants at a specific point in time. It allows for researchers to compare numerous variables at the same time. The hypothetical study outlined in the question stem is not intended to evaluate various variables (choice D is wrong).

5. **A** Persons with cataracts had significantly lower scores in five of the seven domains listed in the table. Therefore, they did have significantly lower scores in most domains (choice A is correct). Persons with uncorrected refractive error had significantly lower scores in six of the seven, or most, domains (choice B is true and can be eliminated). According to the figure, persons with glaucoma had significantly lower scores in six out of the seven domains

included in the sample (choice C is true and can be eliminated). Persons with DR had significantly lower scores in all domains; therefore, they had significantly higher scores in no domains (choice D is true and can be eliminated).

SOLUTIONS TO PRACTICE PASSAGE 3

1. **A** Absolute poverty is when individuals do not have access to basic necessities such as clean water, food, and healthcare (choice A is correct). Cyclical poverty usually lasts for a transient period of time and is related to the overall state of the economy (choice B is wrong). Relative poverty refers to the idea that some persons may not be able to attain the average standard of living within a given society, but it does not indicate absence of the basic necessities (choice C is wrong). Situational poverty arises as a result of a change in circumstances, which may be related to health, environmental, or personal issues, among others. The question stem does not indicate a change in circumstances, and it emphasizes that the family has always struggled to make ends meet (choice D is wrong).

2. **C** In the poorest areas of the world, many people cannot afford screens, air-conditioning, or other luxuries that might protect them from being bitten by mosquitoes. Moreover, access to reliable healthcare is often limited in such regions (choice C is correct). While many people may be unable to take precautionary measures, reliable healthcare is limited in these areas (choice A is wrong). Most people in these areas do not have access to reliable healthcare, regardless of whether it is easy for them to remove waste and debris that may attract mosquitoes (choice B is wrong). People may become aware of the implications of Zika through the media or through friends and family, and general awareness of the existence of endemic diseases remains high even in relatively poor regions (choice D is wrong).

3. **B** In this scenario, the independent variable, which can be manipulated or controlled, is whether or not the subject receives the vaccine. There are two conditions for the independent variable: vaccine and placebo fluid. Therefore, the independent variable is the type of fluid given, not one of the two conditions. The dependent variable is the type of health outcome observed (choice B is correct). Vaccine and vaccine efficacy are both conditions, not variables (choices A, C, and D are wrong).

4. **C** The peripheral route is most effective when the audience may be distracted from, has little motivation about, and may be unable to fully comprehend the message being delivered. Since the ad is given during a sporting event that is likely to be the main focus of the audience's attention and viewers are unlikely to contained specialized knowledge in epidemiology, the peripheral route is more likely to be influential than the central route, which requires more attention, focus, and capability to understand than the peripheral route. A member of a sports team indicating use of a specific regimen uses almost no technical knowledge, and this type of ad depends mainly on source characteristics such as identification with the speaker (choice C is correct). Attractiveness of the model is a source characteristic. However, intricacies that depend on type of measure and region are message characteristics that are unlikely to resonate with the audience in this context (choice D is wrong). Use of statistics would be more effective for the central route of processing (choices A and B are wrong).

SOLUTIONS TO PRACTICE PASSAGE 4

1. **D** Self-efficacy denotes a strong belief and confidence in one's competence and ability to do well on a certain task (choice D is correct). Self-esteem, which is sometimes confused with self-efficacy, is related to one's perception and evaluation of personal worth or value, and is not related to a specific task (choice A is wrong). Self-actualization, which is at the top of Maslow's hierarchy of needs, is the idea that one must realize his or her full potential and discover meaning beyond the self (choice B is wrong). Self-consciousness simply refers to having an awareness of one's self (choice C is wrong).

2. **C** Conflict theory focuses on the inequality of resources within society, viewing society as being in constant competition over limited resources. The themes described in the question stem relate directly to this struggle over resources (choice C is correct). Symbolic interactionism emphasizes the relationships between society and individuals. It centers on communication and how information is transferred via words and symbols (choice A is wrong). Functionalism focuses on how each part of society is specialized with a unique function, noting that all parts work together to form a whole (choice B is wrong). Social constructivism looks at how reality is shaped and constructed by human beings (choice D is wrong).

3. **D** Situational attribution occurs when the individual attributes his, her, or someone else's behavior to external causes rather than to internal ones. Jane is performing poorly in practice, but her teammates blame her struggle on personal issues, or external causes (choice D is correct). Dispositional attribution, in contrast to situational attribution, occurs when the individual attributes his, her, or others' behaviors to internal causes. Sharon assumes that the other driver is inconsiderate, an internal cause (choice A is wrong). Jason's coach believes the player is being lazy, which is another internal cause (choice B is wrong). Alex's coach calls him a vulgar name, inferring that he or she attributes Alex's shortcomings to internal causes (choice C is wrong).

4. **C** The three variables discussed in the study were whether or not students were athletes, students' year in college, and levels of optimism. The results showed that final-year athletes had higher levels of optimism than final-year non-athletes. The findings thus suggested that there may be a relationship between athletic participation, year, and optimism levels (choice C is correct). Income level was addressed in the passage, but it was not a variable considered in the study (choice A is wrong). Gender was mentioned in the passage, but it was not mentioned in the study (choice B is wrong). The study suggested that self-efficacy led to increased optimism levels. However, the year (there was no significant difference in optimism levels of first-year athletes and non-athletes) appeared to have impacted optimism levels (choice D is wrong).

5. **A** The social facilitation effect is usually associated with the individual performing learned tasks well in the presence of others. However, if tasks are new or complex, the individual may actually perform worse in the presence of others. The question stem indicates that Christina is performing a new, complicated routine. Since she has not yet mastered it, she performs poorly in the presence of her mother and trainer (choice A is correct). Normative social influence involves the individual trying to comply in an attempt to gain the approval of others and avoid rejection. The question stem does not indicate whether Christina was seeking approval (choice B is wrong). Social loafing refers to the idea that individuals may exert less effort when working in groups. Christina was performing alone (choice C is wrong). Social dysfunction occurs when a practice or process has negative consequences on and may reduce the stability in a society.

SOLUTIONS TO PRACTICE PASSAGE 5

1. **D.** Experimenter bias is present when the researcher's expectations improperly influence the results of the study. In this case, the researcher, *after* being given the critical information about the various groups, watched the video recordings and interpreted the group interactions. Due to his knowledge of groupthink theory, he may have been more likely to interpret a particular statement to be an instance of mindguarding when offered by a member of a more cohesive group (choice D is correct). Demand characteristics are cues given to subjects, usually inadvertently and subconsciously, that suggest the hypothesis and indicate how those subjects are expected to behave. While demand characteristics are a possible manifestation of experimenter bias, the design of this particular study did not afford the researcher the opportunity to exert influence upon the subjects. Moreover, any information given to the researcher regarding the characteristics of the respective groups was received *after* the discussions were recorded. While the presence of the camera itself may have affected the subjects' behavior, there was no indication of the specific hypothesis or theory under investigation; nothing occurred that would cause subjects to behave in accordance with the principles of groupthink (choice A is wrong). External validity refers to the extent to which a study's findings can be generalized to other situations and to other people (e.g., controlled laboratory experiments often have poor external validity because the situations created are artificial and do not reflect how people behave in the real world). This study, however, would have high external validity; participants were merely observed.

2. **C.** The actor-observer bias is the tendency to attribute others' behavior to internal or dispositional factors, while attributing one's own behavior to external or situational factors. In this instance, "D" views the violent attack by the other perpetrators as indicative of a cruel and callous nature, while his own participation resulted from external coercive pressure (choice C is correct). The in-group bias refers to the tendency to favor members of one's own group. In this case, "D" is not favoring an "in group" above outsiders, he is simply excusing his own conduct while condemning that of the other individuals who participated in the attack (choice A is wrong). The bystander effect deals with the behavior of witnesses in emergency situations; the likelihood that a victim in need will receive assistance is inversely proportional to the number of individuals present at the scene. This phenomenon does not deal with attributions (choice B is wrong). The just-world hypothesis is the idea that people typically deserve what happens to them. "D"'s views as to whether or not anyone involved in this scenario was deserving of his or her fate are unknown (choice D is wrong).

3. **B.** A meta analysis of self reported measures would contain two flaws related to studying the specific phenomenon. Firstly, a meta analysis is likely to miss out on the specific group effects in play since the specifics of each study and interaction would average out over extremely large samples. Secondly, self-reported measures are unlikely to be effective as a way of exploring a phenomenon with negative connotations such as groupthink (choice B is correct). A laboratory experiment is the preferred method of scientific inquiry because it offers the greatest degree of control. While the external validity, or ability to generalize the results to the real world, might be an issue for a groupthink experiment, the ability to manipulate and control for variables would allow for causal inferences and would nonetheless be the superior research design (choice A would be an effective method and is therefore wrong). Naturalistic observation involves closely scrutinizing the behavior of individuals or small groups in a natural setting without any manipulation of variables (the study described

in paragraph 2 employs this approach). This would allow the researcher to document and examine a group decision-making process in depth in order to analyze it for aspects of groupthink (choice C would be an effective method and is therefore wrong). A case study is a highly thorough and in-depth analysis of a particular individual, small group, or event and would also allow for the detection of a groupthink process. The historical examples of groupthink mentioned in paragraph 1 would be considered case studies (choice D would be an effective method and is therefore wrong).

4. **D.** Reinforcement involves an attempt to increase the likelihood that a target behavior will be repeated by systematically manipulating its consequences; positive reinforcement involves the presentation of a stimulus that is pleasurable or desirable to the subject, while negative reinforcement involves the removal of an unpleasant or undesirable one. In contrast, punishment involves an attempt to decrease the likelihood that a target behavior will be repeated; positive punishment involves the presentation of an undesirable stimulus, while negative punishment involves the removal of a desirable one. Harsh criticism from one's colleagues would be an unpleasant and undesirable consequence for most people, and offering such criticism in response to dissent is therefore a form of positive punishment (choices A and C are wrong). Shaping involves ultimately achieving a target behavior on the part of the subject by positively reinforcing approximate successions of that goal. In this case, the group members wanted "J" to agree with the consensus and offered lavish praise (which is desirable to most people) every time that he agreed with them on a minor point until he eventually changed his overall opinion (choice B is wrong; choice D is correct).

SOLUTIONS TO PRACTICE PASSAGE 6

1. **D** The representative heuristic suggests that people have a preconceived idea for what something or someone must look like or be like and make their assumptions based on that preconception (choice D is correct). The availability heuristic, as described in the passage, is when a person makes a judgment based not on facts or statistics, but instead based on the information seen or heard most recently (choice A can be eliminated). The confirmation bias is a problem-solving obstacle that says if one has a preconceived idea about how something is, that person will only look for evidence to confirm that belief, rather than looking for evidence to disprove or even look objectively for alternative responses (choice B can be eliminated). A mental set is another problem-solving obstacle that says people tend to have fixed ways handling different problems so that it becomes difficult to think of alternative ways to solve them if the mental set no longer works (choice C can be eliminated).

2. **C** The researchers' hypothesis stated "that there will be specific risk perception effects, related to the theme of the films, only because the films would make specific risks more salient, that is, that nuclear disaster and the power of fire would stimulate more perceived risk." This would mean the figures for both general and personal risk were positively correlated with the movie viewing and not negatively correlated (choice C is correct, choices A and B are wrong). Additionally, the numbers would all have to be statistically significant. The hypothesis did not distinguish between general and personal risk (choice D is wrong).

3. **D** Cognitive functioning is a complex and integrated process but must involve executive planning and memory to some capacity. The regions most closely associated with these processes are the prefrontal cortex for executive function and the hippocampus for memory (choice D is correct). Sensory information is critical for thought processes as a foundational aspect of all experiences, however, it is not implicated in higher level executive functioning, which integrates raw sensory information (choices A, B, and C are wrong).

4 **A** General risk for the Towering Inferno shows a negative correlation (–0.37) with two asterisks, signifying that the p-value (the measurement of statistical significance) is less than 0.01, meaning that the likelihood of these numbers happening by chance is even lower, a 1% chance, than those with a p-value less than 0.05, a 5% chance (choice A is correct). The figure for general risk to relaxation for the China Syndrome (0.14) has no asterisks and thus that figure is not statistically significant (choice B is wrong). The figure for personal risk to activity level for the Towering Inferno (–0.42) is higher numerically than choice A but has only one asterisk, indicating a slightly greater likelihood that the figure might be a result of chance (choice C is wrong). The figure for the general risk to relaxation for the Towering Inferno (–0.32) with one asterisk is both a smaller negative correlation and has a higher p-value than A (choice D is wrong).

5. **B** The three components of emotion are the physiological, the behavioral, and the cognitive. In choice B, the participants recognize the danger in the moment, which is the cognitive interpretation, their respiration increases, which is the physiological component, and they scream, which is the behavioral component. In choice A, the participants are experiencing two physiological components, increased heart rate and sweating, and one cognitive component, but there is no behavioral response (choice A can be eliminated). In choice C, all three responses—increased respiration, sweating, and increased heart rate—are physiological only (choice C can be eliminated). In choice D, the participants experience the cognitive component, but experience two behavioral responses without a physiological component (choice D can be eliminated).

NOTES

NOTES

NOTES

NOTES

NOTES

NOTES

NOTES

NOTES

NOTES

NOTES

China (Beijing)
1501 Building A,
Disanji Creative Zone,
No.66 West Section of North 4th Ring Road Beijing
Tel: +86-10-62684481/2/3
Email: tprkor01@chol.com
Website: www.tprbeijing.com

China (Shanghai)
1010 Kaixuan Road
Building B, 5/F
Changning District, Shanghai, China 200052
Sara Beattie, Owner: Email: sbeattie@sarabeattie.com
Tel: +86-21-5108-2798
Fax: +86-21-6386-1039
Website: www.princetonreviewshanghai.com

Hong Kong
5th Floor, Yardley Commercial Building
1-6 Connaught Road West, Sheung Wan, Hong Kong
(MTR Exit C)
Sara Beattie, Owner: Email: sbeattie@sarabeattie.com
Tel: +852-2507-9380
Fax: +852-2827-4630
Website: www.princetonreviewhk.com

India (Mumbai)
Score Plus Academy
Office No.15, Fifth Floor
Manek Mahal 90
Veer Nariman Road
Next to Hotel Ambassador
Churchgate, Mumbai 400020
Maharashtra, India
Ritu Kalwani: Email: director@score-plus.com
Tel: + 91 22 22846801 / 39 / 41
Website: www.score-plus.com

India (New Delhi)
South Extension
K-16, Upper Ground Floor
South Extension Part-1,
New Delhi-110049
Aradhana Mahna: aradhana@manyagroup.com
Monisha Banerjee: monisha@manyagroup.com
Ruchi Tomar: ruchi.tomar@manyagroup.com
Rishi Josan: Rishi.josan@manyagroup.com
Vishal Goswamy: vishal.goswamy@manyagroup.com
Tel: +91-11-64501603/ 4, +91-11-65028379
Website: www.manyagroup.com

Lebanon
463 Bliss Street
AlFarra Building - 2nd floor
Ras Beirut
Beirut, Lebanon
Hassan Coudsi: Email: hassan.coudsi@review.com
Tel: +961-1-367-688
Website: www.princetonreviewlebanon.com

Korea
945-25 Young Shin Building
25 Daechi-Dong, Kangnam-gu
Seoul, Korea 135-280
Yong-Hoon Lee: Email: TPRKor01@chollian.net
In-Woo Kim: Email: iwkim@tpr.co.kr
Tel: + 82-2-554-7762
Fax: +82-2-453-9466
Website: www.tpr.co.kr

Kuwait
ScorePlus Learning Center
Salmiyah Block 3, Street 2 Building 14
Post Box: 559, Zip 1306, Safat, Kuwait
Email: infokuwait@score-plus.com
Tel: +965-25-75-48-02 / 8
Fax: +965-25-75-46-02
Website: www.scorepluseducation.com

Malaysia
Sara Beattie MDC Sdn Bhd
Suites 18E & 18F
18th Floor
Gurney Tower, Persiaran Gurney
Penang, Malaysia
Email: tprkl.my@sarabeattie.com
Sara Beattie, Owner: Email: sbeattie@sarabeattie.com
Tel: +604-2104 333
Fax: +604-2104 330
Website: www.princetonreviewKL.com

Mexico
TPR México
Guanajuato No. 242 Piso 1 Interior 1
Col. Roma Norte
México D.F., C.P.06700
registro@princetonreviewmexico.com
Tel: +52-55-5255-4495
+52-55-5255-4440
+52-55-5255-4442
Website: www.princetonreviewmexico.com

Qatar
Score Plus
Office No: 1A, Al Kuwari (Damas)
Building near Merweb Hotel, Al Saad
Post Box: 2408, Doha, Qatar
Email: infoqatar@score-plus.com
Tel: +974 44 36 8580, +974 526 5032
Fax: +974 44 13 1995
Website: www.scorepluseducation.com

Taiwan
The Princeton Review Taiwan
2F, 169 Zhong Xiao East Road, Section 4
Taipei, Taiwan 10690
Lisa Bartle (Owner): lbartle@princetonreview.com.tw
Tel: +886-2-2751-1293
Fax: +886-2-2776-3201
Website: www.PrincetonReview.com.tw

Thailand
The Princeton Review Thailand
Sathorn Nakorn Tower, 28th floor
100 North Sathorn Road
Bangkok, Thailand 10500
Thavida Bijayendrayodhin (Chairman)
Email: thavida@princetonreviewthailand.com
Mitsara Bijayendrayodhin (Managing Director)
Email: mitsara@princetonreviewthailand.com
Tel: +662-636-6770
Fax: +662-636-6776
Website: www.princetonreviewthailand.com

Turkey
Yeni Sülün Sokak No. 28
Levent, Istanbul, 34330, Turkey
Nuri Ozgur: nuri@tprturkey.com
Rona Ozgur: rona@tprturkey.com
Iren Ozgur: iren@tprturkey.com
Tel: +90-212-324-4747
Fax: +90-212-324-3347
Website: www.tprturkey.com

UAE
Emirates Score Plus
Office No: 506, Fifth Floor
Sultan Business Center
Near Lamcy Plaza, 21 Oud Metha Road
Post Box: 44098, Dubai
United Arab Emirates
Hukumat Kalwani: skoreplus@gmail.com
Ritu Kalwani: director@score-plus.com
Email: info@score-plus.com
Tel: +971-4-334-0004
Fax: +971-4-334-0222
Website: www.princetonreviewuae.com

Our International Partners

The Princeton Review also runs courses with a variety of partners in Africa, Asia, Europe, and South America.

Georgia
LEAF American-Georgian Education Center
www.leaf.ge

Mongolia
English Academy of Mongolia
www.nyescm.org

Nigeria
The Know Place
www.knowplace.com.ng

Panama
Academia Interamericana de Panama
http://aip.edu.pa/

Switzerland
Institut Le Rosey
http://www.rosey.ch/

All other inquiries, please email us at
internationalsupport@review.com

31901060138130